Violence and Abuse Issues

After centuries of being considered a private matter in most societies, violence and its profound effect on the health, mental health, and social well-being of victims and their families, as well as on the assailants themselves, has started to take center stage as a public issue of worldwide concern.

Health and social service providers are in pivotal positions to provide preventive and restorative services to those affected by violent and abusive behaviour. This comprehensive textbook presents theoretical background and practical strategies for doing so, providing a solid knowledge base for good practice in this area. It emphasizes the interdisciplinary aspects of violence and victim/survivor care and addresses violence over the life span, covering:

- child sexual and physical abuse
- sexual assault of adults
- battering and emotional abuse of intimate partners
- elder abuse
- perpetrators of violence and abuse
- violence in learning and work environments
- vicarious trauma and self-care
- interconnections between various forms of violence, including socially approved violence in the media and in war.

This text is an essential resource for qualified practitioners wanting to learn more about this area and for students starting out in health and social care. Each chapter includes case studies and thinking points, and suggestions for application in practice settings. A companion website provides materials for students and educators, enabling the inclusion of violence issues in an already busy curriculum.

Lee Ann Hoff is a nurse-anthropologist and crisis specialist. She has published widely and is the author of the award-winning textbook *People in Crisis*. She has extensive experience as an educator, consultant, clinician, and crisis service manager.

Violence and Abuse Issues

Cross-cultural perspectives for health and social services

Lee Ann Hoff with contributions from Bonnie Joyce Hallisey, Magueye Seck and Marilynne Bell

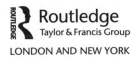

Routledge
Taylor & Francis Group

LONDON AND NEW YORK

First published 2009
by Routledge
2 Park Square, Milton Park, Abingdon, Oxon, OX14 4RN

Simultaneously published in the USA and Canada
by Routledge
270 Madison Avenue, New York, NY 10016

Routledge is an imprint of the Taylor & Francis Group, an informa business

Typeset in Garamond
by Pindar NZ, Auckland, New Zealand
Printed and bound in Great Britain
by TJ International Ltd, Padstow, Cornwall

British Library Cataloguing in Publication Data
A catalogue record for this book is available from the British Library

Library of Congress Cataloging-in-Publication Data
Hoff, Lee Ann.
Violence and abuse issues : cross-cultural perspectives for health and social service / by Lee Ann Hoff ; with contributions from Bonnie Joyce Hallisey, Magueye Seck and Marilynne Bell,.
    p. ; cm.
  Includes bibliographical references.
  1. Violence—Cross-cultural studies. 2. Offenses against the person—Cross-cultural studies. I. Title.
  [DNLM: 1. Violence. 2. Cross-Cultural Comparison. 3. Sex Offenses. HM 1116 H698v 2009]
  HM1116.H64 2009
  362.88—dc22   2008054631

ISBN10: 0-415-46571-0 (hbk)
ISBN13: 978-0-415-46571-7 (hbk)

ISBN10: 0-415-46572-9 (pbk)
ISBN13: 978-0-415-46572-4 (pbk)

ISBN10: 0-203-87562-1 (ebk)
ISBN13: 978-0-203-87562-9 (ebk)

To victim/survivors, their advocates, and professionals worldwide: May you never abandon the mission of violence prevention, but also take care of yourselves as you stay the course on advancing the right of all to be free of violence and abuse from intimates, family, strangers, and the state.

Contents

Illustrations

Tables

Figures

Exhibits

Acknowledgements

This book would not have been possible without the inspiration from the young people I have met in my work. Some have been impossible, some incredible, and all have, in so many different ways, illustrated the complexities inherent within exploitative relationships. For those young people, their friends, families and carers who have suffered (through intimidation, violence, torture or murder), I intend this book to raise awareness to the damage that sexually exploitative relationships can cause.

One of the most important resources for young people who have experienced sexual exploitation is a sustained relationship with a practitioner. Indeed, many of the services have depended upon the determination and resilience of many workers who have struggled to keep their services going against all sorts of odds. They, with members of the National Working Group for Sexually Exploited Children and Young People (NWG) have, as friends and colleagues, informed and developed my thinking.

In particular, Nasima Patel has been with me from the start, with sustained friendship, a clarity in thinking and a helpful insistence that child protection remain high on every agenda. Sheila Taylor has, with the motto "where there's a will there's a way", shown me the import- ance of keeping sexual exploitation in the thinking of all child care policy and practice service providers. Marilyn Haughton has always upheld the importance of the voice of the child with a sense of humour second to none. She has shown me how education can be taken to young people whom others might have abandoned. Ann Lucas has demonstrated how change can be brought about within statutory services while Julie Harris and Paula Skidmore have maintained the importance of good, thorough academic scrutiny, reaching out to research difficult topics with a calm, sensitive and imaginative approach. Jo Phoenix has been a consistent strength, always achieving the daunting challenge of really translating theory into practice, helping me to balance awareness of the young person's agency within their experiences as victims, questioning an uncritical culture of risk and bringing intelligence into all debate. I feel indebted to Jo for helping me to move through different processes from my start as a practitioner to now. Sue Jago has brought clarity of thinking in the policy agenda for sexually exploited children and young people. She has demonstrated, and helped me to understand, how policy can be developed through a relationship between young people, the work carried out by their practitioners and the policy writers. These people, and others such as Mandy from Leeds; Wendy Sheppard from Middlesbrough; Sara Swann who really was, with Tink Palmer, a pioneer for this work; Irene Iveson, who raised awareness of parents and families needs after the tragic murder of her 17 year old daughter, Fiona; Aravina from Coalition Against Removal of Pimping (CROP) has continued to keep parents and families needs in mind, Martin Houghton-Brown and Charlie Hedges whose work on missing children has been so important, have helped to raise the profile of the needs of sexually exploited children and young people through their work.

The book draws heavily on research work I carried out with Mary Williams and Christine Galvin in 2002 funded by the Joseph Rowntree Foundation (JRF) and Middlesex University. Charlie Lloyd from the JRF provided support and encouragement for the work to be completed.

I also want to say a particular thank you to colleagues at Bedfordshire University: David Barrett, John Pitts and Margaret Melrose have been central to the development of my work. Their writing, their friendship, their critical appraisal of my work and their support as colleagues has, with others from the department and faculty at Bedfordshire led by Ravi Kohli and Michael Preston-Shoot respectively, developed one of the best team of colleagues that I have had the privilege in working with.

Throughout all of my work in this area, Professor Susanne MacGregor has been there as a mentor and role model. Her leadership in academic settings, in social policy, her thought and care on all areas of work that she is involved with have been an inspiration.

Most importantly, I would like to thank my family, including my two daughters who are amazing. They have patiently supported me through PhD, research projects and a working life, kept me laughing and pushed me on, despite the odd comment about a school lunch box with a mouldy bread sandwich! They have encouraged my work through every step of the way. Finally, my partner, John Coleman has extended my horizons. With a "keep focused" motto, a willingness to be a listening ear and a critical reader he has made this book possible.

Preface

Writing this book has been one of the most challenging tasks of my professional career – at personal, social and political levels. While I was already established as a mental health clinician in the crisis field and embarking on doctoral research two decades ago, an esteemed professor in my university department questioned (disparagingly) why I chose the topic of "woman abuse" as a serious subject of study. Nevertheless, I plowed ahead with support from other distinguished faculty, only to make this discovery from literature reviews and experience as a volunteer in a women's shelter: Clinicians and researchers like myself were viewed as "part of the problem" (as in "victim-blaming"), not part of the solution to the plague of violence against women.

As a card-carrying member of these professional establishments, and from my experience as a volunteer in a women's shelter, I used the tools of my own clinical and academic trades to examine findings that supported the common view of attributing violence and abuse to the presumed "psychopathology" of the victim/survivors themselves as well as their abusers, or to cultural norms deeply embedded in gender bias. My profoundly enriching interdisciplinary studies across several academic experiences aided me in pulling together what I hope is a coherent whole of the threads comprising the fabric of this book. When Erin Pizzey wrote *Scream Quietly or the Neighbors will Hear*, she "opened the window" in England that had spawned the "battered women's movement." Now, decades later, professionals and the lay public widely agree that interpersonal violence is not just a private domestic secret, but is a public health issue encompassing the broader arena of children, offenders, traffickers, and state-sponsored violence, for which offenders are accountable.

Along the way toward the book's core message I was inspired by a mentor, medical sociologist Sol Levine's term, "creative integration." This theoretical approach led to my bridge building efforts across disciplines, cultures, geographic boundaries, and the spectrum of violence as it touches individuals, families, the wider community, and nations. Included were efforts to close some of the theory-research-practice gaps that can inhibit progress on this urgent topic. In this process I was greatly aided and supported by Canadian governmental initiatives and the Institute for Applied Psychology (ISPA) in Lisbon, Portugal, feminist scholars and activists, and many others. Together, these visionaries were central in my bringing this work to fruition and to embracing two factors pivotal toward achieving the book's aim: "The personal is political" and, progress on this urgent topic is heavily dependent on *collaboration* among ourselves, *not* the competitive and controlling relationships that underpin interpersonal violence and abuse.

My conviction about these principles was a firm buffer against many personal and professional obstacles. It included the determination never to assume a "victim" role, and never lose sight of the millions of victim/survivors worldwide in much worse straits than my own – hence my preferred term, victim/survivor.

Now, evidence reveals that academic questions about the "legitimacy" of this subject matter have finally been laid to rest – as documents from the World Health Organization and elsewhere attest to the centrality of health professionals to make a difference in stemming the worldwide tide of violence. This book is the multi-year result of my resolve to keep "swimming upstream" against considerable odds. And my hope is that it might assist others faced not only with individual crises from whatever source, but also for all who continue to believe that despite historical and current evidence to the contrary, our future in the world community will benefit from our collaborative efforts to find non-violent solutions to our personal, social, and political conflicts.

Audience

Complementing the interdisciplinary theory, research, and practice underpinning this book, its primary audience includes students, faculty, and practitioners among these groups whose mission typically implies *understanding* the complexity of violence prevention and the challenge of providing appropriate services to victim/survivors and assailants:

- Health and mental health practitioners across disciplines
- Social service providers
- Criminal justice teachers and advocates, and police
- Pastoral counselors
- Applied social scientists – especially in sociology and anthropology

Other readers may include victim advocates who pioneered in offering crisis care and social services – typically in NGO (non-governmental organizations) and volunteer capacities – before health and mental health professionals became actively involved. These experts may benefit from the book for its illustration of the collaborative relationships that should exist between health professionals and front-line workers as the ideal in the practice arena with victim/survivors and perpetrators. Since many people have either direct or tangential awareness of violence in their families or community, interested lay readers might also gain insight from the book about what should be expected professionally in the care and treatment of victim/survivors and perpetrators.

Appreciation – Contributors

While the journey toward completing this work was fraught with obstacles large and small, the book would never have seen the light of day without the help of many along the way. I herewith thank you one and all, but with deep regret that your hidden and selfless work on behalf of victim/survivors and violence prevention is often unnoticed and/or unacknowledged in the larger arena – sometimes out of respect for requested privacy. These individuals include victim/survivors themselves, many students, research participants, professionals and others who have shared their stories with me, but who cannot be publicly revealed in this book. The cases are real but disguised to protect persons' identity.

Here are the names and affiliations of those who can be named, beginning with the book's foundation in Ottawa, Ontario, Canada, 1992:

Dr. Margaret Ross, who wrote the successful grant proposal, and Dr. Denise Alcock, who offered me a Visiting Professorship at the School of Nursing, Faculty of Health Sciences, University of Ottawa, for completing this book's forerunner: *Curriculum Guide for Nursing: Violence against Women and Children.* (Hoff & Ross, 1993).

Dr. Betty Cragg and other faculty at the School of Nursing who supported this effort in ways large and small. Other faculty in Ontario's 41 schools of nursing also supported the *Curriculum Guide* and revealed in follow-up surveys their need of more preparation on violence issues as a prerequisite for adequate teaching on the topic.

Joan Simpson, MSW, Health Canada, Mental Health Division, Health Services Directorate, who commissioned the extension of the *Curriculum Guide for Nursing* for expansion to include other health professionals in *Violence Issues: An Interdisciplinary Curriculum Guide for Health Professionals* (Hoff, 1994).

The many health professionals, academics, and students who granted individual interviews, participated in focus groups and workshops across Ontario and other Canadian provinces for implementation of teaching and service strategies using the interdisciplinary curriculum guide.

Kazimiera Adamowski, MSW, an early key informant and steadfast supporter of the inter-disciplinary focus of this book, based on her pioneering work at a rape crisis center and at the Ottawa General Hospital Emergency Department where she established clinical and training protocols for physicians and nurses, and who joined me for workshops on these topics at the Beijing 1995 UN Women's Forum and in The Philippines. There and beyond, she helped with engaging potential international contributors to the envisioned expansion of the Health Canada interdisciplinary curriculum guide to cross-cultural perspectives for the book. Special thanks to Kazimiera also, for assistance with developing ancillary training materials on violence issues – some of which are cited in the book's web site.

Victim/survivors and their advocates across Ontario, other Canadian provinces, and inter-nationally: Israel (Ruth Rasnick); the Philippines; Portugal – ISPA and Women's Association Against Violence – AMCV (Jose Ornelas, Maria Joao Vargas-Moniz, Susana Maria, Margarida Martins, Fatima Jorge Monteiro, Raquel Cardoso); South Africa (Zubeda Dangor and colleagues at NISAA); China (Han Li – A Canadian-Chinese researcher) – and all others who supplied materials from interviews, support, and counseling experiences relevant to the book's aim.

Special thanks go to Joy Adams-Jackson (Australia), and to Glenda Dubienski (Canada) who shared stories from their current clinical and humanitarian aid work among indigenous populations, and who reviewed parts of the manuscript.

Closer to home in Boston, special thanks go to Eliza Hutchinson for assistance with liter-ature review. I also thank Alexandra Weber and Carolyn Drew-Benedict at the International Institute-Boston for assisting with examples of refugees and victims of torture; Bonnie Joyce Hallisey with examples of refugees from Haiti and Vietnam; Magueye Seck for examples from his work in Cambridge, Massachusetts and in Africa with perpetrators of violence; and David Adams and Susan Cayouette for permission to share their pioneering work with the Emerge offender program in Chapter 10. Special thanks also go to police officers in Buffalo, NY, Los Angeles, and Boston, who not only taught me about self-protection in potentially dangerous "ride-alongs" but also helped lay the foundation for a key element of crisis work: The linkages and necessary collaboration between criminal justice and mental health professionals in life-threatening situations.

In South Dakota, at the Pine Ridge Reservation, special thanks go to Thomas Shortbull, President of Oglala Lakota College, and Marilyn Pourier for initial contacts about violence and abuse among a Native American population, the Lakota Sioux. Interviews and extensive conversations with Karen Artichoke, Norma Rendon, and Heath Deucheneaux about the Cangleska (Medicine Wheel) program for abused women and perpetrators were central to capturing what mainstream providers need to know about the context of abuse and violence afflicting indigenous populations world-wide. I also thank Cangleska staff for permission to reprint the Medicine Wheel and Unnatural Power & Control figures in Chapter 8.

Last but not least, my heartfelt thanks go Marilynne Bell, MD, Bonnie Joyce Hallisey, LICSW, and Magueye Seck, PhD, who joined me as Chapter contributors for this book, and who remained steadfast through the last phases of production, including contributions to the book's web site.

Finally, very special thanks to my editor, Grace McInnes, whose wisdom, vision and belief in the book's mission kept me focused; assistants Eloise Cook and Khanam Virjee who ever so graciously never let me forget a deadline; Camille Lowe who navigated us through final stages; Nick Ascroft who made sure everything came together; and the entire Routledge team who have supported and kept me on target throughout trans-continental ramifications of production. It has been my pleasure to work with you! I am also deeply grateful to those who have offered endorsements of the book, and to my faithful friends and family who have stood by with support and patience through all this work.

About the Authors

Lee Ann Hoff, PhD, is a nurse-anthropologist and crisis specialist, and the founding director of the Life Crisis Institute based in Boston. Dr. Hoff has extensive experience as an educator, consultant, clinician, and crisis service manager. Her major publications include the award-winning book, *People in Crisis: Clinical and Diversity Perspectives*. 6th Ed. (2009, Routledge, NY) and *Battered Women As Survivors* (1990, Routledge, UK). Currently, Dr. Hoff is Research Consultant at the University of Massachusetts Lowell; Adjunct Professor, University of Ottawa, Faculty of Health Sciences; and Visiting Professor, ISPA (Institute for Applied Psychology), Lisbon, Portugal. Dr. Hoff is a member of several professional organizations and is active in peace and anti-violence movements.

Marilynne Bell, PhD, is a primary care and family practice physician in Halifax, Nova Scotia. Her background includes clinical protocol development for physicians on assessment and treatment of intimate partner violence and sexual assault, and medical school curriculum materials on violence issues. Besides her private medical practice, Dr. Bell is a clinical supervisor of medical students from Dalhousie University in Halifax.

Bonnie Joyce Hallisey, MSW, LICSW, is a highly experienced clinical social worker at Kit Clark Senior Services in Boston where her practice includes counseling and advocacy with high risk immigrant groups. She is also a Senior Lecturer in sociology and psychology at Curry College in Milton, Massachusetts.

Magueye Seck, PhD is a professor in criminal justice and applied sociology at Curry College, in Milton, MA. Dr. Seck's experience includes research on perpetrators of violence in relation to substance abuse, counseling with court-referred offenders at Emerge (a pioneer in offender service programs), and international work on violence prevention and emigration crises among African refugees. His special interests include violence, social justice, and social policy.

See Online Resources for more information about the Authors

Lee Ann Hoff
Boston, Massachusetts, USA
May 2009

Part I

Overview, theoretical perspective, and essential content

Part I lays the foundation for all remaining chapters. As an international public health issue with profound implications for the health and mental health of individual victim/survivors and their assailants, Chapter 1 presents forerunners to this book, its interdisciplinary scope and particular relevance for public health and front-line providers, and a brief review of unfinished business on this topic in the global community. Chapter 2 summarizes the contributions that grassroots advocates and many professionals have made to our understanding of this issue, and reaffirms the importance of collaboration to replace discipline-specific turf wars that can compromise the progress needed by a united front on the urgent global epidemic of violence. These interdisciplinary offerings constitute the book's theory framework, assumptions, values, beliefs, and the social structures that figure strongly in the origins of violence and abuse, and which are essential in violence prevention and helpful responses to both victims/survivors and perpetrators of violence. Chapter 3 follows with evidence-based essential content proposed for the education of front-line health and social service providers who, for optimal results, need to collaborate across disciplines in the best interests of victim/survivors as well as perpetrators of violence and abuse.

1 Violence prevention and victim/survivor care

An international public health issue

- Background and overview
- Purpose and scope
- Disciplinary and interdisciplinary issues
- Unresolved issues in global perspective
- Cross-cultural approach to education on violence issues

After centuries of definition as a private matter in most societies, violence and its impact on women, children, and the assailants themselves have taken center stage as a public health and social issue of worldwide concern. In virtually every country, violence and oppression against women remains firmly rooted – women and children are the major victims of male aggression and homicide both inside and outside the home – and the greatest risk for women and children is from men they know (UN Population Fund, 2000; US Department of State, 1998; WHO, 2004). Increasingly, countries such as the United States and Canada, and international bodies such as the United Nations (UN), the World Health Organization (WHO), and the International Council on Women's Health Issues are declaring physical and sexual abuse as a violation of human rights.

One of the major domains of social life is health and its preservation. It therefore follows that health and social service providers are in key positions to teach violence prevention and provide preventive, healing, and restorative services to those affected by violent and abusive behavior among intimates, family members, and others. Yet, the survivors of trauma and abuse, along with their advocates, have been the major players in bringing this poignant topic to international attention. Criminal justice professionals followed with activism and reform on the issue; while health professionals were the last influential group to lend their voice to the effort (Hoff, 1991).

During recent decades, many volumes have been written by social science and health professionals on the topic, and diverse professional and community groups have devoted vast time and energy to prevent violence and abuse and alleviate its devastating effects on victims. This includes the offer of shelter or refuge for those in imminent danger, as well as inclusion of victimization assessment in routine health assessment protocols. Yet, attention to the topic in formal curricula preparing health professionals is incidental rather than systematic (Ross *et al.*, 1998; Woodtli, & Breslin, 1996, 2002).

Thus, for example, the American Association of Colleges of Nursing (AACN, 1999) has only recently issued a Position Paper on this topic as essential content in nursing curricula. In 2004, the WHO produced a handbook to aid health professionals in documenting and preventing interpersonal violence, and encouraged implementation of its recommendations based on resolutions for adoption by these WHO members: The World Health Assembly, the African Union, and the World Medical Association (WHO, 2004). While this document focuses on the all-important topic of prevention (in public health terms, vulnerable *population* groups, primarily women and children), this book complements such violence prevention efforts in concert with the *clinical practice* facets of secondary and tertiary levels of care, where attention is on detection and treatment of *individuals already injured or abused,* and efforts toward psychological recovery and prevention of re-abuse. (See Part IV: Online resources, for further information.)

The nature of this topic, deeply embedded as it is in social structures and cultural values, suggests an upward crawl toward change and reform in how health and social service professionals are prepared to deal with this worldwide plague and its implications for the health of individuals, families, the economy, and entire nations. Despite much progress, this book focuses on the serious work that lies ahead, particularly for health and social service educators and future providers who depend on their basic preparation for effective practice in this challenging arena. Whether acknowledged or not by providers, most victim/survivors appear sooner or later in healthcare settings with manifest or latent symptoms of victimization by violence and sexual abuse. When this happens later rather than early in the course of recovery from abuse, the difficult healing process is often unnecessarily compounded.

Background and overview

The impetus for this book is situated in two major initiatives – one national, the other a series of international events. As a nation dedicated to leadership in world peace and non-violent conflict resolution, provincial and federal governments of Canada sponsored a number of initiatives directed to violence prevention and the particular role of health and social service professionals in the care of victims.

In 1992, the Ontario Ministry of Colleges and Universities funded the development of curriculum materials on violence for faculty use in three higher education programs: Early Childhood Development, Law, and Nursing. Recognizing the important role in violence prevention and the care of victims played by these disciplines, the intent was to design discipline-specific curriculum guides for educators in higher education to systematically address this issue in their curricula. In developing the *Curriculum Guide for Nursing* (Hoff, & Ross, 1993), the forerunner to this book, it quickly became apparent that effective nursing practice in this health issue demanded collaboration with other disciplines, for example, medicine, social work, and psychology. In short, a comprehensive approach to the topic cuts across disciplines – albeit with specific functions among particular disciplines.

As the *Curriculum Guide for Nursing* went to press, Health Canada – following sponsorship of earlier initiatives on the issue – conducted a nation-wide interdisciplinary consultation process focused on collaborative strategies among health professionals on behalf of persons and families traumatized by violence and abuse. This process underscored the *vital link* between effective practice and the educational programs preparing various health professionals in pre-service, graduate, and continuing education programs.

A major result of these consultations was Health Canada's commission of *Violence Issues: An Interdisciplinary Curriculum Guide for Health Professionals* (Hoff, 1994). Soon after its publication, the UN sponsored the 1995 Women's Conference and Forum in Beijing. At this conference, attended by some 36,000 people from all corners of the globe, there were numerous workshops and speak-outs on all forms of violence against women – battery, sexual assault, and rape as the spoils of war. However, at this conference the very low visibility of health professionals dedicated to violence prevention and care of victims was disproportionate to the enormous and often *untapped potential* of health providers to make a difference on this topic. However, during two workshops targeted specifically to health professionals and networking throughout the conference (Hoff, & Adamowski, 1995) we established a network of international collaborators dedicated to expanding and adapting the Canadian *Curriculum Guide* for use cross-culturally. This book – addressing *public health* and *clinical* facets in tandem – is the result of that effort and perseverance against great odds.

The thoughtful reflection by many concerned players on these major Canadian projects and the Beijing conference underscored a central tenet of violence and abuse as it concerns health professionals: Violence detection, prevention, and the care of survivors – in society and among intimates and family members – in essence is *an interdisciplinary, community concern*. Nevertheless, while recognizing role blurring in certain instances and the need for collaboration among healthcare workers, members of particular disciplines must first master the distinct role of their professions on behalf of survivors in the overall mosaic of a community's healthcare system. A second revelation from these projects was a characteristic uncovered among *all* professional health education programs: despite widespread recognition of the serious impact of violence and abuse on individual victims and a nation's health, attention to the topic heretofore has been *incidental* rather than *systematic* (with perhaps a few exceptions) in the education of health professionals.

Although most violence among intimates and against family members occurs "behind closed doors," the survivors of interpersonal violence and abuse – whether attacked in public or private – will almost invariably come in contact with a health or mental health professional, either for treatment of acute injury, because they are at risk of injury from violence, or as a result of the long-term emotional/mental or physical damage ensuing from abuse. Clearly, then, all healthcare providers are in strategic positions to prevent violence, detect risk and/or victimization of vulnerable groups (especially women and children), and provide service to survivors of abuse as well as their assailants.

Health professionals' unique role derives from their numbers, the variety of their practice locations, and their influential contact with potential victims from birth to death. Their central place in this poignant facet of life is also grounded in the fact that the healthcare system is *a major domain of social life*, along with economic, religious, political, legal, and educational institutions. While every citizen has a role to play in eliminating the worldwide plague of violence against women and children, the *particular power of health professionals to make a difference* on this issue cannot be overstated. Not only can health professionals ease the profound suffering of victims, but their efforts can favorably affect assailants, entire families, and society as a whole.

A caveat is in order here. Health professionals in primary care and emergency settings are often the first point of contact around violence and abuse – either for treatment of physical injuries (whether or not acknowledged), or for medical ailments with no clear biomedical cause but which often signify the damaging sequelae of abuse on overall health status (Bensman *et al.*, 1992; Hoff, & Morgan, in press; Sugg, & Inui, 1992). This pattern of behavior in seeking healthcare underscores the importance of collaboration between front-line health providers (usually physicians and advanced practice nurses) and the usual next level of service – consultation from and referral to social service or mental health professionals who follow up with a comprehensive assessment and service plan for victim/survivors.

Depending on the agency, ideally this follow-up service is provided by social workers or crisis specialists trained in the particular needs of victimized persons (see Part IV: Online resources). Accordingly, this book assumes the vital collaboration between health and social service professionals if victim/survivors are to be adequately served. In short, a "both/and" rather than "either/ or" model is espoused, not only because it usually results in better outcomes for particular clients, but also as a model of a cooperative vs. competitive approach to an urgent life issue. As one abused woman observed in her job as a nursing assistant, competitive power dynamics between physicians and nurses did nothing to increase her trust of these same professionals to understand or respond empathetically to the abuse of power she suffered in her marital relationship (Hoff, 1990).

Purpose and scope

The dual and related purposes of this book are:

1 To provide evidence-based rationale and data for health and social services educators to move beyond current curricular deficits and embrace "violence issues" and their health and social impact as *essential* content for future health and social service practitioners.
2 To provide a practical resource for students and faculty toward implementing this urgent educational goal and enhancing the enormous potential of these professionals to make a difference on the human rights issue of violence and abuse.

This book is *not* a substitute for the basic texts that prospective teachers must master on particular topics such as incest, depending on the curriculum level. Rather, it provides an overview of the field and parameters of practice and distinctions between *generalists* (e.g. primary care physicians, social service caseworkers, and nurses who are often the first contact in the front lines with an already injured and abused person or someone at risk of the same), and *specialists* (i.e. mental health professionals prepared for delivering the long-term follow-up care needed by some victim/survivors). It is intended as a resource for busy educators, trainers, students, and those already in practice to assess their readiness to address this sensitive topical area, and to take advantage of interdisciplinary cross-cultural resources that enrich teaching and reduce the need to "re-invent" wheels. It includes principles and experience-based precedents established by survivors and their advocates, plus those of various professional bodies recommending the inclusion of violence-related content in the curricula preparing future health professionals. The book enlivens the abstract nature of the topic through stories of survivors; from these stories key concepts, attitudinal factors, and skills are delineated for application in diverse practice settings. Some of this content is enhanced with online resources and exercises for fine-tuning practice skills.

Because the problem is urgent and pervasive, and because the needs of victims and assailants are complex, this book emphasizes the *interdisciplinary* facet of violence and victim/survivor care, while not losing sight of the distinct roles of particular disciplines. Additionally, it addresses violence over the life span: child sexual and physical abuse, sexual assault of adults, battering and verbal abuse of intimate partners (especially women), elder abuse, and the interconnections between various forms of violence, including human trafficking and/or State-sponsored or socially approved violence in the media, etc. Finally, while recognizing the need for specialty books on abuse, this book's focus is intended to address the *interconnections* between the many forms of interpersonal abuse among intimates, family members, and strangers (aided and abetted in media images). Another focus is the *context* of abuse in centuries-old social structure and cultural values that have kept this worldwide problem alive against concerted efforts to put it aside as an anachronism in any civilized society. As such, it is designed to assist a total *curriculum and health system response* to the issue. This assumes the importance of all practitioners mastering the *knowledge, attitudinal stance, and skills* regarding violence issues that are essential for comprehensive service to victim/survivors. It also means not reserving attention to this topic only to the particular interests of individual faculty members or practitioners who may feel ready to teach on the subject.

Despite the often untapped potential and goodwill of health professionals, the topic of violence presents a greater than average challenge to most educators and clinicians charged with teaching and role modeling on this practice issue. Besides the usual complexities of psychosocial healthcare, violence is linked to values and structures which touch everyday life and social interaction that many consider sacrosanct although dangerous to some, especially women and children.

This book's intent is to aid faculty, students, and clinicians in the health and social service professions to address violence prevention and the care of abused clients in a manner that is:

- comprehensive in scope;
- sensitive to the sociocultural, political, and psychological roots of violence;
- attentive to new insights regarding survivor needs as they emerge in everyday life and community practice settings;
- humane, caring, and skilled in professional service delivery;
- linked effectively with the work of grassroots programs for survivors.

Though directed primarily to pre-service undergraduate and graduate educational programs, this book is relevant to all human service workers concerned with the care of children, women of all ages, assailants, and the family as a whole.

As with any subject newly introduced for comprehensive curriculum coverage in under-graduate or graduate educational programs, this topic must be adapted to the background of students, including such factors as age and exposure through experience or an undergraduate elective. The recommendations presented can also be applied in in-service education programs for those whose formal education and clinical placements did not systematically address the topic of violence and abuse. The online resources listed in Part IV offer detailed examples for curriculum development and continuing education programs.

Because caregivers' contact with victims, survivors, and perpetrators encompasses many situations through the life span, the major categories addressed are:

- child physical and sexual abuse, including children witnessing violence;
- violence against and between intimate partners, including gay, lesbian, bi-sexual and transgendered persons;
- sexual assault/rape by intimates, dating partners, strangers;
- victims of torture and human trafficking;
- abuse of older adults, including financial exploitation;
- abuse of those in special risk categories – people with disabilities; those who hold visible and immigrant minority status; indigenous populations;
- assailants/perpetrators and assessment for risk of assault/homicide;
- abuse by professionals (e.g. therapists, other health professionals, clergy) in a power position vis-à-vis the client;
- abuse of caregivers in interpersonal and structural contexts such as the workplace, and the interface of such abuse with the care of other victims, as in vicarious traumatization.

Overall, the intent is to assist faculty, students, and practitioners with delineating the *essentials* as well as *limitations* of particular disciplinary roles in this urgent healthcare issue.

Disciplinary and interdisciplinary issues

While this book is comprehensive in scope and in the number of human service professions it addresses, implementation of its recommendations will vary widely according to discipline. The landscape of this topic is fraught with claims, counter-claims, fragmentation, accusations, and disavowals of whose responsibility violence prevention and the care of victims is. For example, the American Psychological Association asserts that it is the appropriate body to set and enforce standards for batterers' programs (Bennett, & Piet, 1999). Others would assign such responsibility to the courts or public health departments. Unless resolved in the best interests of clients, professional differences can result in fragmented service which, in the case of violence, can take on life or death proportions.

Adversarial vs. contextual, collaborative approaches to this topic serve as a barrier to progress in urgently needed educational and service program designs. Controlling behavior among service providers can also mirror the very *power tactics* that are at the heart of the abuse and violence and that should be eradicated or at least ameliorated. If we are fighting among ourselves, it is easy to lose sight of the fact that millions of women and children worldwide are victimized and most of the assailants are men they know (Adams, 2007; PAHO, 1994; Yllo, 1993). Some of the contemporary power struggles among educators and providers contrast sharply with norms of traditional peoples whose customs included community-based supportive rituals and collaborative responsibility for individuals and families in crisis or passing through major transitions (Bird *et al.*, 2002, Hoff *et al.*, 2009; van Gennep, 1960 [1909]).

Although violent attack – by family member, intimate, or stranger – almost invariably carries criminal sanctions, its adverse health sequelae are widely assumed. Now that national and international bodies have proclaimed violence as a grave public health issue; now that the health implications of social behaviors like interpersonal violence are undisputed scientifically, it is no longer a question of *whether* health professions students should be prepared to address this problem (Hoff, 2000). Rather, the question is: *how* can this task be addressed *systematically*, and what are the *differential responsibilities* for victim/survivor care and arenas for *collaboration* among various health and social service professionals?

Violence prevention and the care of traumatized persons is everybody's business, though the parameters of particular professionals' responsibilities vary. Put another way, health professionals today can be seen as "ritual experts" (substitutes for the wise elder or healer in traditional societies) whose task is to assist victim, assailant, and children in "contemporary rites of passage" to a violence-free life (Hoff, 1990). The delineation of individual and collaborative tasks to achieve this end is a major complex goal of this book.

For example, physicians, nurses, dental practitioners, and physiotherapists are most frequently the first to encounter a person suffering traumatic injury from abuse. Pharmacists may see survivors attempting to "self-treat" with drugs; occupational therapists, physical therapists, and rehabilitation counselors treat the immediate and sometimes long-term disabling effects experienced by some victim/survivors; school nurses and counselors daily encounter distressed students; clinical social workers, mental health counselors, and psychologists are most frequently in roles of follow-up counseling or psychotherapy. However, *all* must know the basics, including identification, empathetic support, and referral, and some must know the details of crisis intervention and follow-up treatment.

The book assumes two basic tenets about interdisciplinary collaboration on this and other sensitive health practice areas:

1   Effective, un-defensive practice that includes a feeling of competence and security with

other disciplines demands *prior grounding* in one's own discipline.

2 Simultaneously with such grounding, students' observation and experience in various practice settings must include *models of interdisciplinary collaboration* by professionals who can demonstrate their own unique roles as well as how to deal with interdisciplinary issues such as role blurring and competition for turf.

Unresolved issues in global perspective

Since launching the concept of this book through networking at the 1995 Women's Conference and Forum in Beijing, author collaborators and many others have developed and conducted education and training courses across the globe on violence issues. This includes national and regional efforts documented in Canada, the Philippines, Portugal, South Africa, the United Kingdom, and the United States. Yet, in analyzing the stories of victim/survivors and their advocates across cultures, it is sobering to realize how many issues remain unresolved and how much work is still to be done. Through the phases of developing this book, many urgent but unresolved issues in communities across cultures have continued to surface. Following are those issues and practices that have particular relevance for health and social service professionals:

1 In some schools, teachers abuse children physically and mentally under the guise of "discipline." Despite public education efforts, a female victim of dating violence may hear this response from other girls: 'if her boyfriend hit her, she must have deserved it.'

2 Healthcare services in many countries are unequally available and various segments of service are fragmented or poorly coordinated. There is a need for "one-stop health service centers." Short of such centers, the general public needs information about where appropriate services are available to actual and potential victims. In the Philippines, for example, a "Violet Ribbon Campaign" included countrywide public service announcements on television; a violet ribbon worn by any health provider signifies that the person has had special training in working with victim/survivors of abuse. This campaign was launched in concert with a one-week training conference for medical and nursing faculty who had attended the Hoff/ Adamowski workshops at the UN conference in Beijing. Similar sessions were conducted in Botswana and South Africa in 1994, and since then have been broadened through the tireless work of the NISAA Institute for Women's Development in Johannesburg, South Africa. Through the GBV (Gender-Based Violence) Prevention Network, NISAA and other activists and practitioners are committed to violence prevention in the Horn, East, and Southern Africa. Comparable programs in Russia and Portugal also inspired the development of this book. In Nairobi at the 1985 UN Women's Conference and Forum, a Sudanese physician's riveting presentation (complete with anatomical models) of the damaging effects of female genital mutilation (FGM) inspired literary (Walker, 1992), content in this book, and other writing and medical policy on this topic (see Chapters 2 and 13).

3 In some cultures, traditional healers and elders play a significant role in resolving marital and family disputes. It is important for health professionals to recognize these traditions and collaborate with lay and other healers in the best interests of those needing service.

4 Members of societies with strong patriarchal values tend to deny the existence of child sexual abuse, treat women as subordinates, and often blame the victim when evidence is overwhelming. Across cultures worldwide, some women are killed in an effort to maintain traditional male power and control.

5 Health professionals need gender sensitivity training. At McMaster University in Hamilton, Ontario, Canada, such training is incorporated in the curricula of all health sciences programs.

6 The law or cultural values are sometimes used to maintain male dominance, and in many instances violence-related disputes and charges drag on in courts for years.

7 Some countries have no national, regional, or local system of secure refuges for victims terrorized or threatened with their life at home. And indeed, even if such refuges existed, women in extremely isolated rural areas might be reluctant to use them at the cost of future isolation from the extended family network that might result.

8 Across cultures, despite laws and widespread public education programs in some, there is a tendency to excuse perpetrators on grounds of psychopathology and/or their own histories of abuse as children.

9 While recognizing the importance of focusing on the needs of victim/survivors rather than their assailants, long-term prevention of violence and sexual assault must include programs for abusers. While exasperated advocates may suggest: "Put them in prison and throw away the key," this is not a realistic response, first because all human beings have basic rights, and second, because there is progress in developing programs globally that emphasize accountability for behavior and opportunities to learn non-violent responses to conflict (see Chapter 10). At the primary prevention level, all would-be parents should be prepared to avoid sex role stereotyping in child-rearing – a deeply embedded practice signifying the power of a patriarchal value system that upholds male superiority, aggression, and control.

10 In societies that have only begun to address the issue of preparing health professionals to address violence issues, concerned persons ask: "Where do we start?" This question gets at the central purpose of this book; that is, it presents key issues and a framework for understanding them, and offers basic principles and examples from across cultures that faculty, agency-based trainers, and practitioners can consider without having to reinvent the wheel. The online resources in Part IV are designed to accompany the text and can be adapted to distinct features and learning needs in specific communities.

One result of cross-cultural efforts with the potential for helping many is the vision to develop a consortium of universities offering (through online networking support) a certificate program called "Violence, Crisis, and Human Rights" (see http://www.crisisprograms.org for current developments). The primary focus of this initiative is to prepare expert practitioners, educators, and consultants to systematically address violence and abuse issues as encountered in the health and social service sectors of diverse communities. Through Internet and distance learning strategies, new partnerships can be developed and strengthened worldwide. The forerunner to this project was initiated by Professor Jose Ornelas and piloted with students and practitioners (psychology, social work, nursing) in Lisbon, Portugal at the *Instituto Superior de Psicologia Aplicada* (ISPA) between 2000 and 2003; it was then incorporated into a European Masters Degree Program (Hoff, 1999). Building on this model, City University in London launched a similar educational program, which has also evolved into a Masters degree with the title "Violence, Society, and Practice." (See Part IV for basics and links to this program.)

Cross-cultural approach to education on violence issues

This book emphasizes an experiential or "emic" approach to learning. Applied to violence prevention and the identification and care of abused persons, the emic approach demands that would-be helpers aim to capture empathetically the realities of the victimization experience from the *perspective of the victim/survivors themselves*.

The book's emic perspective implies attention to the distinct and varied cultural contexts in which violence and abuse occur. It also recognizes that despite varied contexts, there are certain commonalities across cultures in respect to violence and abuse. It also *grounds theoretical analysis in the experience of real people* who have been abused – as expressed in their stories from research and clinical scenarios. Thus, regardless of ethnic or religious heritage, and given our common humanity, physical and sexual abuse is *universally* experienced as personally traumatic – *not right, something that should not have happened* – regardless of how a particular violent episode may be treated in criminal or other courts. Thus, the "rule of thumb" expression connects to the centuries-old contention (which has since been discredited) around a law in England and the United States that at one time allowed the beating of one's wife as long as the switch was no thicker than the man's thumb (see http://en.wikpedia.org/wiki/Rule_of_thumb; Martin, 1976). Contemporary understanding across cultures, therefore, and upheld by international (and most national) courts, affirms the humane purpose of this book: to prevent violence, protect the innocent, and find non-violent approaches to the tensions, conflict, and differences that are endemic to the human condition regardless of place, religion, or deeply embedded cultural values.

The book therefore contains ethnographic data from the following cultural settings: Africa, Australia, Canada, Central and South America, China, First Nations people, immigrant and refugee groups, Israel, Portugal, the Caribbean, and the United States, as well as some published resources. Initial collaboration included several more countries, but financial and other barriers prevented their contribution to the final product. The stories, dilemmas, successes, and barriers encountered in these settings (from individual interviews, focus groups, and clinical experience) are shared as an aid to understanding and action on behalf of diverse clients. Survivors' stories and providers' accounts of best practice on their behalf as told here are central to building bridges between lay and professional visions of violence and sexual abuse and what it does to people.

Entering this terrain is very challenging for the survivor who discloses, and the provider who listens and offers to help – especially if for complex reasons the victimized person is not immediately ready or able to follow through. But it is also immensely rewarding, as attested by survivors as well as those of us inspired by their courage and strength, to see them move beyond "victimhood" and rebuild their lives without violence. Clinical and research experience affirms the healing power that survivors note: telling their painful stories is worth it if it helps other people – a lesson revealed in the therapeutic side-effects of the research process and emulated in the aims of this book. For example, battered women are not just helpless victims, but "survivors" who can escape violence with available supports (Hoff, 1990).

From these sources we describe commonalities across cultures in the experience of abuse, for example, the fear and social isolation described by victims from Africa to Europe, North America, and Asia, and the intersection between interpersonal violence today among tribal groups and the history of slavery and colonization of indigenous people. The accounts also reveal the need of sensitivity to the unique history, culture, and political realities of particular societies in which abuse occurs. For example, the emotional healing of a sexual assault victim is often tied to prosecution of the assailant and receiving a public message that justice has been done on the victim's behalf. But in a poor country that lacks modern laboratories for analyzing forensic evidence such as DNA, a victim may be hard put to move on emotionally from the traumatic ordeal. The dictum "Delayed justice is no justice" seems to apply here.

The book's cross-cultural examples capture *four basic assumptions*: (1) globalization and the narrowing of geographical boundaries through cyberspace, international travel and educational exchanges, and the increasing cultural, political, and economic linkages among societies in the global village; (2) recognition of the *commonalities* across cultures in the experience of violence and what professionals and others need to know to help victim/survivors and their families; (3) recognition of the *differences* between various cultural groups and the need to reconcile the universal human rights principle of a violence-free life with the unique circumstances of particular communities and ethnic groups; (4) respect for the fact that survivors themselves and their grassroots advocates were the first to bring this poignant issue to international public attention; health professionals who joined the effort later must therefore not lose sight of the need for continued collaboration with these groups and the first-hand knowledge and hard-earned expertise they bring to the topic.

Identifying information about survivors described here has been altered to protect privacy. Some, on a first reading of these stories, may feel overwhelmed, a response akin to "culture shock." While acknowledging limitations of the written word, such a reaction can enhance the reader's empathy with survivors who live with the realities expressed here and shared for the benefit of health providers. It also signals the importance of self-care and a collaborative approach to this topic. Besides presenting the "inside" reality of survivors, the book also tries to capture the "inside" world of health and social service practitioners. It recognizes that the work of violence prevention and victim care can exact a toll on providers, and that peer support and teamwork are crucial if health professionals are to avoid cynicism, burnout, and withdrawal out of disillusionment and self-protection (see Chapter 12).

The book generally avoids a "how to" approach in favor of presenting general principles arising from these diverse ethnographic sources, including the experience of community experts working with victims of all ages. Our hope is that the illustration of these principles in diverse communities will be useful beyond the particular countries represented here. Another focus is on the complexities of this service domain, for example:

- multicultural issues;
- the interface of violence with other healthcare factors such as substance abuse, psychopathology, or chronic pain;
- the presence of abuse in the personal history or work setting of caretakers expected to assist victims;
- political issues such as historic tensions between medicine and nursing, and the relationship between traditional staff hierarchies and a comprehensive, interdisciplinary approach to care;
- the intersection between refugees of State-sponsored violence and victimization by sexual assault as the "spoils of war".

These complexities may be difficult to unravel, particularly for students and someone who is new to teaching on this topic, and/or who encounters them in practice without adequate preparation to handle effectively.

Finally, the book complements – rather than replicates – major resources already published for particular disciplines, for example, the WHO (2004) *Handbook for the Documentation of Interpersonal Violence Prevention Programmes*. Also, the *Family Violence Clinical Guidelines for Nurses* (CNA, 1992) is a useful document, but it is not intended as a substitute for systematic classroom and clinical instruction on the topic. *Violence Education: Toward a Solution*, published by the Society of Teachers of Family Medicine (Hendricks-Matthews, 1992), contains substantive theoretical content and some course development suggestions for family medicine (a major player in the interdisciplinary landscape), and thus supports the major purpose of this book: to provide a succinct aid to *interdisciplinary* curriculum development and practice across the spectrum of violence and the life span of survivors of abuse.

This book therefore may encourage the person who may view the horrific problem of violence as "too big for me" to do anything that can make a difference. And indeed, when considering, for example, that rape as the "spoils of war" has gone on for many centuries, it may seem reasonable to conclude that one individual's effort makes no difference. Yet, if everyone reaches the same conclusion it can serve not only as an excuse to do nothing ("Why should I bother ... nothing changes"), but it also becomes a self-fulfilling prophecy – that is, no one objects (or not enough object to make the powerful listen), so it is basically "business as usual" over the centuries. Yet, there are hopeful signs in what some describe as the "hunger" of young people signing up for volunteer service and seeking out ways to give back and shape the world and its problems they will inherit.

In the United States, for example, the AmeriCorp volunteer organization reported a 69 percent increase in applications, while Steven Culbertson of Youth Service America, following the historic election of Barak Obama, said: "I want you to fall in love with the problems of the world and help me solve them, not shun them" (Helman, 2008). With hope – not cynicism – and communal commitment, such waiting-to-be-tapped young energy can also help stem the tide of global violence. Some pioneers and current workers in this field may be close to burnout on this issue (see Chapter 12). But with youth energy, the powerful tool of the Internet for building community, plus world bodies like the International Criminal Court in The Hague prosecuting crimes against humanity, there truly is reason to be hopeful rather than cynical about stemming the global plague of violence and working toward its prevention.

On the smaller stage, however, we all can make a difference in everyday life with such personal steps as refraining from violent language or hitting a child. When time and other supports are minimal, these individual efforts can make a difference, while recognizing that the broader social change strategies addressed in this book are also necessary for reducing the global epidemic of violence. The following might serve as a mantra for keeping hope and courage alive in this very challenging work.

Vision for international development

A vision without a task is but a dream.
A task without a vision is but drudgery.
A vision with a task can change the world.
(From the Mount Abu Declaration, India, 1989)

References

AACN – American Association of Colleges of Nursing. (1999). *Position Paper: Violence as a Public Health Problem*. Washington, DC: AACN.

Bennett, L., & Piet, M. (1999). Standards for batterer intervention programs: In whose interests? *Violence against Women*, 5(1), 6–24.

Bensman, A. S., Winters, J., & Kizilos, P. (1992). The effects of childhood trauma upon adult recovery from injury and illness. *Minnesota Medicine*, 75, 11–13.

Bird, M., Bowekaty, M., Burhansstipanov, L., Cochran, P. L., Everingham, P. J. & Suina, M. (2002). *Eliminating Health Disparities*. Santa Cruz, CA: ETR Associates.

CNA – Canadian Nurses Association (1992). *Family Violence Clinical Guidelines for Nurses*. Ottawa: CNA.

Helman, S. (2008, 24 November). Youth propels a push toward volunteerism. *Boston Globe*, p. A 1, 8.

Hendricks-Matthews, M. (ed.) (1992). *Violence Education: Toward a Solution*. Kansas City, MO: Society of Teachers of Family Medicine.

Hoff, L. A. (1990). *Battered Women as Survivors*. London and New York: Routledge.

Hoff, L. A. (1991). Human abuse and nursing's response. In P. Holden & J. Littlewood (eds.), *Nursing and Anthropology*, pp. 130–47. London and New York: Routledge.

Hoff, L. A. (1994a). *Violence Issues: An Interdisciplinary Curriculum Guide for Health Professionals*. Ottawa: Health Canada, Health Services Directorate (in English and French).

Hoff, L. A. (1994b) Comments on race, gender and class bias in nursing. *Medical Anthropology Quarterly*, 8(1), 96–9.

Hoff, L. A. (1999). Keynote address: Violence, power and gender issues – a graduate certificate program. Launching Conference. Lisbon, Portugal: ISPA.

Hoff, L. A. (2000). Interpersonal violence. In C. E. Koop, C. E. Pearson, & Schwarz, M. R. (eds.), *Critical Issues in Global Health*, pp. 260–71. San Francisco: Jossey-Bass.

Hoff, L. A., & Adamowski, K. (1995). Workshops: 1. Emergency Medical Service: Victims of Battering and Sexual Assault. 2. Education of Health Professionals on Violence Issues. UN Women's Conference and Forum 1995, Beijing.

Hoff, L. A., Hallisay, B. J. and Hoff, M. (2009). *People in Crisis: Clinical and Diversity Perspectives*. (6th edn). New York and London: Routledge.

Hoff, L. A. and Morgan, B. (in press). *Psychiatric and Mental Health Essentials in Primary Care*.

Hoff, L. A., & Ross, M. (1993). *Curriculum Guide for Nursing: Violence against Women and Children*. Ottawa: University of Ottawa.

Martin, D. (1976). *Battered Wives*. San Francisco: Glide Publications.

PAHO (2003). *Violence against Women: The Health Sector Responds*. Washington, DC: PAHO.

Ross, M., Hoff, L. A., & Coutu-Wakulczyk, G. (1998). Nursing curricula and violence issues: A study of Canadian schools of nursing. *Journal of Nursing Education*, 37(2), 53–60.

Sugg, N. K. & Inui, T. (1992). Primary care physicians' response to domestic violence: Opening Pandora's box. *Journal of American Medical Association*, 267(23), 3157–60.

United Nations Population Fund. (2000). *The State of World Population 2000, Chapter 3. Ending violence against women and girls: A human rights and health priority*. Geneva: United Nations Population Fund.

US Department of State (1998). *Overview to Country Reports on Human Rights Practices for 1997*. Washington, DC: Bureau of Democracy, Human Rights, and Labor.

Van Gennep, A. (1960). *Rites of Passage*. Chicago: University of Chicago Press. [French edn. 1909.]

Walker, A. (1992) *Possessing the Secret of Joy*, Orlando: Harcourt Brace.

WHO – World Health Organization (2004). *Handbook for the Documentation of Interpersonal Violence Prevention Programmes*. Geneva: WHO.

Woodtli, A., & Breslin, E. (1996). Violence-related content in the nursing curriculum. *Journal of Nursing Education*, 35, 367–74.

Woodtli, A., & Breslin, E. (2002). Violence-related content in the nursing curriculum: A follow-up national survey. *Journal of Nursing Education*, 41(4), 340–8.

Yllo, K. (1993). Through a feminist lens: Gender, power, and violence. In R. J. Gelles, & D. R. Loseke (eds.), *Current Controversies on Family Violence*, pp. 47–62. Newbury Park, CA: Sage.

2 Theoretical framework and assumptions

Lee Ann Hoff and Magueye Seck

- A psychosociocultural perspective
- Definition of violence
- Violence as a human rights violation
- Violence in and beyond the family
- Victims and survivors
- Violence, values, and culture
- Victim-blaming
- Clients' experience and empowerment as base
- Incidence of abuse: facts/myths
- Violence and learned behavior
- Social theory and constructs of gender and race
- Conflict analysis, gender roles and male liberation
- Critique of feminist philosophies: relevence to violence prevention
- Social support in victim/survivor care
- Understanding racial violence
- Teamwork and preventive focus
- Collaboration in building theory, public health policy, and responsive health services

A psychosociocultural perspective

Among the many volumes on violence issues, most authors reveal a focus on the discipline of the writer, for example, psychology, sociology, or criminal justice, while acknowledging contributions from others. Understandably then, there has been considerable debate about language, the terms used to define the problem, and the theoretical underpinnings of abuse and violence (Boddy, 1998; Dobash, & Dobash, 1979; Gelles, & Loseke, 1993; Hoff, 1990; Segal, 1987). Since the intended audience for this book reflects the interdisciplinary practice facet of the topic itself, we integrate the diverse theoretical underpinnings of the topic in a psychosociocultural perspective. As such, we therefore try to transcend the academic and practice "turf wars" to an approach affirming our belief that "we are all in this together" and that the best projected outcome for clients and ourselves is to work toward common goals – keeping in mind that very often we are in substantive agreement on issues that really matter. Put another way, we really do need one another on this urgent topic. (See literature on the Conflict Tactics Scale and how research findings (Straus *et al.*, 1980) were used to defuse public support of programs for battered women on grounds that women were "statistically" equal to men in incidents of abusive behavior, but minus the footnote that most women's violence was in self-defense and was not life-threatening and did not result in serious physical injury.)

Since this book's intended audience reflects the interdisciplinary practice facet of the topic itself, its eclectic but integrated analytic framework draws on concepts from crisis theory, victimology, sociocultural analysis, and life event research, especially the contributions of feminist scholars and the community activists who brought the issue of violence to public attention in the first place (Burgess, & Holmstrom, 1974; Herman, 1981; Hoff, 1990; Martin, 1976; Pizzey, 1977; Schechter, 1982). Our analyses, our observations, and direct work with victims and perpetrators, and the ideas and stories of numerous collaborators were central to developing this book. And as activists and educators of health and social service professionals, we assume as our own this visionary ideal of renowned sociologist C. Wright Mills who has profoundly informed our work: "It is the political task of the social scientist ... continually to translate personal troubles into public issues, and public issues into the terms of their human meaning for a variety of individuals" (Mills 1959, p. 187).

Basic to critical theory, oral history, and complementary feminist analysis is the importance of making explicit one's values. We therefore acknowledge the importance of epidemiological and sociological survey data and quantitative analysis in making public the devastating health, emotional and social consequences of violence. But since violence and its outcomes are affected by personal and deeply embedded values, the theoretical premises of this book are drawn primarily from stories like that of Erin Pizzey (1977) and other survivors, their advocates, and caretakers, and from qualitative research, clinical experience with victim/survivors and perpetrators – our own work (Hoff, 1990; Seck, 1995), as well other pro-feminist writers.

In her research, Shulamit Reinharz (1979) laid the groundwork for questioning the purported "objectivity" of researchers by highlighting how research findings are affected by the relationship between the person, the problem, and the method. Research with abused women, however, revealed a fourth important factor – theory (Hoff, 1990). That is – assumed claims to scientific objectivity notwithstanding – the researcher's theoretical framework does, in fact, influence how the research is conducted and the findings are reported. And as we have seen, such "findings" have severely compromised the interests and welfare of those researched. Thus, as social scientists and clinicians (the person), doing qualitative research (the method) with victims and perpetrators of violence (the problem), we ground this book on interdisciplinary theory. Further, we define the persons who have shared their stories with us as "collaborators," *not* as research "subjects" – a term that underscores a researcher's presumed authority and a concept central to defining violence, that is: an abuse of power (Hoff, 1990; Oakley, 1981a, 1981b). Put another way, this book speaks to who we are, the urgency of the topic, and the most convincing methods and concepts to convey its mission. Coincidentally, our observations and the stories of victim/survivors and perpetrators complement the major teaching methods among health and social service professionals: critical observation of their patients/clients, and case studies from the field and people's everyday lives – in this case, the *context* of violence and abuse across the life cycle, through deprivation and wars, refuges, and the reserves of aboriginal and segregated people.

Accordingly, we present several assumptions, key concepts, and major theoretical sources that have informed our work and the development of this book. In doing so, to paraphrase C. Wright Mills, we recognize the intersections of biography within history and society. We avoid grand theorizing and obscure languages. We present facts and figures in the context of a comparative, historical, and interdisciplinary framework that is clearly and explicitly sensitive to social justice. Through careful joining of research, theory, and practice, we strive to make the world a better place (Mills, 1959).

Definition of violence

Although influenced by cultural, psychological and political factors, violence is a *social* act. At its most basic, interpersonal violence is not merely an instinct-driven response. Rather, it is primarily the chosen action of human beings who *may* be mentally deranged and therefore excusable (see Chapters 10 and 11), but who generally know a society's rules regarding right and wrong behavior – a universal value governing societies across the globe over the ages.

It is critical to define these layers: What is "interpersonal," and what is "violence"? Violence constitutes behavior for which the perpetrator is *accountable* to the moral community. This definition is important because it goes deep into various aspects of both individual and institutional levels and the problem of victim blaming.

Historically, violence has sometimes been excused as a "cultural norm"; the term "cultural relativism" describes such a misplaced attribution (see the "Violence, values, and culture" section below). Another interpretation defines violence as an inevitable outcome of aggressive instincts, or, an expectable result of mental illness, and therefore excusable. However, these traditional definitions are still alive and used to explain violence (Friedman, 2006; Hoff *et al.*, 2009). In Boston, Massachusetts, for example, despite progress in judicial education and reform, public controversy raged for weeks as recently as the year 2000 around a judge's sentence of probation instead of jail time for an offender who admitted kidnapping and attempting to rape a child; the explanation offered was that some people act out in an "aberrant way" in stressful situations.

Today, however, most violence scholars reject analytic frameworks such as sociobiology which serve to maintain violence as a private matter originating primarily from innate sources. Instead, violence is now widely interpreted in psychosociocultural and feminist terms; i.e. as a predominantly social phenomenon with far-reaching effects on personal and public health worldwide (Burstow, 1992; Everett, & Gallop, 2000; Hoff *et al.*, 2009; ICWHI, 1992; MacLeod, 1989; National Clearinghouse on Family Violence, 1991; US Department of Health and Human Services, 1986; Seck, 1995; Stark, & Flitcraft, 1996; Wendell, 1990; Yllo, & Bograd, 1987). That is the position taken in this book. In such a framework, violence – in most instances – constitutes behavior learned in a milieu permeated with social inequalities based on age, gender, race, ethnicity, etc. and in a cultural context rife with images of violence and physical force portrayed as the dominant modes of conflict resolution and in which depictions of accountability for violence are rare.

Violence consists of exerting physical force and power over another – usually with the intent of controlling, disempowering, and/or injuring the other. Though violent abuse has serious implications for physical and mental health, it is not in itself a medical phenomenon except in the few instances in which a person is found to be "insane" – a legal term designating a person's mental incapacity (and therefore excusability) while behaving violently (Monahan, 1981; Monahan, & Steadman, 1994; VandeCreek, & Knapp, 2001). Nor is violence merely a criminal justice phenomenon. Rather, it crosses legal, ethical, and healthcare domains, and society's major institutions, thus rendering it a complex issue with moral, sociocultural, political, and personal ramifications.

Physical violence is almost invariably accompanied by verbal abuse. For example, regular verbal threats of abuse or killing cause no immediate *physical* trauma, but clearly strike terror and fear for one's life in the heart of the intended victim. This book clearly recognizes the damaging effects of verbal abuse generally, its frequency during conflict between intimate partners, the particular traumas of racial or ethnic slurs, and the taunting of lesbian, gay, and transgendered people or those with disabilities. Such verbal abuse is rooted in bias, fear, and/or hatred, and is often followed by threats or acts of physical violence. Persistent psychological abuse, even without physical attack, can devastate a person emotionally and lead to serious health problems. Also, verbal abuse usually precedes physical abuse. However, in order not to underestimate the life-threatening nature of some violence, it is important to distinguish verbal insults, for example in a dating relationship, from sexual or other life-threatening assault at knife or gunpoint.

The terms "abuse" and "violence" are used interchangeably in this book, though abuse – especially sexual – does not always entail physical injury. For example, an incest victim, after several years of abuse, may have no visible injuries, but most surely she or he is "violated" and almost invariably suffers severe emotional trauma (Herman, 1981). As battered women often say: "It is easier to heal from the physical wounds than the emotional ones," though the two are linked. Without satisfactory healing of such deep-seated emotional wounds, serious physical and mental health problems are often the unfortunate result (Everett, & Gallop, 2000). One way many cope with the trauma of abuse is by dependence on psychotropic drugs, especially in the absence of appropriate support at crisis points, and follow-up counseling or psychotherapy (Hoff *et al.*, 2009).

Violence as a human rights violation

We have moved from defining violence as a private matter, a family problem, a medical illness, or a cultural norm, to the currently dominant view of violence as a social act and public health issue worldwide. A human rights perspective directed to the global epidemic of violence is pivotal in the United Nations (1996b) report on the 1995 Beijing Declaration and Platform for Action.

The UN convention on eliminating all forms of discrimination against women also situates the issue in a human rights framework. Progressively, more countries such as the United States, France, Canada, Senegal and international bodies such as the UN, the World Health Organization (WHO), and the International Council on Women's Health Issues are declaring interpersonal violence as a human rights issue (Delport, 2007). In 2003, signaling the importance that the UN attached to addressing violence against women, the UN General Assembly mandated the preparation of an in-depth study on all forms and manifestation of violence against women. The *Secretary-General's Study on Violence against Women* (UN, 2006) revealed many disturbing facts about violence against women in general, and the issues with the *perpetrators of violence* in particular. The aims of the study included:

- highlighting the persistence and unacceptability of all forms of violence against women;
- strengthening the political commitment and joint efforts of all stakeholders to prevent and eliminate violence against women;
- identifying ways and means to ensure more sustained and effective implementation of State obligations to address all forms of violence against women;
- increasing State accountability.

The study revealed these major facts:

- Violence against women is severe and pervasive throughout the world.
- Many women are subjected to sexual, psychological and emotional violence by an intimate partner.
- More than 130 million girls have been subjected to female gender mutilation/cutting.
- Women experience sexual harassment throughout their lives.

- The majority of the hundreds of thousands of people trafficked annually are women and children.
- Violence against women in armed conflict frequently includes sexual violence.
- Women who are subject to violence are more likely to suffer physical mental and reproductive health problems.
- Domestic violence and rape account for 5 percent of the total disease burden for women aged 15–44 in developing countries.
- Violence before or during pregnancy has serious health consequences for mother and child.
- Women who have experienced violence are at higher risk of contracting HIV.
- Violence against women may prevent women from full economic participation and may hinder employment opportunities.
- Girls who have experienced violence are less likely to complete their education.
- The direct costs of violence against women are extremely high (Delport, 2007).

These points underscore the fact that interpersonal violence is not *just* a "women's issue"; rather, it is a global human rights issue that is increasingly capturing the attention of world leaders, executives of corporations who see the economic toll of violence among employees, and religious leaders, most of whom no longer condone abuse of wives on the spurious grounds of maintaining marital bonds at the expense of victims. A human rights perspective emphasizes the accountability of perpetrators along with opportunities for them to learn non-violent approaches to interpersonal conflict; appropriate health and social services for victim/survivors; and principles of restorative justice. This includes eliminating the abuse of power at the highest levels, as in State-sponsored violence.

The challenge remains: how? We believe that education about theory, values, and cross-cultural exchange regarding prevention and successful intervention efforts provide a good start. Worldwide, we find the widespread belief that some people have the right to control others, with some cultures justifying violence and all forms of aggression, or glorifying violence that devalues certain members of society. A fundamental premise in addressing this human rights issue is this: put a philosophy of *caring* at the center of practice, as suggested in examples throughout this book, and commit oneself to continuing education on this urgent topic. Suggested responses to these challenges to health and social service workers when encountering beliefs that aid and abet violence (but may be different from one's own) are elaborated in Chapter 3.

Violence in and beyond the family

In most communities worldwide, one's greatest risk of attack is from family members (Hoff, 2000). However, the term "family violence" obscures the reality that most perpetrators within the family are heterosexual men, and most victims are women of all ages and children (Finkelhor *et al.*, 1983). "Family violence" also deflects attention from the sociocultural roots of abuse which extend beyond the family to deeply embedded cultural values and traditional social structures which particularly disempower women and children. Further, "family violence" excludes some major forms of violence: physical and sexual assault by an acquaintance or stranger; sexual exploitation by therapists and other professionals; rape as the spoils of war; and the traffic of women and children in the international sex trade arena. Socialization in child-rearing, education, youth culture, employment practices, and family ideology are all central in defining interpersonal violence.

Victims and survivors

The term "victim/survivor" is preferred, and refers here to a variety of persons regardless of relationship to assailant – family member, intimate, therapist, co-worker, acquaintance, stranger, patient/client. "Victim/survivor" is intended to acknowledge explicitly one's victimization, but simultaneously convey an abused person's potential for growth, development, and empowerment; i.e. a status beyond the dependency implied by "victim" (Mawby, & Walklate, 1994; McCullough, 1995).

An emphasis on growth beyond "victimhood" to "survivor" status is underscored in a contemporary climate in which some individuals, under criminal trial for violent acts, use their history of victimization as grounds for "temporary insanity" pleas and excusability for violent behavior. Certainly, those who have been deeply wounded by abuse deserve an appropriate social and healthcare response. While so responding, however, it is crucial to acknowledge the inherent freedom, resilience, and indeterminate nature of human beings, their resiliency, and capacity to rise beyond tragic circumstances – *particularly if they receive social support* (Antonovsky, 1987; M. Hoff, 2005). These points apply regardless of the gender of either the assailant or survivor.

Current international attention to the abuse and victimization of women and children is due primarily to the work of survivors themselves, community-based and criminal justice activists, and women's studies scholars, with health professionals joining later. The field now is often referred to as "victimology" (Campbell, & Humphreys, 1993; Hoff *et al.*, 2009; Russell, 1990). The insights and practice protocols of these pioneers are fundamental in developing complementary programs in health and social service agencies which traditionally have underserved victim/survivors of abuse. Rather than duplicating such protocols, this book incorporates them as major resources for various healthcare professionals.

Violence, values, and culture

There is wide variation cross-culturally in ideas about interpersonal violence and the roles of men and women. Professionals, like other members of a cultural community, are informed by deeply embedded beliefs, myths, and traditions concerning women, marriage, the family, and violence (Canadian Panel on Violence against Women, 1993; Hoff, 1990; Kurz, & Stark, 1988). As a result, despite claims of neutrality and objectivity, research, theoretical formulations, and practice protocols on behalf of victim/survivors are value-laden.

It is useful, therefore, to consider several key concepts that underpin our understanding of violence and its effects on diverse groups. *Ethnicity* is tied to the notion of shared origin and culture. In multicultural societies such as the United States and Canada, ethnic identities can shift and change based on power distribution and factors like language, skin color, religion, or country of origin, while some groups may define themselves as *bicultural* within a dominant culture of a particular society (Loustaunau, & Sobo, 1997). If we do not know another's cultural heritage, we should explore with sensitivity and a non-judgmental attitude. *Ethnocentrism* is the emotional attitude that one's own ethnic group, nation, or culture is superior to that of others. Exaggerated ethnocentrism can lead to prejudice, bias, and discrimination toward others based on their ethnic or religious identity, e.g. "Jews are greedy," or "Blacks are lazy," "Mexicans are dirty," "Muslims are religious fanatics." *Stereotyping* refers to an unvarying pattern of thinking and pigeonholing a person or group in a box that disallows for individuality, critical judgment, and basic respect for people different from oneself – thus putting a damper on positive care outcomes.

Cultural relativism is a more complex concept. First, it requires that instead of prejudging others, we should consider various actions, beliefs or traits within their cultural *context* in order to better understand them. Cultural relativism presents particular difficulties with respect to violence and in healthcare practice. That is, some cultural practices may be harmful to physical and emotional health and welfare. It allows outsiders to ignore or dismiss certain human rights violations such as woman battering as "relative" to particular cultures, as in the expression, "That's just part of their culture."

A dramatic and controversial example illustrating cultural relativism is female genital mutilation (FGM), which, in one folk language, is called *tahara*, or "purity," implying that girls and women who have not undergone this procedure are "impure." In some cultures, female genital mutilation is a rite of passage. However, the term itself (FGM) is controversial – considered by Boddy (1998, p. 80), for example, as a decontextualized term that obscures its meaning in specific cultures. As a result, some have substituted the more neutral term "cutting" for mutilation. Until recently, FGM has been excused under the guise of a "cultural norm." Instead of the "cultural relativism" illustrated by such a stance, we accept for this book the WHO definition of FGM as a human rights violation; WHO has urged abolishing the ritual because of its harmful effects on women's reproductive health and sexual expression (WHO, 1994). (See Chapter 13 for further discussion of FGM and surgical restoration of "virgin status".)

In a related vein, the importance of female virginity and marital fidelity is upheld by the custom of "honor killings" carried out by the "offended" husband or male family member. Though legally forbidden in most societies and not approved by Islamic religious tradition, "honor killing" has been accepted with minimal punishment for perpetrators. These killings occur in mostly in the Middle East, although three such killings have been reported in the American states of Georgia, New York, and Texas (Dryta, 2009; Jacoby, 2008; Vandello, & Cohen, 2008). The instances for honor killings include: when a woman engages in extra-marital sex, has been raped, or has engaged in any action viewed as a violation of chastity norms. She is thus labeled as "unclean," and thereby brings disgrace to a family's "honor" – judgments used by male relatives to justify killing her.

At the heart of these killings is the "double standard" regarding male and female sexual expression. In essence, the cultural value of "purity" is attached to women but not men, and is by no means limited to Islamic societies. In Christianity, this double standard dates back many centuries at a time when illiteracy was common and major moral teaching was done through preaching and art forms. For example, in an architectural gem of a church in Italy – resplendent with sculptures and mosaics – all the martyrs (Christianity's most honorable form of death) are depicted as male, while all the virgins are depicted as female. This is not to say that male martyrs perhaps were also virgins, or that some female virgins were also martyrs.

But the power of symbols for conveying values enduring across many centuries to the current era is illustrated in the following question raised about the widespread contemporary acceptance of male promiscuity: If men are not expected to control pre-marital sexual expression to the same extent prescribed for women, but still desire a "virgin" bride, where are all the virgins supposed to come from? Clearly, this double standard crosses religious boundaries as well as male/female boundaries, as indicated in this quip by a contemporary American Jewish woman (age 29, in a society where the majority of both men and women willingly "lose" their virginity before age 19) who was "saving" her virginity until she found a Jewish husband. When her friend asked if her betrothed was also a virgin, she laughed, saying "Somebody has to know what they're doing!" Acceptance of male dominance is also evident among contemporary American brides who are "given away" to the groom by their father, apparently with no awareness of this custom's origin in the ancient cultural norm of the "patriarch" (owner of wives, children, animals, and the estate) transferring ownership of his daughter to another male. Tolstoy's classic novel *Anna Karenina* reveals the tragic results of Anna's extra-marital love – losing her children, and her suicide.

This double standard and male ownership of women reverberates across generations to the present era. Contemporary women threatened with their lives by abusive partners are familiar with this declaration of "ownership": "If I can't have you, nobody can," while current news stories about murders of female partners frequently cite male jealousy and murderous rage because of a woman's choice to divorce and/or find a new partner (see Adams, 2007).

The double standard and "cultural norm" excuse for indifference to violence is also revealed in language, for example: "Boys will be boys," and this statement excusing promiscuity or even rape: "Once a man is aroused, he cannot stop himself" – a demeaning judgment suggesting men's inability to control sexual expression, and thereby implying an inferior moral stature than that accorded women. Here is another example of language revealing beliefs: after noting repeated episodes of violence against a Native woman, the frustrated observer says "That's the way they are ... What can you do?" Such a remark fails to connect personal trauma to the tragic political oppression and forced social isolation endured by aboriginal people (LaRocque, 1994; Wakegijig, & Jenkins, 1992). Such thinking that reveals "cultural relativism" also obscures the reality of pre-reservation life among the Lakota Sioux, for example, when wife-beating was rare, taboo and a violation of harmony, moderation, and the deeply embedded Sioux value of equality between adult men and women (Mousseau, 1989, p. 8).

In a similar vein, most adults in Western societies believe it is impossible to rear a child without at some point using physical discipline, despite research documenting the negative results of this approach to child rearing (Gil, 1970; Greven, 1990). Children in traditional cultures are not just the responsibility of their parents; they are considered the responsibility of the clan, the entire community – their care not confined to individual parents whose parenting abilities vary (Brendtro *et al.* 1990; Mandamin, 1993). (See Chapter 8.)

Additionally, some people still believe that women who are raped have somehow "asked for it." As one informant said: "Some don't believe the survivor's reality ... that is one of the worst things they can do." Unfortunately, the legacy of disbelieving victims is still alive. This is particularly dangerous in the case of innocent children who most often cannot defend themselves. In some treatment settings, survivors may face double jeopardy in that traditional psychiatric theories distort the reality of sexual abuse. For example, the primary problem of abuse may be obscured under a diagnosis of "borderline personality disorder" (Everett, & Gallop, 2000). Such a diagnosis effectively discredits victim/survivors who are brave enough to disclose a victimization history during psychiatric assessment and treatment, and affirms the value and power placed on biomedical models and psychiatric nomenclature (Becker, 1963; Burstow, 1992; Cooksey, & Brown, 1998; Goffman, 1963; McHugh, & Clark, 2006; Mitchinson, 1993; Stuhlmiller, 1997; Warshaw, 1989).

Another deeply embedded value concerns the centuries-old acceptance of rape (and its rare prosecution) as the "spoils of war." Only recently has this crime been addressed in the International Criminal Court at The Hague as an international example of a violation of human rights (see Chapter 6).

Victim-blaming

One major result of health professionals' acceptance (until recently) of mainstream values about violence is the blaming of victims for their plight, a legacy embedded in the psyches and attitudes of abused clients as well as their caretakers (Hilberman, 1980; Rieker, & Carmen, 1986; Ryan, 1971). One incest survivor asked: "Am I guilty for loving my father? It was up to my dad to draw the line .... He was the adult in control."

The commonality of self-blame and depression among victims is linked to society's tradition allocation of accountability for violence to victims rather than their assailants (Caplan, 199. Cloward, & Piven, 1979; Jones, 1980; Mawby, & Walklate, 1994; Stanko, 1990). A battered woman's query: "How can I please my husband? .... I did everything he demanded" varies only slightly from the counselor's classic question: "What did you do to provoke him?" In other words, victims tend to blame themselves because they have first been blamed by others. The issue of victim-blaming implies the ironic expectation that battered wives – to stop the abuse and/or escape death itself – take up the role of fugitive, along with continued responsibility for children, while her assailant often goes on with life as usual (Hoff, 1990). In the past few decades, community activists and feminist scholars have challenged the notion of victim-blaming. Consequently, there have been some qualitative changes in attitudes and particularly in the US media, since the famous case of O. J. Simpson and Nicole Brown in 1994. Blaming the victim has now entered into the general arena of intellectual discourse – clinical and legal.

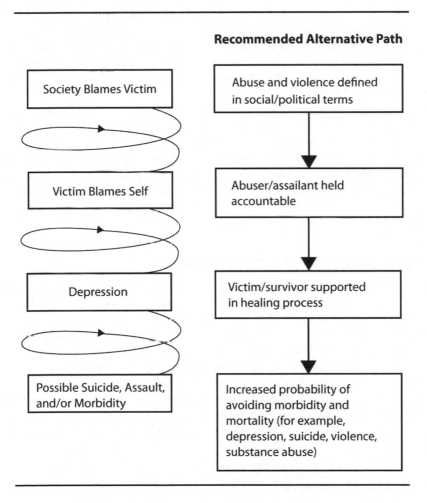

Figure 2.1 Abuse, the downward spiral, and alternative path.
Source: Hoff, *et al.* (2009, p. 49).

Recent mandatory arrest laws are a new twist on the tradition among Native American people in the US: if a man battered his wife, *he* had to leave, *he* couldn't marry again, couldn't lead or take part in a war party or hunt, or own a pipe (Mousseau, 1989, p. 13). Canadian men's National White Ribbon Campaign similarly illustrates that wife abuse is not merely a women's issue, but a community responsibility. (See Chapter 10, the example of Emerge and men's action internationally to stop male violence.)

A "downward spiral" emanating from culture and rigidly defined social roles illustrates what happens in the victim-blaming process if it is not interrupted at its source or as soon as possible: When it is the individual victim/survivor against society, its values and policies about accountability for violence, a victim/survivor typically will suppress the emotional pain of abuse and violence, with self-blame and depression easily following. Unless the downward spiral is interrupted – preferably through grassroots prevention efforts, societal change strategies, and holding perpetrators accountable – morbidities, further violence, and even suicide or murder may result (Hoff *et al.*, 2009, Chapter 2).

The deeply embedded process of victim-blaming is compounded by the influence of "medicalization," that is, the tendency to interpret life's problems – whether medical or not – in a medical framework (Hoff *et al.*, 2009, Chapter 12). In the case of violence, this means ascribing a psychiatric diagnosis to the victim (e.g. depression or borderline personality disorder, in the DSM[1] nomenclature) and excusing the assailant (e.g. temporary insanity), thus alleging psychopathology and obscuring the sociopolitical roots of the problem (Caplan, 1993; Cooksey, & Brown, 1998; Stark *et al.*, 1979).

It also may mean "adding insult to injury" from the original violence by treating it as evidence of psychopathology, and therefore excusing accountability for violence and abuse – a misguided approach that benefits neither victim nor perpetrator – and which loses an opportunity for perpetrators to learn non-violent responses to life stressors. But for the advocacy of feminist psychologists and psychiatrists, the diagnosis "rapism" (vs. defining rape as the crime it is) would have been included in the DSM (see Chapter 10). And as a result of widespread political activism from many progressive groups, "homosexuality" no longer appears in the ever-expanding roster of diagnosable mental "illness".

Clients' experience and empowerment as base

To be relevant, health service and education protocols on behalf of victim/survivors must be grounded in the realities and complexities of the victimization experience. As a battered woman stated in response to the question of what health providers might do to help: "Come to a shelter, listen to our stories, learn how to be with us. We don't expect you to do it for us, but just be there to help when we finally decide to leave." Health educators on this topic must therefore immerse themselves – at least vicariously – in the unique and tragic world of victimization as a way to lend credibility to their teaching. Key to survivors' empowerment is a partnership with them which recognizes that they are in charge of their healing and do not expect to be rescued. Such immersion, however, also suggests the need for attention to self-care by providers as a means of avoiding burnout and cynicism when facing the multifaceted challenges of working in this field (see Chapter 12).

Incidence of abuse: facts/myths

Statistically, most violence worldwide is perpetrated against women of all ages, children (girls and boys), and other men by heterosexual males (homophobia notwithstanding). Contrary to widely held fears of attack by strangers, the majority of victims know their abusers. Nevertheless, some women abuse their male partners; and mothers physically abuse children in numbers approximately equal to that of abusive fathers, stepfathers, and/or boyfriends. This figure is misleading, however, considering that mothers typically spend much more time with children than fathers do and their abuse is not as injurious physically (Martin, 1983). Similarly, lesbian and gay partners are not immune to violence (Renzetti, 1992). Yet, among couples, the most serious injuries are inflicted by male abusers, and in the majority of instances of female violence, the occasion is *self-defense*, and usually no medically serious injury results from their violence (Johnson, 1998). Furthermore, when women do resort to violence, more serious abuse or murder by their male partners often follows (Adams, 2007; Browne, 1987; Campbell *et al.*, 2003), thus countering the common myth of violence as an acceptable or necessary response to violence.

These facts contradict the alleged "gender neutrality" of violence and should be kept in mind while acknowledging the recent and troubling embrace of violence by girls and women. This book also underscores the double jeopardy of those experiencing social and physical isolation rooted in prejudice, inaccessibility of service, and geopolitical or religious factors, e.g. Native people, immigrant or racial minorities, gender oppression based on alleged religious grounds, people with disabilities, lesbian women, rural women and children, and those displaced and/or attacked during State-sponsored violence.

Violence and learned behavior

The incidence of violence by girls and women in both heterosexual and lesbian relationships is increasing. While this issue has not been extensively researched, it does suggest evidence of women's widespread adoption of aggressive behaviors traditionally engaged in by men. It also supports the concept of violence as "learned behavior," equally available to boys and girls, men and women, that can be (for those inclined to violence) displaced by *learning non-violent approaches* to conflict resolution, traditionally the domain of women (Ruddick, 1989). In other words, despite sociobiologists' claims, conflict is endemic to the human condition, but violence is not (Dobash, & Dobash, 1979; Gailey, 1988; Hoff, 1992).

This important concept lends a note of optimism to an otherwise grim subject, and strengthens a fundamental premise of this book:

* Boys and girls, women and men can learn non-violent as well as violent responses to stress and conflict.
* Health professionals (and students aspiring thereto) can learn compassion and crisis intervention with victims.
* Human service providers can learn about shared responsibility among disciplines and can teach clients and the public about violence prevention.
* Healthcare workers can learn non-violent responses when they themselves are abused in work settings.
* Health educators with traditional backgrounds can emphasize an interdisciplinary, community-focused response to victim/survivors and perpetrators.

Social theory and constructs of gender and race

According to the sociologist Talcott Parsons (1951), gender differences help to integrate society, at least in its traditional form. Although "structural functionalism" is now largely discredited among social theorists, we note it here in respect to traditional social role theory as a factor explaining gender-based violence. Parsons believed that a complementary set of roles links women and men into family units that in turn build a larger society. Over many generations, a sex-based division of labor became institutionalized, built into the structure of society and taken for granted.

Parsons' view stresses the theory of complementarity (instrumental and expressive) by which gender integrates society, both structurally, in terms of what people do, and morally, in terms of what they believe. Critical analysis of this view argued that Parsons' analysis ignores personal strains and the social costs produced by rigid gender roles, and legitimizes the status quo, which may not be functional for either women or men (Seck, 1995). Many field observers would agree that sex role stereotypes have been one of the greatest challenges in the fight against male violence.

Conflict analysis, gender roles and male liberation

Social conflict analysis and gender stratification takes a closer look at the issues of male violence against women by underlining inequality. This analysis points directly to the inequality of men and women not only in a social context, but also politically, and economically – a view shared by many contemporary writers and policy analysts on male violence (Schechter, 1982; Adams, 2007; Gil, 1970; Hartmann, 1981), and one shared by most feminists (Seck, 1995).

Their view is that women are a "minority" power group and men benefit from the unequal relationship, which is perpetuated by sexism and sexist ideology. In other words, violence has its sources in gender inequality. Allocation of rigid gender roles, which in fact continues to legitimize male violence and male aggression against women worldwide, is something that health and social service providers everywhere must be concerned about. Although many feminists view sex role theory as limited and often dangerous, there are others who strongly believe that sex role has a positive function. Interestingly, historical observation of the facts shows a gradual weakening of the men's liberation movement in the 1970s and 1980s. Consequently, on one hand, the progressive wing of the men's liberation formed a pro-feminist movement which held the notion of gender relation and power. On the other hand, the conservative wing maintained their anti-feminist view founded upon rigid sex roles. Sawyer (1970) asserts that a fuller concept of humanity and characteristics such as strong and weak, active and passive, are not the province of only one sex.

Critique of feminist philosophies: relevance to violence prevention

Sawyer's work on male liberation invites our critique of feminist philosophies and their impact on women and violence prevention.

In university and college classrooms (mostly women) in the US and Canada, if one opens a session on feminism and its relationship to violence with these questions: "Do you ever refer to yourself as a feminist? If not, why not? Can men be feminists?" a typical response includes snickers and questioning looks that imply, "Are you kidding? In no way could I identify with those crazy man-hating women!" Any men in the class appear afraid to speak up regardless of what opinions they may hold. Follow-up questions and likely responses might include: "Do you think women and men should be paid equally for the same job?" (yes). "Are you against male partners beating their wives?" (yes). "Do you think rape victims should be blamed for the attack?" (no). "Do you think men and women should share in child-rearing and the other unpaid work of society?" (yes).

Typically, the responses to questions like these suggest a need for feminist analysis, while beginning "snickers" suggest widespread stereotypes about what "feminism" is. This scenario also reflects the opportunities that young and other women in Western societies enjoy, thanks largely to the hard work of "troopers" in the "third wave of feminism" to advance the rights of women on many fronts – the home, in paid jobs, educational, political and other institutions. Despite these advances, many millions of women in poor countries eke out a living on as little as US$2.00 per day, and are the major civilian casualties – including rape of themselves and girl children – of primarily "men's wars."

We therefore present a brief overview of feminist philosophies, with this basic definition: "feminism" means taking gender into account regarding daily life, social and other theories, research methodology, and professional practice. Broadly, there are five main branches of feminist philosophy: Liberal, Radical, Marxist, Socialist, Psychoanalytic. What these philosophies share in common is their activism to end violence against women. In this overview we draw on, and recommend for further reading, especially the works of Segal (1987, 1999), Chodorow (1978), Miller (1976), and Smith (1982). We also ascribe to Bergman's (1991) relational perspective citing the overall disadvantages for male psychological development of all boys in male-dominant societies in which (unlike for girls) boys get very little practice in the relationship and empathy arena – thus for some, laying a foundation for male violence.

Liberal: Counter-intuitively, this is the most conservative branch of feminist thought. While advocating for equal wages, for example, it raises few questions about hierarchical social structures that indeed show a few women sharing advantages with men at the top, but which leave a majority of women (especially in poor countries) at serious disadvantage economically. The privileged women in these top positions can afford homemaker and nanny services, usually offered at low wages and minimum job security by young women of color (often immigrants).

Radical: A source of many myths and stereotypes about feminism; e.g. "All feminists are lesbians and hate men." The truth is, some lesbian women do not subscribe to feminism, and most have male friends, while some feminist women have loving and satisfying relationships with men who also advocate for women's rights and equality. Radical feminism argues for separatism for women, and comes close to "essentialism" and biological determinism in its assumption of the natural, inborn, or "essential" superiority of women – the opposite of Freud's thesis regarding innate female "inferiority."

Marxist: Defines women as a class while omitting gender and cultural values. Thus, in societies built on Marxist theory, women as a class indeed earn salaries equal to men's, but suffer similar gender and culture-based interpersonal violence (battering and rape) as do women in capitalist societies.

Socialist: Moves beyond Liberal, Radical, and Marxist analysis and emphasizes the intersection between gender and class. It complements critical theory in its emphasis on unveiling unconsciousness of gender, race, class, sexual identity or other non-dominant status as factors in discrimination among both consumers and providers of healthcare and social service. It offers powerful grounds for various disadvantaged groups to work collaboratively toward equality for all, and to avoid divisive arguments about who is more or less oppressed.

Psychoanalytic: Complements socialist feminism in its redefinition of Freudian theory regarding the purported inferiority inherent in the female sex lacking a penis. It asserts that women's social disadvantage is *socially constructed* rather than biologically determined.

With our definition of feminism, and in the context of "labeling theory" we do not limit ourselves to a *single* way of identifying who we are as in, "Hear me, I am a feminist!" Rather, we frame our identity and analysis of violence through the lens of "socialist feminism," critical sociocultural theory, our professional health and social service practice, our personal history, family identity, and more.

Combating gender-based violence is not only necessary for the rights of women but for communities around the world to strengthen themselves economically and politically. Combating gender violence also means understanding the perpetrators, and preventing their attacks in the first place (see Chapter 10). Thus, health and social service professionals have the enormous task of enhancing their understanding of gender-based violence and particularly its impact on women and children. Many scholars now agree with the definition that violence in most instances constitutes behavior learned in a milieu permeated with social inequalities based on age, gender, ethnicity, etc., and on images of violence and physical force as the dominant modes of conflict resolution (Carlsson-Paige, & Levin, 2008).

Social support in victim/survivor care

The American Sociological Association (ASA) provides the following explanation: "Medical sociology is the subfield which applies the perspectives, conceptualization, theories, and methodologies of sociology to phenomena having to do with human health and disease. As a specialization, medical sociology encompasses a body of knowledge which places health and disease in a social, cultural, and behavioral context" (Weiss, & Lonnquist, 2006). In the vast medical sociology literature, central to victim/survivor care is the concept of social support, the resources available for dealing with problematic conditions of life, particularly those that overwhelm the individual's own coping ability. Included in social support are three kinds: first, emotional support (feelings of comfort, respect, love, caring, and concern); second, cognitive support (information, knowledge, and advice); and third, material support (products or services to assist in handling specific problems) (Weiss, & Lonnquist, 2006).

Understanding racial violence

On the meaning of race, no sociologist has written more than W. E. B. Du Bois. Phil Zuckerman (2004) wrote in his analysis of race that unlike Marx, Durkheim, Weber, Lenin, Gilman, Veblen – or Simmel, Mead, or Comte – Du Bois focused on race, and that contemporary social theorists should recognize this critically important fact about Du Bois and race: he keenly recognized that racial issues are supremely important and pivotal to how human beings experience the world – in matters of health, wealth, literacy, religion, and crime, as well as in political interactions at city, State, and international governance levels.

Du Bois's most important contribution was his ability to link his racial and class analysis together. He was extremely critical of Karl Marx's shortcomings on racial analysis. For Du Bois, Marxist class analysis completely ignored the color line. He insisted that race is a social construction, involving matters of economics, history, politics, heritage, and culture much more than simple biology or physicality. In fact Du Bois was the first sociologist to argue explicitly that race could not be reduced to merely a scientific category or biological determinant (Zuckerman, 2004).

In order to understand the concept of social support, its presence or absence, and how it relates to violence in America, one must understand the history of the civil rights movement in America. The civil rights movement began a long time ago – as early as the seventeenth century, Blacks and Whites, slaves in Virginia and Quakers in Pennsylvania, protested the barbarity of slavery. Nat Turner, Sojourner Truth, Frederick Douglass, William Lloyd Garrison, John Brown, and Harriet Tubman are but a few of those who led the resistance to slavery before the Civil War. After the Civil War, another protracted battle began against slavery's legacy – racism and segregation. But for most Americans, the civil rights movement began on May 15, 1954, when the Supreme Court handed down the *Brown v. Board of Education of Topeka* decision out-lawing segregation in public schools. "The court unlocked the door, but the pressure applied by thousands of men and women in the movement pushed that door open wide enough to allow Blacks to walk through it toward this country's essential prize: freedom" (Williams, 1987).

There have been painful recorded stories of the slave trade and its links to the violence and crimes against Blacks for over 300 years, ranging from violent laws and policies of segregation and discrimination. But one story that left an indelible mark is the Tuskegee Syphilis Experiment, and the secrecy around it which today continues to incite interest in the teaching of sociology, law, policy, medicine, ethics, and nonviolence. Much has been written about the Tuskegee Syphilis Experiment. For 40 years between 1932 and 1972, the US Public Health Services (PHS) conducted an experiment on 399 Black men in the late stages of syphilis. The violence, the crime, the policy, and the secrecy around this experiment go far beyond any psychological or biological explanations of human behavior (Jones, 1993).

In 1972, when the experiment was brought to the attention of the US national media, news anchor, Harry Reasoner, described it as an experiment that "used human beings as laboratory animals in a long and inefficient study of how long it takes syphilis to kill someone" (Jones, 1993). By the end of the experiment, 28 of the men had died directly of syphilis, 100 were dead of related complications, 40 of their wives had been infected, and 19 of their children had been born with congenital syphilis. How had these men been induced to endure a fatal disease in the name of science? Even the Surgeon General of the United States participated in enticing the men to remain in the experiment, sending them certificates of appreciation after 25 years in the study.

It is a great irony that the experiment's name comes from the Tuskegee Institute, the Black university founded by Booker T. Washington. Its affiliated hospital lent the PHS its medical facilities for the study, and other predominantly Black institutions as well as local Black doctors also participated. A Black nurse, Eunice Rivers, was a central figure in the experiment for most of its 40 years. It takes little imagination to blame racist attitudes of the White government officials who ran the experiment, but what can one make of the numerous African Americans who collaborated with them? (Jones, 1993).

Paulo Freire's classic work, *Pedagogy of the Oppressed* (1989), offers one explanation for African Americans' collaboration in this experiment in his concept of *oppressed group behavior*. That is, when an individual or group feels – and in fact IS powerless relative to the powerful groups who are responsible for unfair laws and unequal distribution of resources, etc. – "taking it out on one another" is one unfortunate result (as in Black-on-Black violence or the "lateral" abuse of fellow nurses in the healthcare hierarchy). Also, collaboration with one's oppressors may be a survival tactic, especially when facing threat of punishment, loss of job, etc. for failure to cooperate (see Chapters 8 and 11). Further, Freire's concept also sheds light on the question of why some battered women stay in abusive relationships (or may even collude in covering up an abuser's crimes) under threat to her life and economic livelihood.

The WHO's Declaration of Helsinki (1964) specified that "informed consent" was needed for experiments involving human beings. Similar concerns were noted by W. E. B. Du Bois when he said during his investigation of the negro conditions in Philadelphia: "I trust that this study with all its errors and shortcomings will at least serve to emphasize the fact that the Negro problems are problems of human beings; that they cannot be explained away by fantastic theories, ungrounded assumptions or metaphysical subtleties. They present a field which the student must enter seriously, and cultivate carefully and honestly" (Du Bois, 1899, Chapter V).

Today, based largely on the Tuskegee case and its inexcusable ethical breaches, all qualified academic and clinical researchers – most often university-affiliated – know about the tragic Tuskegee Experiment. To proceed with research involving human beings, they are required to conform with clearly stated ethical norms protecting the persons who consent to participate in the research. Following government guidelines and policies, these norms are strictly enforced by a review board usually titled "Human Subjects Review Committee" and attached to any institution that sponsors research and/or receives financial support for a research project. In the United States, all research team members (including graduate students) must pass an ethics test administered by the government as a condition of participating in a federally funded research project.

Teamwork and preventive focus

Last in our theoretical framework – but as the book's title implies, not least, as in other high risk, stressful work – healthcare providers cannot expect to provide appropriate service if working alone with a highly individualistic or biomedical focus. Since violence is essentially a *social* phenomenon, a collaborative approach, including the biopsychosocial parameters of the situation, is paramount. Consider, for example, the prevention of further abuse in the case of an infant severely injured and in critical medical condition as a result. The mother was sexually molested as a child, and now lives with a highly controlling boyfriend. She failed to bond with her infant. A comprehensive team approach would help the abused and abusive mother to heal and prevent further damage to the child: the social worker would work with the overburdened mother and deal with mandated reporting; the physician would treat the injured child and assure follow-up; the nurse would assist with treatment of the child and case coordination, including possible referral for follow-up physical therapy for the child and counseling for the mother. (The distinctive and complementary functions of particular disciplines are illustrated in Chapter 3, Table 3.1.) Through such teamwork health providers can promote:

- non-violent conflict resolution to replace centuries-old aggressive norms;
- teaching non-violent childrearing, a preventive focus, and immersion in the everyday lives of people in their community;
- interdisciplinary collaboration to replace traditional turf wars.

Child-rearing, education, and learning to reach such goals must be grounded in the realities of victims' and students' lives if health professionals are expected to contribute to violence prevention and provide service for survivors of abuse. Such a reality-based approach was central to developing this book.

Collaboration in building theory, public health policy, and responsive health services

As noted in Chapter 1, survivors themselves and their advocates were the prime movers in bringing this issue to public attention. They continue – often against great odds – to work as volunteers or for low pay to establish refuges, to change outmoded laws that collude in protecting abusers rather than their victims, and to obtain financial support for their efforts. Healthcare institutions, on the other hand – even in poor countries – wield proportionately much greater influence among government representatives and various power brokers who can either facilitate or oppose change in oppressive laws and the allocation of resources.

Thus, for example, the 1995 Beijing Declaration and the Platform for Action produced by government representatives of United Nations Member States is not a legally binding document; rather, implementing its recommendations regarding violence against women, for example, depends on *voluntary* action by Member States which in turn depends on the political influence of non-governmental organizations (NGOs), other grassroots community groups, and some professional groups (e.g. progressive sections of the American Public Health Association and Doctors Without Borders). Significantly, the primary players in drafting the document are members of NGOs which historically have had to struggle for a voice among policy makers, governmental agencies, and foundations which control the purse strings that support necessary services.

These grassroots groups, which include the contributors to this book, cite the challenge of trying to influence professionals in the often fragmented healthcare sector that injured victims of abuse must depend on for treatment. Some of these healthcare professionals have listened to victimized persons and their advocates and have joined their efforts to effect change in healthcare and criminal justice systems that would result in more informed and responsive providers. Later chapters in this book highlight such efforts with examples from around the world. Here, though, we emphasize several guiding principles:

1 Unfortunately, there is more than enough work to go around; competition for this work only mirrors the very power and control tactics so central in abusive situations. Collaboration produces more fruitful results in both human and financial terms.
2 Some grassroots groups have observed that when health professionals do take an interest in the issue of violence, they also like to take control and "professionalize" the process of working with victim/survivors and their assailants. This not only results in fragmentation of effort that ill-serves those needing service, but also discredits the work of often unrecognized advocates and front-line crisis workers (Hoff, & Morgan, in press).

It is a given that if a rape victim, for example, chooses to press criminal charges against the assailant, medical and forensic specialists are required to obtain and examine evidence. But if the medical professionals performing these procedures are not trained in the emotional and social implications of sexual assault, further victimization can occur. Advocates from rape crisis centers have compensated for this deficit to some extent by accompanying a rape victim to an emergency medical facility. The support of such advocates is critical in countries where, even today, some professionals with enormous power and influence do not believe that sexual assault has occurred if there is no evidence of physical injury, or that penetration must occur to count as childhood sexual abuse. In some countries, public health and nursing professionals have addressed this problem by training Sexual Assault Nurse Examiners (SANE) to staff all hospitals that holistically treat sexual assault victims (see Chapter 13 for illustrations).

While most health professionals have good intentions, there is an urgent need to recognize and collaborate with community-based groups whose wisdom and skills have been the mainstay of assisting victims. So important is this principle, that "grassroots/professional collaboration" was a criterion for contributors to this book. Ethnographic examples in later chapters underscore the importance of such collaboration and the negative outcomes that can result in its absence.

References

Adams, D. (2007). *Why do They Kill? Men Who Murder Their Intimate Partners*. Nashville: Vanderbilt University Press.

Antonovsky, A. (1987). *Unravelling the Mystery of Health*. San Francisco: Jossey-Bass.

Becker, H. (1963). *Outsiders: Studies in the Sociology of Deviance*. New York: Free Press of Glencoe.

Bergman, S. (1991). Men's psychological development: A relational perspective. Working Paper No. 48. Wellesley, MA: Stone Center, Wellesley College.

Boddy, J. (1998). Violence embodied? Circumcision, gender politics, and cultural aesthetics. In R. E. Dobash, & R. P. Dobash (eds.), *Rethinking Violence against Women*, pp. 77–110. Thousand Oaks, CA: Sage.

Brendtro, L. K., Brokenleg, M., & Van Bockern, S. (1990). *Reclaiming Youth at Risk*. Bloomington, IN: National Educational Service.

Browne, A. (1987). *When Battered Women Kill*. New York: Free Press.

Burgess, A., & Holmstrom, L. L. (1974). *Rape: Victims of Crisis*. Bowie, MD: Robert J. Brady Company.

Burstow, B. (1992). *Radical Feminist Therapy: Working in the Context of Violence*. Newbury Park, CA: Sage.

Campbell, J. C. (ed.). (1998). *Empowering Survivors of Abuse: Health Care for Battered Women and Their Children*. Thousand Oaks, CA: Sage.

Campbell, J. C., & Humphreys, J. H. (1993). *Nursing Care of Survivors of Family Violence*. St. Louis: Mosby.

Campbell, J. C., Webster, J., Koziol-McLain, J., & McFarlane, J. (2003). Risk factors for intimate partner femicide. *American Journal of Public Health*, 93, 1089–97.

Canadian Panel on Violence against Women (1993). *Changing the Landscape: Ending Violence, Achieving Equality*. Ottawa: Minister of Supply and Services.

Caplan, P. (1993). *The Myth of Women's Masochism* (2nd edn.). Toronto: University of Toronto Press.

Carlsson-Paige, N., & Levin, D. (2008). *Taking Back Childhood: Helping your Kids Thrive in a Fast-Paced, Media-Saturated, Violence-Filled World*. New York: Hudson Street Press.

Chodorow, N. (1978). *The Reproduction of Mothering: Psychoanalysis and the Sociology of Gender*. Berkeley: University of California Press.

Cloward, R. A., & Piven, F. F. (1979). Hidden protest: The channelling of female innovation and resistance. *Signs: Journal of Women in Culture and Society*, 4(4), 651–9.

Cooksey, E. C., & Brown, P. (1998). Spinning on its axes: DSM and the social contruction of psychiatric diagnosis. *International Journal of Health Services*, 28(3), 525–4.

Delport, E. (ed.) (2007). *Gender-Based Violence in Africa: Perspectives from the Continent*. Pretoria: Centre for Human Rights.

Dobash, R. P., & Dobash, R. E. (1979). *Violence against Wives: A Case against the Patriarchy*. New York: Free Press.

Dryta, M. (2009). Hassan arraigned in beheading of wife; denied bail as potential flight risk. *The Buffalo News*, 14 March, pp. D1, 2.

Du Bois, W. E. B. *The Philadelphia Negro*. New York: Lippincott, 1899.

Everett, B., & Gallop, R. (2001). *Linking Childhood Trauma and Mental Illness: Theory and Practice for Direct Service Practitioners*. Thousand Oaks, CA: Sage.

Finkelhor, R. J. Gelles, G. T. Hotaling, & M. A. Straus (eds.), *The Dark Side of Families: Current Family Violence Research*, pp. 293–304. Beverly Hills: Sage.

Friedman, R. A. (2006). Violence and mental illness – How strong is the link? *New England Journal of Medicine*, 355 (November 16–13), 2064–6.

Gailey, C. (1988). Evolutionary perspectives on gender hierarchy. In B. B. Hess, & M. M. Ferree (eds.), *Analyzing Gender: A Handbook of Social Science Research*, pp. 32–67. Newbury Park, CA: Sage.

Gelles, R. J., & Loseke, D. R. (eds.) (1993). *Current Controversies on Family Violence*. Newbury Park, CA: Sage.

Gil, D. (1970). *Violence against Children*. Cambridge, MA: Harvard University Press.

Goffman, E. (1963). *Stigma*. Englewood Cliffs, NJ: Prentice-Hall.

Greven, P. (1990). *Spare the Child: The Religious Roots of Punishment and the Psychological Impact of Physical Abuse*. New York: Alfred Knopf.

Hartmann, H. (1981). The family as the locus of gender, class and political struggle: The example of housework. *Signs: Journal of Women in Culture and Society*, 6, 366–94.

Herman, J. (1981). *Father-Daughter Incest*. Cambridge: Harvard University Press.

Herman, J. (1992). *Trauma and Recovery: The Aftermath of Violence*. New York: Basic Books.

Hilberman, E. (1980). Overview: The 'wife beater's wife' reconsidered. *American Journal of Psychiatry*, 137, 1336–47.

Hoff, L. A. (1990). *Battered Women as Survivors*. London: Routledge.

Hoff, L. A. (2000). Interpersonal violence. In C. E. Koop, C. Pearson, & M. R. Schwartz (eds.), *Critical Issues in Global Health*, pp. 260–71. San Francisco: Jossey-Bass.

Hoff, L. A. (1992). Review essay: Wife beating in Micronesia. *ISLA: A Journal of Micronesian Studies*, 1(2), 199–221.

Hoff, L. A., Hallisey, B., & Hoff, M. (2009). *People in Crisis: Clinical and Diversity Perspectives* (6th edn.). New York and London: Routledge.

Hoff, L. A., & Morgan, B. (in press). *Psychiatric and Mental Health Essentials in Primary Care*.

Hoff, M. (2005). Resilience: A paradigm of promise. Unpublished Master's thesis. Fargo: North Dakota State University, Department of Counselor Education.

ICWHI – International Council on Women's Health Issues (1992). Congress statement. Environment, daily life and health: Women's strategies for our common future. Copenhagen: Danish Technical University.

Jacoby, J. (2008). '"Honor" killing comes to the US.' *Boston Globe*, 10 August, p. A11.

Johnson, H. (1998). Rethinking survey research on violence against women. In R. E. Dobash, & R. P. Dobash (eds.), *Rethinking Violence against Women*, pp. 23–51. Thousand Oaks, CA: Sage.

Jones, A. (1980). *Women Who Kill*. New York: Holt, Rinehart & Winston.

Jones, J. (1993). *Bad Blood: The Tuskegee Syphilis Experiment*. New York: Free Press.

Kurz, E., & Stark, E. (1988). Not-so-benign neglect: The medical response to battering. In K. Yllo, M. Bograd (eds.), *Feminist Perspectives on Wife Abuse*, pp. 249–66. Newbury Park, CA: Sage.

LaRocque, E. D. (1994). *Violence in Aboriginal Communities*. Ottawa: Royal Commission on Aboriginal People.

Loustaunau, M. O., & Sobo, E. J. (1997). *The Cultural Context of Health, Illness, and Medicine*. Westport, CT: Bergin & Garvey.

Luhrmann, T. M. (2000). *Of Two Minds: The Growing Disorder in American Psychiatry*. New York: Alfred A. Knopf.

McCullough, C. (1996). *Nobody's Victim: Freedom from Therapy and Recovery*. New York: Clarkson Potter/Publishers.

McHugh, P. R., & Clark, M. R. (2006). Diagnostic and classificatory dilemmas. In M. Blumenfeld, & J. J. Strain (eds.), *Psychosomatic Medicine*, pp. 39–45. Philadelphia: Lippincott Williams & Wilkins.

MacLeod, L. (1989). *Wife Battering and the Web of Hope. Progress, Dilemmas and Visions of Prevention*. Ottawa: National Clearinghouse on Family Violence, Health and Welfare Canada.

Mandamin, C. (1993). Child abuse among First Nation people. Panel presentation at Curriculum Implementation Workshop, Sudbury, Ontario.

Martin, D. (1976). *Battered Wives*. San Francisco: Glide Publications.

Martin, J. (1983). Maternal and paternal abuse of children: Theoretical and research perspectives. In D. Finkelhor, R. J. Gelles, G. T. Hotaling, & M. A. Straus (eds.), *The Dark Side of Families: Current Family Violence Research*, pp. 293–304. Beverly Hills: Sage.

Mawby, R. I., & Walklate, S. (1994). *Critical Victimology*. London: Sage.

Miller, J. B. (1976). *Toward a New Psychology of Women*. Boston: Beacon Press.

Mills, C. W. (1959). *The Sociological Imagination*. London: Oxford University Press.

Mitchinson, W. (1993). The medical treatment of women. In S. Burt (ed.), *Changing Patterns: Women in Canada*, pp. 391–415. Toronto: Stewart, McLelland.

Monahan, J. (1981). *The Clinical Prediction of Violent Behavior.* Rockville, MD: National Institute of Mental Health.

Mousseau, M. (1989). *The Medicine Wheel Approach to Dealing with Family Violence.* West Region Child and Family Services, Inc.

National Clearinghouse on Family Violence. *FVC – Family Violence in Canada.* (1991). Ottawa: Health and Welfare Canada.

Oakley, A. (1981a). Interviewing women: A contradiction in terms. In H. Roberts (ed.), *Doing Feminist Research*, pp. 30–61. London: Routledge & Kegan Paul.

Oakley, A. (1981b). *Subject Women: Where Women Stand Today – Politically, Economically, Socially, Emotionally.* New York: Pantheon Books.

Pizzey, E. (1974). *Scream Quietly or the Neighbors Will Hear.* Middlesex, England: Penguin.

Reinharz, S. (1979). *On Becoming a Social Scientist.* San Francisco: Jossey-Bass.

Renzetti, C. M. (1992). *Violent Betrayal: Partner Abuse in Lesbian Relationships.* Newbury Park, CA: Sage.

Rieker, P., & Carmen (Hilberman), E. (1986). The victim-to-patient process: The disconfirmation and transformation of abuse. *American Journal of Orthopsychiatry*, 56, 360–71.

Ruddick, S. (1989). *Maternal Thinking: Toward a Politics of Peace.* Boston: Beacon Press.

Russell, D. (1990). *Rape in Marriage* (rev. edn.). New York: Collier Books.

Ryan, W. (1971). *Blaming the Victim.* New York: Vintage Books.

Sawyer, J. (1970, March 8). On male liberation. Workshop presented at the Women's Liberation Teach-in. Chicago: Northwestern University.

Schechter, S. (1982). *Women and Male Violence.* Boston: South End Press.

Sciolino, E., & Souad, M. (2008, June 11). Muslim women and virginity: 2 worlds collide. New York: *New York Times*, p. 1, A13.

Seck, M. (1995). Substance abuse among male batterers. Doctoral dissertation research. Ann Arbor, MI: UMI.

Segal, L. (1987). *Is the Future Female? Troubling Thoughts on Contemporary Feminism.* London: Virago Press.

Segal, L. (1999). *Why Feminism? Gender, Psychology, Politics.* New York: Columbia University Press.

Smith, J. (1981/82). Sociobiology and feminism: The very strange courtship of competing paradigms. *Philosophical Forum*, 13, 226–43.

Stanko, E. A. (1990). *Everyday Violence: How Women and Men Experience Sexual and Physical Danger.* London: Pandora.

Stark, E., & Flitcraft, A. (1996). *Women at Risk: Domestic Violence and Women's Health.* Thousand Oaks, CA: Sage.

Stark, E., Flitcraft, A., & Frazier, W. (1979). Medicine and patriarchal violence: The social construction of a 'private' event. *International Journal of Health Services*, 9, 461–93.

Straus, M. (1983). Ordinary violence, child abuse and wife-beating: What do they have in common? In D. Finkelhor, R. J. Gelles, G. T. Hotaling, & Straus, M. A. (eds.), *The Dark side of Families: Current Family Violence Research*, pp. 213–34. Beverly Hills: Sage.

Straus, M. A., Gelles, R.J., & Steinmetz, S. K. (1980). *Behind Closed Doors: Violence in the American Family.* New York: Anchor.

Stuhlmiller, C. M. (1995). The construction of disorders: Exploring the growth of PTSD and SAD. *Journal of Psychosocial Nursing*, 33(4), 20–3.

Tilden, V. P., *et al.* (1994). Factors that influence clinicians' assessment and management of family violence. *American Journal of Public Health*, 84(4), 628–39.

UN – United Nations (1996a). *Report on the World's Women 1995: Trends and Statistics.* New York: UN.

UN (1996b). The Beijing Declaration and the Platform for Action. New York: UN.

UN (2006). *Secretary-General's Study on Violence against Women.* New York: UN.

US Department of Health and Human Services (1986). *Surgeon General's Workshop on Violence and Public Health Report.* Washington, DC: Health Resources Service Administration.

VandeCreek, L., & Knapp, S. (2001). *Tarasoff and Beyond: Legal and Clinical Considerations in the Treatment of Life-Endangering Patients* (rev. edn.). Sarasota, FL: Professional Resource Press.

Vandello, J. A., & Cohen, D. (2008). Culture, gender and men's intimate partner violence. *Social and Personality Psychology Compass*, 2(2), 652–7.

Wakegijig, A., & Jenkins, R. (1992). *Aboriginal Family Violence Consultations.* Toronto: Ontario Federation of Indian Friendship Centres.

Warshaw, C. (1989). Limitations of the medical model in the care of battered women. *Gender and Society*, 3(4), 506–17.

Weiss, G., & Lonnquist, L. (2006). *The Sociology of Health, Healing, and Illness* (5th edn.). Upper Saddle River, NJ: Pearson Prentice Hall.

Wendell, S. (1990). Oppression and victimization: Choice and responsibility. *Hypatia*, 5(3), 15–46.

Wiehe, V. R. (1998). *Understanding Family Violence: Treating and Preventing Partner, Child, Sibling, and Elder Abuse.* Thousand Oaks, CA: Sage.

WHO – World Health Organization (1994). Maternal and Child Health and Family Planning: Traditional Practices Harmful to the Health of Women and Children: 47th Resolution (WHA 47). Geneva: World Health Assembly

Yllo, K., & Bograd, M. (eds.) (1987). *Feminist Perspectives on Wife Abuse.* Newbury Park, CA: Sage.

Zuckermann, P. (ed.) (2004). *The Social Theory of W. E. B. Du Bois.* Thousand Oaks, CA: Pine Forge Press.

Note

1 The DSM is the *Diagnostic and Statistical Manual of Mental Illness*, now in its 4th edition, and while controversial and scientifically questionable (Cookesy, & Brown, 1998; McHugh, & Clark, 2006), it is nevertheless widely accepted even by non-medical clinicians as the "bible of psychiatry" (see Hoff *et al.*, 2009, Chapter 2).

3   CORE content
Essential knowledge, attitudes, and skills

- The concept of CORE content
- Primary, secondary, and tertiary prevention

  — Primary prevention
  — Secondary prevention
  — Tertiary prevention

- General and specific functions of health professionals

  — Knowledge
  — Attitudes
  — Skills

- Illustration of CORE content

This chapter builds on the premise that the issue of violence prevention and victim/survivor care, while essentially interdisciplinary, also has discipline-specific features. It presents certain *generic* components which apply to any and all providers in the health and social service system.

For example, no matter what the discipline, when a service provider hears a victim of rape or battering blame herself, it is basic that the listener provide an *alternative* message to interrupt the misplaced blaming of oneself for the deviant behavior of another: "No, it's not your fault .... No matter what you said, violence is not an acceptable solution to a problem." It says, in effect: "Society cares about the wrongful injury of its members." Such a message has the potential of reversing the legacy of "blaming the victim" which, historically, has permeated health and welfare agencies. This example of client/provider interaction illustrates that psychotherapeutic communication with a victimized person should transcend the professional identity of the provider. Put another way, an empathetic message is more important than the messenger.

This chapter outlines content essential to the *knowledge, attitudes*, and *skills* of health team members on behalf of victim/survivors and assailants. It includes suggestions about the relevance of this content to practice across disciplines. While recognizing a variety of teaching methodologies, recommendations assume the principles of adult learning which emphasize an *interactional and experiential* vs. hierarchical relationship between learner and teacher (Knowles, 1980). Such an approach, allowing ample time for discussion and clarification, is particularly important when addressing the value-laden topic of violence. (See Chapter 13 for illustrations of interdisciplinary practice.)

The concept of CORE content

The notion of CORE content can be used in several different contexts. In formal pre-service professional programs (e.g. a bachelor's degree in nursing or social work) CORE victimology content would be part of a total curriculum. For those professionals already in practice whose formal preparation did not include the content discussed here, these curriculum principles apply in continuing education or in-service programs. The term *curriculum* refers to the complex array of learning activities or a body of courses organized to achieve specific educational goals. CORE curriculum encompasses those courses or learning units *required of all students* graduating from an educational institution, without which the educational goals would not be met.

That said, nursing and medical students face the stark reality of having to master other essential content as well as violence and abuse issues as groundwork for passing national examinations for licensure to practice. Significantly, in 1985, Surgeon General C. Everett Koop (the chief medical officer in the US) convened a national interdisciplinary workshop on violence and public health (US Department of Health and Human Services, 1986). Among the recommendations from this workshop was this one: all publicly licensed professionals should be taught and *examined* on violence content as a *condition of licensure*. Yet, nearly three decades later, many faculty feel either unqualified to teach this content or cannot squeeze it into an already over-crowded curriculum, although it is increasingly recognized by some (Coretta, 2008; Breslin, & Woodtli, 2002; Hamberger, 2007; Hoff, & Ross, 1995).

Moving to the course or unit level, "CORE violence content" refers to the KNOWLEDGE, ATTITUDES, and SKILLS essential to any person working with survivors and assailants, regardless of the discipline, setting, or framework in which she or he learned this content (Hoff & Adamowski, 1998; see also the online resources in Part IV). The concept of CORE content is central to this book's purpose for several reasons:

- It explicates what every healthcare provider needs for appropriate care of abused children, women of all ages, other victims, and their assailants.
- It provides a standard against which existing health professions' curricula and learning activities can be assessed vis-à-vis such care.
- It facilitates examining curricula for the balanced allocation of time and practice activities relative to the nature and complexity of subject matter.

Primary, secondary, and tertiary prevention

Although already implied, the emphasis on CORE content here refers primarily to the knowledge, attitudes, and skills of the *generalist*. Specialists' roles in victim/survivor care are also addressed, however, not only because of their importance in a comprehensive service system, but as an aid for generalists to clarify their own responsibilities and know when to refer to others.

While recognizing the need for various specialists – given the complexity of this healthcare issue – the centrality of *preventing* violence and the serious physical and mental heath impairments that can follow underscores the fact that most abused persons are *first* seen by providers at various entry points to the health and social service system. These entry points include primary, secondary, and tertiary levels of prevention and service. The potential for violence prevention and the treatment and rehabilitation of victim/survivors and perpetrators exists in each of these three facets of health and social service delivery. The concepts of primary, secondary, and tertiary prevention (Caplan, 1964; Hoff *et al.*, 2009; Rutherford *et al.*, 2007) are briefly reviewed here for their particular relevance to violence and its sequelae. They underscore pronouncements and publications of the World Health Organization (WHO) on this topic (WHO, 2002; 2004).

Primary prevention

Consisting of education, consultation, and crisis assessment and intervention, primary prevention is designed to reduce the incidence of violence and abuse, promote growth and development through the victimization and crisis resolution process, and enhance a potential victim's future resistance to abuse. Traditional primary prevention strategies include:

- Eliminate or modify the hazardous situation. For example, an emergency physician, nurse, or social worker helps a battered woman devise a safety plan.
- Reduce the person's exposure to the hazardous situation. For example, a community health nurse or school counselor teaches students non-violent conflict resolution strategies; a family health practitioner teaches parents non-violent discipline skills and how to protect their children from abuse by strangers; occupational and physical therapists teach disabled or frail elderly persons how to protect themselves; an entire community takes measures to ensure the economic and social necessities for effective and safe parenting.
- Reduce the person's vulnerability by facilitating coping ability. For example, a pharmacist observes and teaches about overdependence on tranquilizers during a violence-related crisis and refers the person for counseling; a social worker, psychiatric nurse, family physician or psychologist conducts crisis counseling (including decision counseling) with persons at risk.

Health promotion includes but goes beyond primary prevention by emphasizing the *social context* affecting health and safety. In the spirit of the WHO's Health for All by the Year 2010 program, and with reference to violence, health promotion policies target major social institutions, for example, equal access to health service regardless of economic states and legal protection for vulnerable populations.

Secondary prevention

As the name suggests, secondary prevention (associated with treatment) implies that some form of physical and emotional trauma has already occurred as a result of abuse or violent attack, either because primary activities were absent or because of the person's inability to profit from available services. A major aim of secondary prevention is to alleviate the pain of trauma and shorten the length of time a person may be disabled by abuse. This means detection and treatment at entry points such as primary care and dental centers, and a smoothly coordinated referral system focused on psychological trauma from abuse.

Crisis intervention and counseling are major next steps in achieving this aim and preventing institutionalization and serious emotional/mental dysfunction as sequelae of abuse. For example, health professionals frequently observe that once an abused woman enters the downward spiral to depression (usually because she lacks the social, psychological and financial resources for escape from her abuser), she is more prone than before to desperate crisis resolution tactics like substance abuse, suicide, or killing her abuser. Given the role of front-line health and social service providers in key elements of secondary prevention, Chapter 13 illustrates a Crisis Paradigm and comprehensive care with examples of intimate partner violence and sexual assault.

Tertiary prevention

Tertiary prevention (associated with rehabilitation) aims to reduce the long-term disabling effects of abuse. The unfortunate truth is that this level of prevention is currently relevant in considerable measure because violence by intimates and family members traditionally was regarded as a "private" matter rather than the public health issue all now acknowledge. Also, some health and social service providers may have refrained from talking with clients about concerns stemming from their abuse histories out of the perception that this is a "specialist's job", not theirs. In fact, longer-term psychological rehabilitation is primarily the province of mental health or victim/survivor specialists. But the earliest access to such therapy for most victim/survivors is through trauma centers and primary care routes, rather than years later in response to debilitating depression or other post-trauma symptoms.

When such early access is unavailable, many clients with chronic mental or physical health problems suffer as they do because the *primary problem* – abuse or violent attack – was either untreated altogether or obscured in an earlier era by a medical or psychiatric diagnosis. For example, women who suffered any invasive body trauma through sexual abuse as children may suffer extreme anxiety or panic during dental visits or routine gynecological care. Only recently is abuse and violent attack beginning to appear in official health statistics nomenclature, a symbol of its emergence from "behind closed doors" to public concern; e.g. trauma to women from battering exceeds that from accidents, mugging, and stranger-rape combined.

The history of treating female clients who have histories of abuse primarily for "depression" and/or behaviors ascribed to such diagnostic entities as "borderline personality disorder" is now widely discredited (Burstow, 1992). Increasingly, groups are available in hospital and community settings which offer services tailored explicitly to the needs of abuse survivors. Given current constraints on mental health resources, it is important for front-line providers to maintain workable linkages with such groups. Doing so can prevent recidivism among clients whose problems can ultimately be traced to untreated traumatic injury at earlier points of entry to the health and social service system.

These realities underscore the urgency of including *crisis assessment and intervention* as an integral facet of primary prevention in psychosocial healthcare delivery. Such assessment always includes risk to life – i.e. victimization level, suicide, and assault/homicide (Hoff *et al.*, 2009, Chapter 3). On the other hand, since routine attention to victimization in primary care is only now emerging, it is equally important that practitioners in secondary and tertiary care settings move beyond crisis components of care to evaluate and treat victimization as the root or significant part of many long-standing mental health problems. An issue receiving public and professional examination is "repressed memories" of child abuse attributed to therapist intervention. However, this controversial issue does not negate the importance of believing people's stories of abuse.

The current emphasis worldwide on health promotion and primary care underscores the importance of front-line clinicians in identifying victim/survivors of abuse and preventing the long-term damaging effects of neglect at the time of victimization crisis (Bishop, & Patterson, 1992; Herman, 1992; Hoff *et al.*, 2009; Mandt, 1993; Sugg, & Inui, 1992; WHO, 2004). A re-peated point made by survivors interviewed for this book was that *no one* – nurses, physicians, or others – had asked them about their abuse histories (see Chapter 13).

General and specific functions of health professionals

The CORE content presented here refers to the essentials within the healthcare system, or among diverse providers *as a whole*. It does not imply that each provider among all health disciplines must master each item. The intent, rather, is to delineate the broad parameters of comprehensive service to survivors. While all providers need a general understanding of the "big picture" as outlined here, no single provider is expected to be "all things to all survivors." It is the task of educators from particular disciplines to specify for students which pieces of the whole correspond to their profession's mission (e.g. detection and referral, treatment, or follow-up) while not losing sight of the whole. However, it is legendary that some clients – not only survivors of abuse – "fall through the cracks" of an uncoordinated system because inter-disciplinary collaboration has failed, or because of naive assumptions about "somebody else's" responsibilities for particular tasks.

Accordingly, this chapter is not intended to overwhelm, but rather to provide background for the remaining chapters' ethnographic illustrations and delineation of interdisciplinary and discipline-specific roles. Table 3.1 portrays the "big picture" plus areas of role blurring among various health professionals. It also depicts, in general, the roles of particular disciplines to

Table 3.1 Categories and functions of particular disciplines

Discipline	Function
All health disciplines	General understanding of and alertness to the issue in all facets of practice as background for detection, intervention, treatment, and/ or referral for longer-term psychosocial counseling or treatment. Role modeling non-violence in general behavior, and in client/ provider and interdisciplinary team relationships. Advocacy for violence prevention and victim services in professional organizations and community roles.
1 Medicine, nursing (generalist roles)	Detection, assessment, diagnosis, crisis intervention, treatment, referral for follow-up counseling/treatment. Key roles at entry points in primary, secondary, and tertiary care settings. Primary care physicians may be an entry point in the community. Nursing has key coordinating role in most settings.
2 Dental hygiene, pharmacy	Detection, immediate support and initial steps of crisis intervention, referral.
3 Dentistry, physical therapy (PT)	As in 2 above, plus treatment for maxillo-facial injuries (dentistry), and for chronic pain from injury (PT).
4 Occupational therapy	As in 2 above, with more extensive role in community mental health treatment settings.
5 Psychology, social work (clinical)	Frequently in liaison or consulting role to medicine and nursing; abuse detection and crisis intervention; key role with families and follow-up counseling and/or psychotherapy across the spectrum of health and mental health services.
Graduate specialists	Entry point and follow-up treatment or counseling. May include traditional mental health disciplines (clinical psychology, clinical specialist in psychosocial nursing, psychiatric social work, psychiatry); pastoral counselors with clinical training; family medicine, pediatrics, and women's health specialists (e.g. obstetricians); midwifery; psychiatric nurse practitioners – various specialties.

assure comprehensive service and avoid harmful fragmentation of tasks on behalf of survivors. Thus, for example, dental practitioners' and physical therapists' primary role is to detect signs of abuse, treat and make an effective referral for follow-up counseling; a pharmacist may detect abuse, assess safety, teach about appropriate use of drugs, and refer. While Table 3.1 distinguishes between generalist and specialist roles, it *should not be assumed* that graduate training in itself is sufficient preparation for serving the special needs of survivors if it does not include formal instruction, clinical experience, and supervision along lines suggested here and in the online resources in Part IV.

These generalist/specialist role delineations apply broadly across Canada and the United States, and may vary in title and standards governing professional practice within and across cultures and licensing jurisdictions. For example, in a geographically isolated rural area of Ontario, Canada or North Dakota, USA, the community health nurse may have a broader scope of practice than, say, in Toronto or Boston where many specialists are available.

Knowledge

Essential concepts in the violence field include two broad categories:

1 Concepts *explicitly* concerned with violence, victimization, and its health/mental health implications.
2 *Related concepts* already addressed in a curriculum, but which require explicit elaboration for their relevance to violence prevention and victim/survivor care.

For example, concepts such as stress, trauma, primary prevention, crisis, social change, and cultural variation are not unique to specific disciplines or the care of victimized people. Their inclusion here is to emphasize their particular importance to *this population*, and to adapt established curriculum content to the specific needs of abused women and children and others affected by violence.

Key concepts

As used in this book, the term *key concepts* refers to the theoretical underpinnings to health status and service delivery, as discussed in Chapter 2. Building on that conceptual base, key concepts fall into three categories, with their relevance to practice illustrated throughout the book:

1 The problem, incidence, and sociocultural context:
 • Epidemiological data and demographic correlates of violence and victimization such as age, sex, class, ethnicity, sexual identity, physical ability/disability, immigration status; geographic location.
 • The intersection of violence with economic disparity and other disadvantages such as those based on age, ethnicity, or sexual identity.
 • Family dynamics, role theory, sex-role stereotyping, and the concept of learned behavior.
 • Gender relations, power disparities, feminist analysis, and social change theory.
 • Multiculturalism, cultural relativism, and cross-cultural patterns and differences in violence, victimization, and healing.
 • Stigmatization, bias, and its potential for creating a climate that activates violence potential toward people who are "different".

- Labeling theory and its power to obscure the realities of victimization trauma, especially by psychiatric diagnoses or victim-blaming.
2 Prevention and protection:
    - Primary, secondary, and tertiary prevention of violence and abuse.
    - Ethical/legal issues, e.g. legal protections, limits of legal restraint, mandated reporting, duty to warn potential victims, rights and accountability of defendants.
3 Clinical concepts (all chapters, some more detailed):
    - Traumatic stress of abuse and its implications for self-esteem, health and wellness, e.g. rape trauma syndrome.
    - Dynamics of victimization, including social, cultural, economic, psychological, behavioral, biophysical ramifications.
    - The intersection of violence and victimization with substance abuse and physical health status, e.g. significant numbers of battered women present at entry points with psychosomatic complaints traceable to abuse, while many self-medicate and seek prescription drugs as a coping device.
    - The intersection of victimization with depression, suicidal risk, and other mental health sequelae such as post-traumatic stress disorder.
    - Criteria for identifying victims in health and social service entry points (triage) – Chapter 4.
    - Criteria for assessing victimization trauma – Chapter 13.
    - Criteria for assessing assault/homicide potential – Chapter 11.
    - Crisis intervention and social support strategies with victims, families, and assailants, including appropriate referral for longer-term service.
    - Follow-up counseling or psychotherapy for mental health sequelae – Chapters 9, 10, and 13.
    - Community resources for victims and abusers, especially peer support groups such as for incest, rape, and battery survivors.
    - Team relationships, community-wide networking, and follow-up process.

Immersion in the victimology literature is a primary avenue to mastering essential knowledge about abuse generally, and in specific chapter references and the online resources in Part IV of this book. "Must" reading of these works depends, of course, on previous study and experience, as well particular professional roles. Overall, it is important to acknowledge, for example, as one faculty interviewee did: "I just can't deal with child abuse" etc., and then collaborate for appropriate coverage of the topic by others. However, because abuse victims are ubiquitous in diverse healthcare settings, it is imperative that all faculty possess *general* knowledge of the topic, at least sufficient for detection and referral. Without such knowledge, future practitioners are shortchanged, while health service agencies must add to their work the responsibility of teaching the essentials of victim/survivor care to new graduates.

Attitudes

Attitudes are based on one's knowledge of a topic, as well as on deeply embedded values, whether these values are rooted in myth or fact. The common question, among lay persons and professionals alike, "Why do battered women stay?" itself reflects the traditional belief that it is the *victim's* responsibility to do something about abuse. Given the legacy of victim-blaming, legal loopholes for women who take action, and the real danger a woman faces even with (or sometimes, because of) a peace bond (restraining order), most abused women must still leave their homes to avoid further injury or even death. However, it is a commentary on the powerful influence of attitudes and values on public policy and program planning when we consider that we have not asked instead: "Why are violent men *allowed* to stay?" or, "Why should the victim rather than the assailant be expected to leave?" (Hoff, 1990).

A change in cultural norms regarding violence and its widespread tolerance requires an examination of *personal attitudes* and *citizen inaction* which support a climate of violence. For example, war and corporal punishment are socially approved forms of aggression, while TV violence could not thrive as it does without consumer support. Deeply embedded values regarding aggression create a context in which individuals facing conflict and stress can readily turn to violence as solutions to problems. One male counselor of abusive men finds that the biggest problem is the tradition of "not holding the guys accountable" for their violence. Success with men who batter, he says, assumes a feminist value system which acknowledges the power dynamic in abusive relationships (Adams, & Cayouyette, 2002).

It also implies adoption of traditional values such as equality, harmony, cooperation, and moderation that characterized pre-colonial life among indigenous people. While epidemic rates of violence cross ethnic, class, gender, sexual identity, and national boundaries, all must confront the dramatic fact that rates of violence for many indigenous people *now* greatly exceed those of other groups. Data reflect the reality that a subjugated people *learned* violent ways in domestic life from those who confined them to reserves, introduced alcohol, and essentially destroyed their way of life (Brendtro *et al.*, 1990; Sacred Circle, 2008). This violent pattern is found among many nations – e.g. African countries, Australia, Canada, Micronesia, island nations, and the USA – in which one people, the colonizer, imposed control and their values over another (Hoff, 1992b). A parallel pattern is evident in the domain of gender relations: women, traditionally nurturant and life-preserving, increasingly are choosing the violent competitive approaches to conflict resolution that characterize traditional male behaviors (Ruddick, 1989). A revised learning curve is therefore required: the dominant, the colonizers, the violent, need to adopt the more peaceful behaviors of those whom they oppressed; while the victimized need to eschew the violence they have learned and reclaim their more harmonious heritage.

Since health professionals, like other societal members, are influenced by the dominant values which have spawned and exacerbated the plight of victim/survivors, values clarification is critical to their selection into the professions and preparation in the care of society's abused members. An appropriate attitudinal stance, flowing in part from evidence-based knowledge, lays the foundation for crisis intervention, counseling, and treatment of victims and their assailants. A worker's deeply held values can form barriers to otherwise skillful application of knowledge, if not examined in relation to their potentially negative impact on victim/survivors. For example, a judgmental attitude can effectively neutralize the value of "technically correct" communication with a victimized person. Our values can also influence how we convey respect for a victim's decisions and implement professional ethical and mandated reporting laws regarding intimate partner violence and sexual assault. When compared with knowledge and skills, *attitudinal* and values content presents the greatest challenge for teachers, learners, and practitioners.

In female-dominated professions such as nursing, physical therapy, occupational therapy, and social work, educators note that a significant attitudinal barrier in dealing with this topic is the students' views regarding feminism. As one nurse educator stated: "They seem to equate it with hating men, burning their bra, and lesbianism [1960s stereotypes]. They don't want to appear radical in their thinking .... So I had to go around it in a different way and they were more receptive." As discussed in Chapter 2 and illustrated in ethnographic data throughout this book, gender-based violence is alive and rampant across the globe, but is often intertwined with race, class, sexual identity, and/or religious affiliation. Framing gender issues, then, in concert with other diversity issues is usually more successful, as it avoids casting people as one-dimensional – a labeling process which many resent, since most people are multidimensional in outlook.

In male-dominated professions like medicine, dentistry, and pharmacy, similar dynamics are apparent. Women physicians of feminist persuasion, for example, are challenged with the balancing act of how to include male colleagues in discussion of sensitive gender issues (e.g. perceived and real power differentials between various professionals) while avoiding both alienation and appeasement. Values clarification, then, aims to expose *all* students to a broader conception of gender analysis including progressive concerns with child care, equal pay and parenting, degrading media portrayals of women and nurses, gender and other disparities in the healthcare system, stopping violence, etc. – issues affecting *all* of society, not merely a minority of radical feminists.

Without a climate that promotes discussion of values, myths and stereotypes, some may feel silenced in order to fit into the profession and/or institutions in which they work. For example:

- Most women support equal pay and egalitarian child-rearing – explicit feminist issues.
- Sexual orientation is not feminism.
- Lesbian women are not necessarily feminist.
- Some happily married women embrace feminism but may also be homophobic.
- The majority of victims are women and children.

Therefore, it is crucial that all health professionals (among themselves and with their students) examine anti-feminist and related stereotypes if they are to deliver unbiased care to abused and disadvantaged clients. Stereotypes aside, feminist analysis at its simplest takes *gender* into account when considering theory, practice, and research domains (Hoff, 1990; Keddy, 1993; Keller, 1985; Oakley, 1981; Reinharz, 1992; Segal, 1987, 1999).

Skills

Following is a summary of the major skills required in caring for abused persons:

- Apply the techniques of *formal crisis care*: Identification of risk *before* violence happens, assessment (including victimization trauma and the risk of suicide and/or violence toward others), planning, implementation, evaluation.
- Facilitate a "partnership" approach with survivors, including collaborative decision making in next steps, protection, reporting, etc.
- Communicate – listen actively, question discretely but directly, respond empathetically, and advise and direct appropriately.
- Teach potential victims about conflict resolution, and how to assess assault/homicide potential in domestic, learning, and other environments.
- Make an effective referral if one's role is primarily detection and linkage to other providers, or if a person's psychological needs are longer-term than crisis counseling.
- Teach people how to recognize symptoms of abuse, name the problem and its source, and avoid self-blame.
- Advise an abused woman of legal rights and link her to legal resources which will avoid the traditional practice of "re-victimization."
- Mobilize safety, legal, and community resources effectively, e.g. linkage to children's protective service; arranging admission to a refuge for battered women; finding a translator

for an immigrant woman; linking a rape victim with an advocate; providing support for caregivers as a means of preventing abuse of home-bound older persons.

- Implement agency policy regarding mandated reporting, and keeping accurate records, including dental and other X-rays, so that records cannot be used against a victim, but rather can possibly aid later legal action.
- Use the consultative process, i.e. know *whom* to call under *what* circumstances, and *do it*; review one's referrals and/or interventions with other health and social service providers.
- Complete the crisis care and follow-up referral or treatment steps while withholding judgment and not imposing values on the victim and her or his significant others.
- Provide follow-up counseling to survivors and assailants according to professional mission.
- Advocate for programs and policies that *prevent* violence.

Illustration of CORE content

In attempts to move from incidental to systematic inclusion of violence-related content in health professions' curricula, a typical comment is this: "There's just no time for a course on violence issues." In response, consider this example in relation to CORE content:

A woman is hospitalized for complications of pregnancy. Among risk factors to be considered with this woman are gestational diabetes and abuse by her spouse. Epidemiologically speaking, the risk of gestational diabetes, a medical condition – albeit with psychosocial implications, as is true for any diagnosis – is 2–6 percent; the risk of current or past history of abuse is around 25 percent (McFarlane, 1992; Rodgers, 1994; Stewart, 1993). Each risk factor comprises essential (CORE) content in medical and nursing curricula.

Most nursing and medical educators would concede that gestational diabetes is less complex for student mastery than the issue of intimate partner abuse. Thus, when considering these two content areas in curriculum development, decisions can more easily be made about learning activities against the standard of essential knowledge, attitudes, and skills. Unlike battering, gestational diabetes is not embedded in values and myths which may affect both the practitioner's ability to broach the subject in routine assessment, and the woman's willingness to disclose. Rarely would such factors complicate a physician's or nurse's assessment and teaching around diabetes. Accordingly, this example suggests that curriculum planners allocate relatively less time for diabetes than for partner abuse; in fact, gestational diabetes might be covered in reading and self-directed learning, while intimate partner abuse almost certainly requires teacher-facilitated classroom discussion.

Essential *knowledge* in this example includes:

- incidence rates of battering during pregnancy;
- the ramifications of abuse for the woman herself and its correlation with low-birth weight of her infant;
- victimization assessment strategies, including crisis intervention and possible referral;
- the social-psychological ramifications of abuse.

Attitudinal content includes, for example:

- compassion;
- avoidance of disempowering "rescue" messages;
- recognition of the possible impact on the client/provider relationship if the provider's mother, for instance, was a battered woman or a female provider herself is a battered spouse or was sexually abused as a child.

Skills content includes:

- the application of knowledge and attitudinal stance in a non-judgmental approach to the crisis assessment and intervention process;
- using effective communication and advocacy strategies.

Ideally, CORE content will be incorporated into the licensing examinations of health professionals and the clinical standards guiding accrediting bodies when they evaluate health service programs. See the online resources in Part IV for suggestions within a health service paradigm (Provider, Person/Family, Health, Environment) for teaching and clinical practice around various abuse situations.

References

Adams, D., & Cayouette, S. (2002). Emerge: A group education model for abusers. In E. Aldarondo, & F. Mederos (eds.), *Programs for Men Who Batter: Intervention and Prevention Strategies in a Diverse Society*, pp. 4-1–4-23. New York: Civic Research Inc.

Burstow, B. (1992). *Radical Feminist Therapy: Working in the Context of Violence*. Newbury Park, CA: Sage.

Bishop, J., & Patterson, P. (1992). Guidelines for the evaluation and management of family violence. *Canadian Journal of Psychiatry*, 37, 458–71.

Brendtro, L. K., Brokenleg, M., & Van Bockern, S. (1990). *Reclaiming Youth at Risk: Our Hope for the Future*. Bloomington, IN: National Educational Service.

Caplan, G. (1964). *Principles of Preventive Psychiatry*. New York: Basic Books.

Coretta, C. M. (2008). Domestic violence: A worldwide exploration. *Journal of Psychosocial Nursing & Mental Health Services*, 46(3), 26–35.

Hamberger, L. K. (2007). Preparing the next generation of physicians: Medical school and residency-based intimate partner violence curriculum and evaluation. *Trauma, Violence, & Abuse*, 8(2), 214–15.

Herman, J. (1992). *Trauma and Recovery: The Aftermath of Violence*. New York: Basic Books.

Hoff, L. A. (1990). *Battered Women as Survivors*. London and New York: Routledge.

Hoff, L. A. (1992). Review essay: Wife beating in Micronesia. *ISLA: A Journal of Micronesian Studies*, 1(2), 199–221.

Hoff, L. A., Hallisey, B. J., & Hoff, M. (2009). *People in Crisis: Clinical and Diversity Perspectives* (6th edn.). London and New York: Routledge.

Hoff, L. A., & Ross, M. Violence content in nursing curricula: Strategic issues and implementation. *Journal of Advanced Nursing*, 21(4), 627–34.

Keddy, B. (1993). Feminism and patriarchy in university schools of nursing: An unsettling dualism. Conference address: Women's Issues and Nursing Education. Moncton: Atlantic Region Canadian Association of University Schools of Nursing.

Knowles, A. (1980). *The Modern Practice of Adult Education: From Pedagogy to Andragogy*. Chicago: Association Press/Follett.

Mandt, A. K. (1993). The curriculum revolution in action: Nursing and crisis intervention for victims of family violence. *Journal of Nursing Education*, 32(1), 44–6.

McFarlane, J. (1992). Battering in pregnancy. In C. M. Sampselle (ed.), *Violence against Women: Nursing Research, Education, and Practice Issues*, pp. 205–18. Washington: Hemisphere.

Reinharz, S. (1992). *Feminist Methods in Social Research*. New York and Oxford: Oxford University Press.

Rodgers, K. (1994). Wife assault: The finds of a national survey. *Juristat Service Bulletin*. Ottawa: Canadian Centre for Justice Statistics.

Ruddick, S. (1989). *Maternal Thinking: Toward a Politics of Peace*. Boston: Beacon Press.

Rutherford, A., Zwi, A. B., Grove, N. J., & Butchart, A. (2007). Violence: A priority for public health? Part 2. *Journal of Epidemiology and Community Health*, 61, 764–70.

Sacred Circle – National Resource Center to End Violence Against Native Women (2008). Kyle, SD, Pine Ridge Reservation: Sacred Circle.

Segal, L. (1987). *Is the Future Female? Troubling Thoughts on Contemporary Feminism*. London: Virago Press.

Segal, L. (1999). *Why Feminism? Gender, Psychology, Politics*. New York: Columbia University Press.

Stewart, D. E. (1993). Physical abuse in pregnancy. *Canadian Medical Association Journal*, 149(9), 1257.

Sugg, N. K., & Inui, T. (1992). Primary care physicians' response to domestic violence: Opening Pandora's box. *Journal of American Medical Association*, 267(23), 3157–60.

US Department of Health and Human Services (1986). *Surgeon General's Workshop on Violence and Public Health Report*. Washington, DC: Health Resources Service Administration.

WHO – World Health Organization (2004) *Handbook for the Documentation of Interpersonal Violence Prevention Programmes*. Geneva: WHO.

WHO (2008). *Violence and Injury Prevention and Disability* (VIP). Geneva: WHO.

Woodtli, A., & Breslin, E. (1996). Violence-related content in the nursing curriculum. *Journal of Nursing Education*, 35, 367–74.

Woodtli, A., & Breslin, E. (2002). Violence-related content in the nursing curriculum: A follow-up national survey. *Journal of Nursing Education*, 41(4), 340–8.

Part II

Illustrations of violence issues across cultures

Life stories and applications to clinical practice

Part II includes seven chapters discussing the various faces of violence and abuse – including physical, sexual, and psychological. The ethnographic examples illustrate the continuum of violence, abuse, and neglect from childhood through old age, as well as the similarities and differences in victimization response across cultures. The majority of examples are from family and marital contexts that are deeply rooted in cultural values and gender-based inequalities (Chapters 4 through 7). Tools for early identification of victimization and life-threatening behaviors are presented in Chapter 4, and are relevant to all other chapters in Part II, while a Child Screening Checklist is offered in Chapter 5.

Chapters 8 and 9 focus on political, religious, and socioeconomic factors that intersect with inequalities based on gender, race, ethnicity, and class. Apartheid in South Africa, for example, was justified on religious grounds. Its legacy included the emasculation of African men, widespread disempowerment, military violence, and sexist colonial attitudes that perpetuated stereotyping, objectification, alienation, and abuse of women. Similar oppression of indigenous peoples occurred in North and South America, the Caribbean, Australia, and New Zealand. One major result is horizontal violence, that is, widespread attacks against the most vulnerable among one's *own* group when feeling disempowered vis-à-vis the larger dominant group. These powerful socioeconomic and politically driven forces have exacerbated the damage traced to deeply embedded cultural values regarding women, their "proper" role in the family, and their abuse as mere "commodities" in the sex trade and cross-cultural trafficking of women and girls.

Chapter 10 builds on the increasing recognition that strategies to prevent violence and provide services to all survivors must include attention to the perpetrators of violence and abuse – the majority of whom are men. Much public debate and many policy statements from the United Nations, many States, and NGOs have resulted in some progress on human rights issues worldwide. And clearly, many men have led and are part of this progressive movement. But further action to curb violence and abuse of women must include attention to the deeply embedded values of men's power and control over women, children, and much more – as mirrored in their dominance as heads of most States worldwide, as well as the other major domains of all societies: religion, the economy, the military, healthcare, the arts. More men must use their enormous power and influence to help end the pandemic of violence and abuse.

The examples in these chapters provide a mini-field experience of sorts for entering the world of victimized people and their assailants, and connecting that experience to planning health and social services with them. By listening carefully to survivors' stories – here, in the literature, and in real life situations – we take the first important step in helping.

The next step follows from an understanding of "Here's my role ... here's what we can do together." Culturally sensitive providers who vicariously embrace the reality of their clients' pain can advocate or counsel them in the arduous – and sometimes lifelong – process of re-empowerment and healing. These beginnings shine a light on the road ahead in addressing the complex health and human rights challenges surrounding violence and abuse.

4 Intimate partner and gender-based violence

- International perspective
- Central and South America – the PAHO Study

  – Key concepts and implications for practice

- Case example: wife abuse, child custody, the "Final Blow" (Israel)

  – Key concepts underpinning practice

- Case example: marriage, abuse, and coping (China)

  – Key concepts underpinning practice

- Commonalities and differences cross-culturally
- The power of values and beliefs, and policy implications
- Practice implications for early identification and prevention
- Case example: opening the door (Australia)

While violence takes its toll across the life span, this chapter's focus on abuse and battery of female intimate partners (most often in a publicly recognized marital relationship) is pivotal in its illustration of the interconnections between different forms of interpersonal violence. Women who are verbally and physically abused by their male partners are frequently raped as well. Traditionally, across cultures, marital rape has not been recognized as a legal entity, on the assumption that husbands' sexual access to wives is an entitlement regardless of the wife's consent. Legal and feminist advocacy has changed that situation for married women in some countries.

The continuum of violence is illustrated further in that many women abused by their partners have also suffered physical and/or sexual abuse as children – most often from a father, stepfather, mother's boyfriend, or other male relative. This frequently unacknowledged history of abuse during childhood, and inadequate or totally absent support, usually leaves survivors more vulnerable for later abuse by intimate partners – including sometimes through old age – than may be the case for women without such histories. Further, most of these women have children who either witness the abuse of their mother directly, or at the very least are negatively affected in their emotional and social development by living in the toxic environment of a violent home. In the worst case scenario, some of these women also lose their children – either to the abusive father, or to child protective authorities – in what contributor Ruth Rasnic describes as "The Final Blow."

International perspective

The United Nations Population Fund (2000) reported that violence against women is still firmly rooted throughout the world. The report reveals that at least one in three women are beaten, raped, forced into sex, or abused in other ways – most often by someone they know. The context of such abuse and violence is women's second-class social status worldwide which leaves them disadvantaged educationally and economically. While poor women of color and their children are the most vulnerable, abuse cuts across all class, racial, ethnic, and religious groups (Amowitz, 2004; WHO, 2004; Kim *et al.*, 2007; Paterson *et al.*, 2008; Romans *et al.*, 2007).

In industrialized wealthy countries, immigrant women, their partners, and families may have found some freedoms lacking in the countries they fled, but they bring with them the values that define women's subordinate status across the globe (Handewerker, 1998). In most instances these values intersect with those affecting women in the host country and can be compounded by ideologies in the social service and psychiatric systems they turn to for assistance – that is, if they feel secure in seeking any assistance at all as "guests" in a land where deportation may result if the problem of abuse becomes publicly visible. Regardless of the material wealth or international status of various countries, these ideologies linger in human service settings where abused women may be re-victimized by the system whose mission is to provide service, *not* do further harm (Luhrman, 2000). In short, patriarchal authoritarian norms and continued medicalization of violence and victimization in the new millennium form the context in which control and abuse of women and their children still flourish – despite the groundbreaking work of grassroots community groups to dislodge traditional definitions of such abuse as the "private" business of the family, and society's effort to contain it behind closed doors.

The PAHO Study – Central and South America

This study (Velzeboer *et al.*, 2003) was carried out in 16 communities of 10 countries in Central and South America. It was inspired by the various world conferences on human rights; the 1995 Fourth World Conference on Women in Beijing; the 1979 UN Convention on the Elimination of All Forms of Discrimination against Women (CEDAW); the Inter-Americana Convention on the Prevention, Punishment, and Eradication of Violence against Women (Belem do Para, 1994); and these words of Monserrat Sagot, who with Elizabeth Shrader coordinated the research process: "The obstacles to overcoming family violence are 500 years of culture ingrained through socialization in our children" (Velzeboer *et al.*, 2003, p. xii). The research protocol was titled *The "Critical Path" Studies: From Research to Action*, to highlight the critical path women follow to escape their violent situation (p. 9).

In context of the issues noted in Chapter 2 regarding the language used in discussing violence and abuse issues, the authors of this study adopted "gender-based violence" as the preferred term for the project, based on this definition of violence against women: "... any act of gender-based violence that results in, or is likely to result in, physical, sexual, or psychological harm or suffering to women, including threats of such acts, coercion, or arbitrary deprivations of liberty, whether occurring in public or private life" (UN General Assembly, 1993, cited by Velzeboer *et al.*, 2003, p. 4). It builds on the overview and research data discussed in Chapter 2, and the ecological model cited by Heise *et al.* (1999) that highlights societal norms of male control and rigid gender roles; poverty and social isolation; marital conflict and male control of wealth; and individual factors intersecting with sociocultural ones, for example, alcohol abuse.

The following vignettes from Velzeboer *et al.* (2003) capture the essence of this study's results in the 10 countries:

One of the issues is the machismo in our culture that says a man is the strongest and has to be, in whatever manner, over a woman, and when something does not suit him, he just beats her.

(Justice of the Peace, El Salvador, p. 11)

As most abused women report, the women said that the psychological abuse accompanying physical and sexual abuse was even more painful, and that threats to their children were especially traumatic:

He tells her: "You are stupid [crying], you are worthless and useless," and she was only a year old. Then he tells me: "Look at your baby. She is worthless and stupid; you do not respect her". ... She was only a year old; she couldn't even talk yet; so she just stared at him, taking it all in.

(Guatamala, p. 12)

As pioneering studies in the US also revealed (McFarlane *et al.*, 1992), pregnancy – when a woman is most in need of protection – was often the occasion of first and repeated violence:

I am eight months pregnant and when he comes home, he starts to rail and break up things. He kicked me in my belly, and the water bag burst.

(Belize, p. 13)

Women often stayed in the situation because of social pressure to stay and out of fear and inadequate resources to survive:

My parents told me: "If he is your husband, you just have to put up with the situation; that is the way it is." Then my mother said: "This is how I have suffered with my husband, too."

(Peru, p. 15)

And as with other abused women worldwide, when they became aware of available support they could take the first step on the "critical path" away from the violence, and work toward leaving:

Thank God for those advertisements! When I saw them, I said: "I have to find out more; I have to leave; I have to find out what can be done about this."

(Honduras, p. 15)

Overall, the "critical path" encompassed three key features: (1) response factors: these included the availability and quality of services, how providers represented the services, and the results obtained; (2) motivating factors: information and knowledge; perceptions and attitudes; previous experiences; and support from close people; (3) the woman's decisions and actions taken.

Key concepts and practice implications

Considering these factors, researchers asked the question: Are service providers part of the problem or are they part of the solution? The answer to the question had been addressed in some of the earliest groundbreaking research on gender-based violence at Yale University by Stark, Frazier, and Flitcraft (1979). This sociology-medical team examined a large sample of battered women seeking treatment in a medical emergency service. Their widely cited study uncovered the process whereby the criminal behavior of gender-based violence was redefined by medical professionals as a "private event" accounted for by the victim's presumed psychopathology, while the perpetrator was excused, also on grounds of his presumed psychopathology – one of the classic examples in social science literature of the "social construction" of mental illness (see Cooksey & Brown, 1998; Hoff *et al.*, 2009, Chapter 11).

In "lessons learned" from the PAHO study, researchers built on the provider role question by application of the "Power and Control Wheel" concept. This widely used teaching tool was originally developed by the Domestic Abuse Intervention Project in Duluth, Minnesota, USA, to depict the process and tactics used by perpetrators to maintain the submission and continued vulnerability of their female victims (see Chapter 8 for a detailed description of this concept). Here, the PAHO researchers cite the parallel "Medical Power and Control Wheel" developed by the Domestic Violence Project of Kenosha, Wisconsin, USA. In this model, *healthcare workers can hurt women* by escalating danger and increased entrapment through these actions:

- Normalizing victimization, e.g. through belief that abuse is the outcome of noncompliance with patriarchal control.
- Violating confidentiality, e.g. by calling the police without her consent.
- Trivializing and minimizing the abuse, e.g. not taking seriously the danger she feels, or emphasizing the importance of keeping the family together.
- Blaming the victim, e.g. asking what she did to provoke him, or "Why do you let him do that to you?"
- Not respecting her autonomy, e.g. "prescribing" divorce, couples counseling, or psychotropic medications.
- Ignoring her need for safety, e.g. by not asking "Is it safe to go home? Do you have somewhere to go if the situation escalates?"

On the other hand, *health workers can help women* and facilitate empowerment by:

- Respecting her confidentiality, e.g. building trust through discussion without other family members present.
- Believing and validating her experiences, e.g. by listening and letting her know she is not alone.
- Acknowledging the injustice, e.g. stating that what happened to her is not right, and it is not her fault.
- Respecting her autonomy, e.g. since she knows her circumstances best, respecting her decisions about leaving.
- Helping her plan for future safety, e.g. exploring what she has tried for keeping herself and children safe, and whether she has a place to go if she needs to escape.
- Promoting access to community services, e.g. sharing resources such as a hotline, shelter, support groups and legal services.

Besides the lessons learned from this study on behalf of survivors, the study team addressed the needs of health providers that surfaced in their day-to-day work over the several years of this project, including publication of a self-care guide for health providers working in the domestic violence field (Claramunt, 1999). The needs of providers are discussed more fully in Chapter 12, including the issue of vicarious traumatization.

Case example: wife abuse, child custody, and "The Final Blow" (Israel) [told by a shelter advocate]

The International Social Workers' Organization referred Sarah White to our shelter. Sarah was a young Englishwoman who had married and divorced an Israeli. The couple had two daughters, both of whom were in Sarah's custody when she returned to the UK. The ex-husband, who had threatened to kidnap the children, was denied entry to England.

One day the girls did not return from school. Their father had entered England with a false passport, stalked his daughters and taken them back to Israel. He then began harassing his in-laws, threatening them and their daughter. The family was petrified, and within several years Sarah's parents died. Sarah did not have the strength or finances to start the legal battle in Israel.

We accepted Sarah, a former battered woman, into our shelter – a mother grieving for her living daughters. Shelter life is not easy. It was doubly difficult for Sarah, who was neither Israeli nor Jewish, who was not fleeing from an abuser, for whom everything Israeli recalled her abusive, abducting, ex-husband. The law has its own weird, slow, often uncaring processes. The entire pace of social welfare bureaucracy took its toll with reports and evaluations as to whether the children should or should not see their own mother after close on to four years' separation.

The "loving" father had placed the girls with Israel's Social Services. He would visit them and they spent the weekends with him. The younger child was in a children's home and her sister, in her early teens, in one of the country's excellent schools – a boarding school for many children who come from "problematic" or "broken" homes. Both girls had been fed lies by the father and were thoroughly brainwashed against their mother. After many months of residency at our shelter, Sarah received visitation rights, but only on the premises of the girls' residence, in the presence of a social worker. Those harrowing visits could try the patience of an angel, with the girls spurning their mother as she slowly tried to woo them and win back their love.

Dates for the hearing were so distant that Sarah went back to England to settle some of her affairs and return to her second year at college. Eventually Sarah returned to Israel for the trial which was to determine whether her girls would be returned to her, or if the rift was too great, and to ascertain if removal again would be detrimental to the girls' mental stability. After several months, the judge decided to give her custody of the youngest child only. Her eldest daughter refused adamantly to have any contact with her mother. There was no way she could be made to re-establish relations with her mother. The child gave false testimony about her life in England, her mother's behavior and attitudes; the judge left her in the custody of the father. To those of us in the shelter, the story reeked of incest.

Sarah returned to Britain. After several years, through the International Social Workers' Organization, Sarah's eldest daughter renewed contacts with her mother. The father had removed her to the USA. She had been badly beaten and sexually abused by him, and left for dead on the streets of New York City. After arrest and incarceration, he was evicted from the United States. One day, hopefully, Sarah will write her story. Now all she wants is peace and quiet.

Key concepts underpinning practice

The usual challenges and possible friction points in a "mixed" marriage are exacerbated in a case like Sarah's in which the partners differ not only in religion but in country of origin. Major issues and concepts illustrated by this situation include the following:

* The complexity and barriers that abused women confront in most legal and social service

systems are magnified if the woman is caught between these systems in two different countries. The adage: "Justice delayed is justice denied" seems to apply here. Experience with abused women tells us that, in general, justice delayed or denied impedes the healing process.

- Some judges and social service professionals are still influenced by the patriarchal norms that historically have favored men, even when these men have been shown to have broken laws, for example, presenting a false passport and abducting children, as Sarah's ex-husband did. Class issues also play a role in some of these judgments: most divorced men have more money than divorced wives and are able to employ lawyers to argue their case for custody based on greater material resources – this, despite the fact that (in most of these cases) the father was never the primary caretaker, there is no evidence of the mother's parental incompetence, and the father's intent is to have his new wife assume the role of primary caretaker (Chesler, 1986).

- In this context, awarding child custody on the basis of class or to an abusive father affirms the patriarchal legacy of ownership and control of children regardless of the father's fitness for or record of caring for these children. The education of judges and child protection authorities on this issue has resulted in changed policies in the jurisdictions of some countries which proscribe custody awards to any parent with a criminal record.

- Awarding child custody to an abusive father as was done in Sarah's situation takes advantage of the vulnerability of young children who are used as a weapon against the non-custodial parent. Once done, it is relatively easy for the custodial parent to alienate a child from the absent parent since security needs and fear of abandonment often will dominate in the mind of a child, even in the face of physical and sexual abuse, and the absent parent cannot counter any false allegations.

- The life-threatening outcome for Sarah's eldest child dramatically illustrates: (a) the misguided judgment of the court in awarding custody of the eldest daughter to the father; (b) the shelter staff's intuition that child sexual abuse by the father was an imminent possibility; (c) the advisability of professional health and social service agencies to call on shelter staff for consultation in complex cases like Sarah's, since their experience base is usually much broader than that of many professional providers.

Case example: marriage, abuse, and coping (China) [told by Lin Wong to Han Li, a Canadian-Chinese researcher in British Columbia]

Prior to our marriage, Hu-fang was the sweetest person on earth. I got pregnant the first month after we were married. By the seventh month of my pregnancy, Hu-fang demanded sex every day even when I told him I did not feel like it. My illusion of a marriage started to shatter.

Two weeks after my daughter was born we started a quarrel and he raised his fist at me. Luckily our neighbor stopped him. Although those fierce fists did not hit my fragile body, they hit my heart, broke it and tore it into pieces. I wept all night that night, grieving for my lost dream of a good marriage as well as my fatal mistake of marrying a beast. His loud yelling and angry fists passed me a strong message: He did not love me, not at all. This realization was as cruel as it was true.

From the next day on, I started to speak carefully, making sure not to offend Hu-fang. When he lost his temper and yelled at me, I would pretend not to have heard. Eventually I developed a better strategy to laugh and laugh loudly. At first he was startled at my loud laughter. Then he got used to it and believed that I was really laughing, not being sarcastic.

Our neighbors' children would watch me when I started my scary laughter. They thought I was crazy. Maybe I was. I was not sure anymore.

In the last four years, I had not let Hu-fang kiss me on the lips and I refused him constantly when he wanted to have sex. For him, having sex was a way to get the body relaxed, thus he could get a good sleep. Shortly before he went to sleep he would come to me to demand sex. As time was precious for a surgeon, he usually finished it in five to ten minutes. I had complained to him that I was just starting, but he ignored me. Gradually I lost interest in sex and started to refuse him completely. When his wishes were not granted, he would bump his head on the wall to threaten me. Sometimes he would grab me and bump my head on the wall as well.

"I don't want to live any more. Let's die together," he would murmur desperately. I would start to cry and sit on the sofa with a blanket. He would take my blanket away and let me freeze in the cold winter nights – you know we had no indoor heat when it was -15° Celsius. While I was weeping and agonizing he would fall asleep in five minutes. In order to be away from his loud snores, I would crawl to the sofa in the living room. He would then get up and turn on the light every ten minutes or so to make sure that I did not get any sleep. When he thought that turning the light on and off was not punishing me enough, he would throw shoes at me to make sure that I was miserable.

Sometimes I thought that an animal is better off than me. An animal is allowed to sleep yet I am not. In order to get some sleep, sometimes I would give up and let him have his sex. Then I would weep, and he pretended not to see my tears. Very often, I think that there is not much of a difference between being a prostitute for one person [one's husband] and a prostitute for any person. Yet, the former is perceived as a virtuous woman and the latter is called a rotten woman.

Key concepts underpinning practice

Lin Wong's situation must be understood in the context of Confucian teaching about girls and women. Confucius, one of the two dominant philosophers throughout Chinese history, wrote in his *Law of Conduct*, the famous *Three Character Book for Girls and Women*, that a daughter must obey her father and a wife must obey her husband. The inferior status of Chinese girls and women dictated by Confucius was reinforced by the Yin and Yang doctrine (305–240 BC) which implicates that Yin represents the female gender and Yang the male gender. Yin is negative, weak, passive, feeble-minded, whereas Yang is positive, strong, active, and powerful (Chan, 1963).

According to Confucian teaching, women are born to serve, first their parents, then in-laws and husbands, then male children. They are not supposed to eat at the table, their place is in the kitchen. They are born to obey and to serve and please others. Girls are born cheap, especially if the family is poor. They are not sent to school. It is considered a waste of money to train them – they will marry into another family sooner or later. Girls are sold for money or exchanged for goods.

Although Chairman Mao banned Confucian teaching in schools in 1949, centuries-old cultural norms cannot be eliminated by simple edict. Thus, for example, a Chinese rural girl recently (in the 1990s) chose to drown herself in a village lake because she could not live without disobeying her father. This girl's coping by suicide is embedded in Confucian teaching in which punishment was severe for defying parental authority. To maintain parental dignity, stories are told of parents who had rolled their rebellious daughter in a straw mat, tied the mat up and thrown it into a lake. The life of a woman was worthless if she violated family rules. The parents would not be punished for drowning the daughter. Instead, they would be admired for disciplining their children. The suicides of abused Chinese women can be better understood in this context.

These deeply embedded cultural norms in China are compounded by economic situations and efforts to control population. As China has been mainly an agricultural country, girls and women are not as useful as boys and men in the fields. To worsen the situation for girls and women, the Chinese tradition was set in such a way that a grown-up daughter usually marries out and her children no longer carry her parents' family name (Bloodworth, 1967; Chen, 1971). They cannot be relied on in old age nor can they continue the family name. Daughters usually have no say in the family. Thus, while the status of girls and women improved somewhat after 1949, the deep-rooted traditions remain. Husbands beating wives is considered a normal practice. Since the 1978 one-child policy was enacted, the fate of baby girls is very tragic – abortion of female fetuses and female infanticide abound to maintain the traditional preference for boys and devaluation of women who do not produce them.

Global awareness of violence against wives certainly holds the potential to alleviate situations like Lin Wong's and provide alternatives beyond "walking on eggshells" to avoid blows or stoically enduring the abuse. Yet, health providers in China and those serving Chinese immigrants around the world must recognize the power of ancient Confucian ideology even among contemporary Chinese. Denial of abuse in Chinese culture is still widespread. For example, when North American nursing professors working as visiting scholars in China during the 1990s were asked about the incidence of wife abuse, they replied that to their best knowledge this was not a problem in China. The reality, as in many societies, is that it is not a very *visible* problem. Even in societies like Canada and the United States that have directed vast resources to address the issue, many still either deny its particular impact on women; some women are poorly informed about resources and safety measures; and some immigrant women in particular feel culturally alienated from the resources that exist.

Commonalities and differences cross-culturally

What do the women in these stories have in common beyond their gender and experience of abuse by their male partners? And what might they have in common with abused women worldwide? Perhaps most basic is their love and concern for their children regardless of their personal suffering. Such love is rooted in the parent/child bond and – for mothers – bolstered by the social designation of women in all cultures as society's primary caretakers – of children, their partners, elderly parents and in-laws, often at the considerable sacrifice of self-care. Another commonality is the economic disadvantage of all the women; most of the women in Central and South America were poor; although Lin Wong was married to a surgeon, in China she faced material deprivation, struggling to stay warm in her house. As if the traditional values influencing most criminal justice systems and judicial decisions were not enough, the economic and wage disparities of women worldwide – not to mention the struggle against depression from abuse and its sequelae – serve as barriers and take a serious toll on the attempts of any abused woman who decides to fight for her rights in courts of law. However, mother love and a woman's social role as caretaker were not sufficient to protect Sarah from losing custody of her eldest daughter.

The centrality of male *power and control* is also common cross-culturally. Such control is maintained through verbal abuse, blaming a woman for her partner's angry outbursts, threats of harm, and denigrating the woman in interaction with children and thus alienating them from their mother. In Sarah's case, the abuser's control was enhanced by engaging the courts, other public agencies, or medical psychiatric personnel to support his cause by imputing the woman's unfitness for parenting. Even when there is no objective evidence of a mother's neglect, abuse, or parental unfitness, some attorneys are too ready to accept at face value an abusive husband's allegations about his wife's unfitness.

This situation is not helped by the fact that some women (without objective evidence) allege child sexual abuse by fathers as an inappropriate weapon during bitter divorce proceedings. Public education for women around divorce and professional training on violence issues in the legal community might prevent some of these unfortunate pitfalls. Such misplaced adversarial approaches and the misuse of children in marital conflict only detract from the broader agenda of violence prevention and the protection of children in the dissolution of abusive and other un-happy marriages. Another misguided approach to abuse between marital partners is therapists' agreement to requests for joint marriage counseling sessions before the abuser has acknowledged accountability for violent behavior and a safety plan for the victim is in place (Adams, 2003; Bograd, & Mederos, 1999).

For Lin Wong of China, however, the prospect of taking her case to court was not even a possibility – let alone winning a judgment against her abuser. One of the major outcomes of the controlling behavior of abusive men is the woman's *social isolation*. Typically, the isolation increases as the woman becomes depressed, starts doubting herself and believing the abuser's put-downs, then begins blaming herself for her plight. Psychiatric records in the United States and Canada reveal that a majority of women with mental and emotional problems have a his-tory of abuse that was never addressed before serious depression and other negative sequelae resulted (see Chapter 9, Case example of Leela). Many women with these histories also resort to self-destructive behaviors as a means of coping when social support and healthy alternatives are lacking (Burstow, 1992; Hoff *et al.*, 2009).

Another commonality among abused women cross-culturally is their remarkable capacity to cope and survive against familial and institutional forces that militate against their best interests. Some actions by families and professionals are well-intentioned though misguided, as may have been the case with Sarah (and Leela in Chapter 9). Yet, the women's stress responses to the trauma of abuse and their coping strategies can easily be discredited and/or ascribed to their purported psychopathology, particularly in instances where health professionals have little or no formal instruction on violence topics.

The power of values and beliefs, and policy implications

In all the examples, the control and abuse of women can be traced to beliefs and codes of con-duct emanating from definitions of women's place according to ancient systems of philosophy and religion: Christianity, Confucianism, Hinduism, Islam, and Judaism. In the Middle Ages, Christianity conducted witch hunts against women healers; the Taliban regime in Afghanistan provided a contemporary example of using Islam to justify its oppression and cruel treatment of women.

Each of the major religious traditions is essentially patriarchal, despite moderation and some accommodation in recent times in response to demands of human rights and women's advocacy groups, and UN proclamations regarding violence and discrimination against women. These issues are addressed further in Chapters 8 and 9, which address the particular circumstances of indigenous and immigrant women.

Understanding the concept of "cultural relativism" is central to providers' ability to assist abused women to escape violent relationships and rebuild their lives. Unfortunately, some are still willing to use "culture" or "machismo" as an excuse to look the other way, rather than recognize abuse as a universal human rights violation, regardless of the cultural group in which it occurs. The examples reveal that the power ascribed to family court judges, child protective authorities, and psychiatric providers can easily be misused. Thus, the persons in these systems need to acknowledge their culturally embedded attitudes and that clinical practice is not value-free despite the claims of some. Also central (as the Power and Control Wheel depicts) is recognition that *re-empowerment* (rather than disempowerment through legal imposition) is a central ingredient of justice as well as movement toward a violence-free life for abused women and their children.

Some professional providers may be reluctant to identify themselves as either informed by or sympathetic to feminist perspectives and a critical analysis of widespread discrimination based on gender. Instead, there is ready dismissal of feminism as a monolithic ideology promulgating hatred of men and scorn for traditional family values. Yet, it is a feminist perspective combined with critical social analysis that has revealed discrimination based on gender and *violence against women as harmful not only to women, but to children, the perpetrators themselves, and an entire society that allows or inadvertently supports its continuance*. The absence of such a critical perspective around values informing practice can often result in the misguided use of legal and psychiatric authority in the care and treatment of abused women. A central means of changing deeply embedded attitudes that are more harmful than useful is the widespread inculcation of knowledge about the social, health status, economic, and spiritual toll exacted by violence and abuse of intimate partners and children.

Epidemiological and ethnographic data form the basis of such knowledge. Professionals who cling to a "gender-neutral" approach to the topic are advised to consult peer-reviewed data sources and examine the values supporting claims of objectivity regarding violence and the majority of its victims (see Chapter 2. Feminist and critical social analysts make no claims of being value-free on this topic (Segal, 1999). Rather, they openly acknowledge that the research endeavor itself is value-laden (e.g. in choice of research methods) and make explicit their assumption of violence as a human rights issue, not merely a scientific enterprise (Hoff, 1990; Oakley, 1981; Perilla, 1999; Reinharz, 1992).

In countries where wife-beating is considered "normal" behavior belonging in the "private" domestic arena rather than a "criminal" act demanding accountability by the perpetrator, political action is indicated to hold governments accountable to UN Conventions and the 1995 Platform for Action from the Beijing Women's Conference. One European country has used the UN Convention proscribing discrimination against women on behalf of an abused wife threatened with her life: after failed efforts to gain court-ordered protection from her violent husband, the woman fled her country and sought refuge in a neighboring state. The host country that granted her asylum used the UN Convention as grounds to file suit against the woman's country for its failure to protect one of its citizens from life-threatening danger. See Chapters 8, 9, 10, and 13 for additional examples of services for survivors, their families, and perpetrators, and Table 3.1 for roles of generalists and specialists in health sector practice; see the online resources in Part IV for teaching/learning suggestions.

Practice implications for early identification and prevention

These concepts and openness to exploring controversial issues lay the foundation for the goal of early identification of victim/survivors at various entry points to health and social service agencies. But without established policies and clinical protocols to achieve this goal, clients at risk may remain so by staying in an abusive relationship, and opportunities to prevent further violence go missing as well. The following example shows that the therapeutic relationship and the provider's leadership in asking about safety "planted a seed" for seeking further help, even if a woman is not ready to act on first inquiry.

Case example: opening the door (Australia)

A 23-year-old mother of two small children reported to her case worker that she was experiencing psychological abuse by her male partner. The case worker asked if the client felt safe at home and if there was any specific assistance she could provide. The client declined the offer of assistance. She stated that her family had offered to help if necessary. The case worker accepted the client's position and gave assurances about the availability of future assistance if required. Two weeks later the client re-presented to the case worker and said that things at home were no longer tenable. She was leaving her partner. Since her last visit to community health, her partner had started 'roughing up' the children. She was leaving. This time she accepted the worker's offer of assistance; she sought emergency accommodation, an AVO [protection order], and short-term Centrelink financial assistance. She reported feeling strong and determined, as if she had been relieved of a crushing weight. She had plans to leave the local area and move to a city and complete her university studies.

Based on extensive research on the role of health professionals with women already injured or at risk of abuse, in the 1990s the Joint Commission on Accreditation of Healthcare Organizations (JCAHO) in the United States issued a policy requiring routine inquiry about victimization on admission for health service. As a result of this policy, all health history questionnaires now include a question on injury from abuse. However, if such questions are "patched into" a medical history form for check-off before seeing a health provider, their value is questionable outside the context of a trusted "doctor-patient" or other trusted relationship. But to move beyond a "mechanical" approach to the issue, as Furniss *et al.* (2007) found in their research, nurses want brief clear resources, protocols, and time alone with a patient for addressing intimate partner violence. Exhibit 4.1 was developed from research with abused women (Hoff, 1990; Hoff, &

Exhibit 4.1   Screening for victimization and life-threatening behaviors: triage questions

Have you been troubled or injured by any kind of abuse or violence? (for example, hit by partner, forced sex)

Yes_____No_____Not sure_____Refused_____If yes, check one of the following:

By someone in your family_____By an acquaintance or stranger_____

Describe:

If yes, has something like this ever happened before?

Yes_____No_____If yes, when?_____

Describe:

(continued)

Exhibit 4.1 (*continued*)

Do you have anyone you can turn to or rely on now to protect you from possible further injury?

Yes_____No_____If yes, who?_____

Do you feel so bad now that you have thought of hurting yourself/suicide?

Yes_____No_____If yes, what have you thought about doing?

Describe:

Are you so angry about what's happened that you have considered hurting someone else?

Yes_____No_____

Describe:

Rosenbaum, 1994). See Chapter 13 for an illustration of using triage questions and follow-up victimization assessment in the context of comprehensive care around intimate partner abuse.

Besides identifying risk of victimization and potential suicidal danger, this tool also addresses the fact that some abused women's level of injury or despair has led them to retaliatory violence or even murder of their abusers (Whitaker *et al.*, 2007). See Chapters 4 and 13 for discussion of such a scenario.

References

Adams, D. (2004). Treatment programs for batterers. *Clinics in Family Practice*, 5(1).

Amowitz, L. L. (2004). Human rights abuse and concerns about women's health and human rights in Southern Iraq. *Journal of American Medical Association*, 291(12), 1471–9.

Bloodworth, D. (1976). *The Chinese Looking Glass*. New York: Straus and Giroux.

Bograd, M., & Mederos, F. (1999). Battering and couples therapy: Universal screening and selection of treatment modality. *Journal of Marital and Family Therapy*, 25(3), 291–312.

Burstow, 1992. *Radical Feminist Therapy: Working in the Context of Violence*. Newbury Park, CA: Sage.

Chan, W. T. (1963). *A Source Book in Chinese Philosophy*. Princeton: Princeton University Press.

Chen, K. Y. (1971). *History of Marriage in China* [in Chinese]. Taipei: Taipei Commercial Press.

Chesler, P. (1986). *Mothers on Trial: The Battle for Children and Custody*. Seattle: Seal Press.

Claramunt, C. (1999). *Helping Ourselves to Help Others: Self-Care Guide for Those Who Work in the Field of Family Violence (Gender and Public Health Series 7)*. San Jose, Costa Rica: PAHO.

Cooksey, E. C., & Brown, P. (1998). Spinning on its axes: DSM and the social construction of psychiatric diagnosis. *International Journal of Health Sciences*, 28(3), 525–4.

Dangor, Z., Hoff, L. A., & Scott, R. (1998). Woman abuse in South Africa: An exploratory study. *Violence against Women: An International Interdisciplinary Journal*, 4(2), 125–52.

Dobash, R. E., & Dobash, R. P. (eds.) (1998). *Rethinking Violence against Women*. Thousand Oaks: CA: Sage.

Furniss, K., McCaffrey, M., Vereene, P., & Rovi, S. (2007). Nurses and barriers to screening for intimate partner violence. *American Journal of Maternal Child Nursing*, 32(4), 238–43.

Handwerker, W. P. (1998). Why violence? A test of hypotheses representing three discourses on the roots of domestic violence. *Human Organization*, 57(2), 200–8.

Heise, L., Ellsberg, M., & Gottemoeller, M. (1999). *Ending Violence against Women* (*Population Reports, Series L, 11*). Baltimore: Johns Hopkins University School of Public Health, Population Information Program.

Hoff, L. A. (1990). *Battered Women as Survivors*. London: Routledge.

Hoff, L. A. (1992). Review essay: Wife-beating in Micronesia. *ISLA: A Journal of Micronesian Studies*, 1(2), 199–221.

Hoff, L. A., Hallisey, B. J., & Hoff, M. (2009). *People in Crisis: Clinical and Diversity Perspectives* (6th edn.). New York & London: Routledge.

Hoff, L. A., & Rosenbaum, L. (1994). A victimization assessment tool: Instrument development and clinical implications. *Journal of Advanced Nursing*, 20(4), 627–34.

Kim, J. C., *et al.* (2007). Understanding the impact of a microfinance-based intervention on women's empowerment and the reduction of intimate partner violence in South Africa. *American Journal of Public Health*, 97(10), 1794–802.

Luhrmann, T. M. (2000). *Of Two Minds: The Growing Disorder in American Psychiatry.* New York: Alfred A. Knopf.

McFarlane, J., Parker, B., Soeken, K., & Bullock, L. (1992). Assessing for abuse during pregnancy: Severity and frequency of injuries and associated entry into prenatal care. *Journal of the American Medical Association*, 267(23), 3176–8.

Paterson, J., *et al.* (2008). Maternal intimate partner violence and behavioural problems among Pacific children living in New Zealand. *Journal of Child Psychology and Psychiatry*, 49 (4), 395–404.

Perilla, J. L. (1999). Domestic violence as a human rights issue: The case of immigrant Latinos. *Hispanic Journal of Behavioral Sciences*, 21(2), 107–33.

Reinharz, S. (1992). *Feminist Methods in Social Research.* Oxford & New York: Oxford University Press.

Romans, S., *et al.* (2007). Who is most at risk for intimate partner violence? A Canadian population-based study. *Journal of Interpersonal Violence*, 22(12), 1495–514.

Segal, L. (1999). *Why Feminism? Gender, Psychology, Politics.* New York: Columbia University Press.

Stark, E., Flitcraft, A., & Frazier, W. (1979). Medicine and patriarchal violence: The social construction of a "private" event. *International Journal of Health Services*, 9, 461–93.

Sugg, N. K., & Inui, T (1992). Primary care physicians' response to domestic violence: Opening Pandora's box. *Journal of the American Medical Association*, 267(23), 3157–60.

United Nations Population Fund. (2000). *The State of the World's Population 2000, Chapter 3. Ending violence against women and girls: A human rights and health priority.* Geneva: United Nations Population Fund.

Velzeboer, M., Ellsberg, M., Arcas, C. C., & Garciai-Moreno, C. (2003). *Violence against Women: The Health Sector Responds.* Washington, DC: PAHO, WHO.

Whitaker, D. J., Haileyesus, T., Swahn, M., & Saltzman, L. S. (2007). Differences in frequency of violence and reported injury between relationships with reciprocal and nonreciprocal intimate partner violence. *American Journal of Public Health*, 97(5), 941–7.

WHO – World Health Organization (2002). *World Report on Violence and Health.* Geneva: WHO.

WHO (2004). *Handbook for the Documentation of Interpersonal Violence Prevention Programmes.* Geneva: WHO.

5 Sexual assault and physical abuse during childhood and adolescence

- Overview: child abuse from ancient to contemporary times
- Case example: physical battering, neglect, and abuse – Bobby and his mother
- Case example: Amelia with disabilities (Australia)

  – Key concepts and practice implications
  – Complexities and prevention focus

- Case example: violence and abuse in dating relationships – Jennifer (Canada)

  – Key concepts and practice implications

- Case example: neglect and violence in late adolescence – Kendall (the Caribbean)

  – Sociocultural factors contributing to child neglect and abuse

- Hope and growth potential vs. pathologizing wounded and alienated youth

  – The Circle of Courage
  – The ROPE program: Rite Of Passage Experience

We often hear and read about children and youth as a nation's future, its greatest resource. Yet, juxtaposed against this hopeful message are tragic stories of abuse, neglect, and violence toward the most vulnerable among us. Because of the natural human instinct across cultures to protect and defend innocent children, it is all the more heart-rending to observe the continuation of violence against children.

Overview: child abuse from ancient to contemporary times

The centuries-old biblical expression "spare the rod and spoil the child" persists in the child-rearing practices of some contemporary families. But as De Mause (1975) points out, historically, the "helping mode" of concern for children is quite recent compared with widely accepted infanticide and rampant cruelty toward children in earlier centuries. Also, "adolescence" is a term of recent origin traceable in part to socioeconomic trends that have ushered in the need of a college or technical education for future job prospects and the subsequent prolongation of dependency on parents that is out of sync with their offspring's sexual maturity following puberty.

Contemporary teachers, health and social service professionals, researchers, governmental and non-governmental agencies are dedicated to addressing the special needs of children and adolescents. Despite what is known, however, about the health and social welfare of children; the enormous wealth of some nations that might be dedicated to children; and declarations of the United Nations on the rights of children, across the globe there are pictures of children scavenging for food in shanty towns and garbage heaps, and sniffing glue to assuage their suffering in communities too poor to support them in any modicum of human decency.

Less prominent in the vast literature on the crises and social needs of children and adolescents is the intersection of this topic with other facets of violence, for example, the poverty and abuse of mothers who are the predominant caretakers, or that the rights of children for special protection appear almost as an afterthought as a nation goes to war. Yet, when a soldier dramatically saves a child from the rubble of a bomb's destruction, the scene of this individual action stemming from the natural instinct to protect children regardless of race, class or gender is broadcast around the world. Usually less prominent is analysis of what accounts for the millions of unseen children whose neglected and injured bodies and psyches can be traced to sociopolitical sources and the deliberate decisions of adults.

This chapter addresses the plight of children using examples from economically advantaged and disadvantaged cultures. The focus is on the interrelationship between child abuse and neglect and other facets of violence which demand attention for sensitive, comprehensive, and integrated programs for children and adolescents in contemporary societies (see Havig, 2008). Discussion builds on the concepts of primary, secondary, and tertiary prevention introduced in Chapter 3. This includes education of parents and health and social service providers, as well as tools for early detection of abuse or neglect. One is the Child Screening Checklist integrated into crisis prevention and intervention programs; another is the Circle of Courage that complements the Medicine Wheel philosophy of indigenous peoples; and a third is the ROPE (Rite Of Passage Experience) program that brings adolescents, parents, educators, and entire communities together – thereby offering a metaphorical "rope" that young people need in what for many is a precarious and dangerous "climb" toward adulthood.

Case example: physical battering, neglect, and abuse – Bobby and his mother (Canada)

Bobby, age 7, is brought by his mother, Ms. Sarah Jones (hereafter Sarah) to a local emergency facility for an acute rash. On the course of physical examination and treatment, emergency personnel noted that Bobby had several welts on his buttocks. Following treatment for the rash, while Bobbie was resting, the nurse spoke with Bobby's mother about the welts which she and the physician suspected might have originated from use of a strap to discipline Bobby. Sarah readily acknowledged that she had strapped Bobby several times and went on to say that she has been discussing her general problems with a child protective case worker, but has not told the worker about strapping Bobby. She described her discipline of Bobby as "mild compared with the beatings he took from his father." In fact, one of the reasons she finally left her husband is that she was afraid for the children as well as herself (Sarah's other child is a daughter, age 9). On one occasion Sarah said she was nearly strangled to death, and on another occasion she took after her husband with a meat cleaver but became very frightened when realizing how close she came to possibly killing him. Most of these violent incidents occurred when her husband drank excessively. Sometimes Sarah also drank a lot, thinking if she joined him, maybe she could appease some of her husband's outbursts. Sarah has watched some TV shows on child abuse: "But, you know," she says, "when we grew up you knew .... You misbehaved? You knew you had it coming." Sarah claims she is trying to get hold of herself and stop disciplining Bobby so harshly. She says the worst times are after she has a "disappointing dating relationship with a man and I take out my frustration on my kids." "Sometimes," she says, "instead of hitting the kids, I just let 'em fight, and I sit there and eat or drink too much." Since leaving her husband

Sarah is parenting her two children alone on public assistance, while also attending a vocational training program "in order to better myself." Sarah is interested in a parents' support group her caseworker mentioned, but she has not yet found time to attend. Nor has she ever attended any groups for substance abusers. "Maybe if I went to one of those AA meetings I could find a husband who wouldn't beat me."

Case example: Amelia with disabilities (Australia)

Amelia, a 17-year-old girl with an intellectual disability and a diagnosis of Asperger's syndrome, reported to her psychiatrist during a recent consultation that she was pregnant. The client was living independently with friends in a shared household. She left her family home at 14 years of age. She mentioned casually to the psychiatrist that the baby's father was a neighbor aged 40. She was distressed and anxious because she had made up her mind to have a termination but the father insisted that she keep the baby; he had bashed her when she said she would not keep it. The client did not really like the baby's father and had no intention of carving out a life with him and a child. She believed he was only interested in the baby because as new parents they would receive a significant one-off payment from the government. She accepted appropriate support from the health staff. She took out an AVO (protection order) against the baby's father. A few weeks later she announced to her counselor that she was returning to live with her biological parents in a different town. Her partner called in to the health facility a few days later to register his apparent concern for the client and wanted to know her whereabouts. Staff advised him to take his concerns to the local police.

Key concepts and practice implications

In many respects, Bobby, his mother Sarah, and Amelia are classic examples of the interrelationship between stress, violence, substance abuse, various psychosomatic conditions, parental abuse, older men violating and controlling vulnerable adolescents, and how these factors affect child/adolescent development patterns and parenting roles. The abuse of Bobby and Amelia highlights other concepts underpinning comprehensive service planning for both child and mother, including:

- Myths and facts regarding maternal and paternal child abuse. The first US national survey on violence in the family (Straus *et al.*, 1980) revealed that rates of violence against children were approximately equal between mothers and fathers, but as Sarah's report attests, fathers' abuse is generally more injurious and more often results in a child's death than that of mothers. Though Sarah seems to sense that strapping her child may not be appropriate, she apparently lacks skills in non-abusive discipline. Her behavior supports the widespread belief – held by many other parents as well – that it is not possible to parent children without at some point resorting to physical discipline. Sweden was the first country to enact a national law forbidding the corporal punishment of children, with some other countries, States, and provinces passing similar laws or still debating the issue.
- Although "legal" age of consensual sex varies across cultures, Amelia's exploitation by an older man and his later abuse and control of her pregnancy choice crosses ethical and other boundaries between child abuse, parental protection, and intimate partner violence usually associated with mature adults.
- Women's primary role in child care is still the international norm, while the economic and social supports necessary for the very continuity of society through this essentially unpaid

work is often far from adequate (Kozol, 2000; Waring, 1990).

- The context, climate of violence, and aftermath of intimate partner battering inevitably affects the children. Researchers now consider the witnessing of violence between their parents as a form of child abuse with serious effects on their health and development (Abrahams, & Jewkes, 2005; Groves *et al.*, 1993). If a child witness is developmentally disabled, the psychological risks are compounded by the child's limitations in expression of feelings when abused.

- Beside the economic stress of single parenting, children are also at risk as a mother attempts to meet intimacy and leisure needs while trying to avoid another violent relationship. While Amelia decides against single parenting, others may choose a return to familiar parental support for birthing and nurturing a child at such a tender age when adolescence is not yet over.

- Sarah's self-esteem issues related to battering and substance abuse and her quest for a "new man" to fill the void – absent supportive counseling – are bound to affect her parenting skills with Bobby and his sister.

- The issue of public laws requiring the reporting of child abuse apply here: Do Bobby's injuries technically constitute child abuse? Does the situation warrant a report to child protective services? The general understanding of the law in contemporary societies says "yes," which raises legal, attitudinal, and finely tuned practice questions with mothers like Sarah and her abused children. Amelia's case appears to fall between the cracks, depending on governmental jurisdictions and laws regarding age of consent and a father's rights.

Child protection laws across countries and intra-country jurisdictions intersect with culturally specific problem-solving regarding child-rearing, for example, the sense of *community* responsibility for all children among most indigenous people. Health and social service professionals, as well as teachers and clergy, who suspect abuse are responsible for knowing the law in their particular State or province. This includes the *requirement* to report such abuse and physical injury to their respective government child protective authorities. However, great sensitivity, team collaboration, and clinical assessment skills are fundamental to success in carrying out this responsibility – lest the problem be exacerbated.

As a first step – prior to encountering real life child abuse situations – all professionals involved with children and adolescents must examine their own attitudes, experience, and beliefs about the complex issues involved in child abuse and maltreatment. This entails especially adopting a stance comprising the whole family, not just the abused child or adolescent. Most clinicians and researchers today do embrace an ecological interactive approach that includes the significance of race, class, and gender in understanding as well as preventing child abuse and neglect, and treating those already injured (Everett, & Gallop, 2001).

Complexities and prevention focus

Consider then, for example, this complex scenario faced by a well-intentioned professional: a) a badly bruised child with cigarette burns and other horrific injuries; b) knowledge of the mother's alcohol problem and her few economic options – either acknowledged by a mother like Sarah on assessment, or from previous encounters in emergency medical or social service visits; c) the realization of duty to report and knowledge of parental rights balanced against children's rights; and d) the need to enact a collaborative plan with the parent and professional team without alienating the mother in the process – this through self-awareness and controlling of an attitude of revulsion toward the mother (see Chapter 12). Key practice skills on behalf of Sarah and her children and Amelia include:

• Establishing rapport and trust, and creating the time and space which allowed Sarah to acknowledge her harsh behavior and discuss its context in her own stressful life.
• Victimization assessment of Bobby's injury, and Sarah's past history of battering and assault potential. Structured tools incorporated into protocols requiring routine assessment of victimization and risk to life are helpful in this process (see Exhibit 5.1, Child Screening Checklist, and Table 13.1; Hoff *et al.*, 2009).
• Communicating to Sarah the laws regarding child abuse and the reporting obligation of health workers, without threatening her or losing her trust; similar communication with Amelia regarding her rights and responsibilities under the law, and supporting her in re-engagement of her parents for support.
• Establishing trust with Bobby and letting him know that the way he has been treated is unacceptable, while at the same time not building barriers between him and his mother.
• Engaging Sarah in learning non-violent coping with personal problems and approaches to discipline.
• Collaborating with a child protective worker to implement the required reporting procedure without alienating Sarah.
• Exploring with Sarah community referral sources for her substance abuse problem, and possible extended family support or respite services for child care which might enable her to take advantage of support groups for herself.
• Establishing specific follow-up plans with Sarah, Amelia, and her parents.

At the interdisciplinary level, a physician, midwife, or APN (nurse practitioner) would examine for physical injury and emotional trauma. A social worker would initiate follow-up counseling regarding discipline, other issues, and possible referral for substance abuse and respite care. If no referral is made, the team decides together who will do follow-up counseling – a social worker, family physician, or nurse. Any one of the team members might coordinate the overall crisis management and referral process. Specialists who might serve in follow-up care include a child protective worker, usually a social worker; substance abuse counselor or group; women's health and/or pediatric medical provider; and psychotherapist (any mental health professional) sensitive to gender issues and interaction between substance abuse, psychosocial stress, and survivor issues. Students in this scenario (primarily medicine, nursing, and medical social work) would observe and assist in above tasks, e.g. communicate and spend time with Bobby and his mother Sarah, and Amelia to convey support and build trust.

For student learning and practice in a situation like Sarah's and her children's, it is unlikely that all students could be provided a direct practice opportunity comparable to this case or one in which physical trauma requires extensive follow-up treatment. But several approaches could afford a vicarious learning experience, particularly in maternal/child/family health and related courses in nursing, medicine, physical therapy, occupational therapy, social work, and clinical psychology, for example:

• A formal class session using a film and planned case analysis, and/or guest appearance by a mother with issues similar to Sarah's and Amelia's cases.
• Incorporation of victimization assessment into crisis assessment protocols applied in routine clinical assignments.
• Student journals citing contacts with abused children/women, the concepts/issues

involved, student's feelings, and practice issues encountered, followed by clinical seminar discussion.
- Role playing regarding issues and dilemmas.

Exhibit 5.1 Child screening checklist

Child's full name_____ Gender_____
Date of birth_____

Family relationship concerns:

Does not get along with mother_____ father_____ brother(s) _____ sister(s) _____ refuses to participate in family activities_____ refuses to accept and perform family responsibilities_____ frequently absent parent_____ marital problems/domestic violence_____ rotating "parents" (parents' girlfriends or boyfriends) _____ inadequate child care arrangements_____ family health problems_____ financial insecurity/homelessness_____ family transitions (move, divorce, remarriage, incarceration, death) _____ rejection of child_____ other_____

School concerns:

Poor grades/underachievement_____ lack of motivation/disinterest/failure to do homework_____ frequent absences or tardiness_____ warnings, detentions, suspensions_____ does not get along with students_____ does not get along with teachers_____ other_____

Peer relationship concerns:

Inability to get along with peers_____ lack of friends_____ prefers to be alone_____ prefers to be with adults_____ does not associate with peers_____ not accepted by peers_____ bullied/harassed by peers_____ reluctant to leave parent/home _____ other_____

Dysocial behavioral concerns:

Excessive lying_____ stealing_____ vandalism_____ fire setting_____ aggression/fighting/violence_____ runaway_____ early sexual behavior_____ inappropriate sexual behavior_____ substance abuse_____ court involvement_____ homicidal_____ suicidal_____ other_____

(continued)

Exhibit 5.1 (*continued*)

Personal adjustment concerns:

Temper tantrums_____ easily upset_____ clinging/dependent_____ sleep disturbances_____ nervous mannerisms_____ thumb sucking_____ speech problems_____ eating problems_____ wetting, soiling, retention_____ lacks self-confidence/self-esteem_____ other_____

Emotional concerns:

Loneliness_____ boredom_____ being different_____ frustration_____ anger/hostility_____ anxiousness_____ fearfulness_____ negativism_____ depression_____ other_____

Medical and developmental concerns:

Acute illness_____ chronic illness_____ disabilities_____ allergies_____ accident prone_____ seizures_____ physical complaints_____ lengthy or frequent clinic/hospital visits_____ medication_____ surgery_____ mental retardation_____ other_____

Strengths and assets:

_____

_____

_____

_____

_____

Comments:

_____

_____

_____

_____

_____

Screened by:

_____

_____

_____

Case example: violence and abuse in dating relationships – Jennifer (Canada)

Jennifer, age 16, and Daryl, age 17, have been dating for six months. Before that, Jennifer dated Tim, now age 17, for two years. Jennifer broke up with Tim because he was verbally abusive to her, very controlling, and very demanding sexually. In fact, Jennifer had stopped seeing Tim off and on over the two years they dated, but always went back after his begging and pleading because she "had no one else to talk to who really seemed to love her." Jennifer was clearly not alone in her desperation for love. Tim was abused as a child himself (usually beaten and locked in a closet for misbehavior). On two of these occasions he was treated for a broken tooth and a ruptured eardrum which the emergency physician and dentist each traced to abuse. Upon referral from both the physician and dentist, Tim's parents saw a family counselor, but refused to return after two sessions. Although Jennifer was very emotionally dependent on Tim, what really scared her into breaking up was getting a diagnosis of Chlamydia after several bladder infections. Jennifer had never been that interested in sex, and worried about getting pregnant because Tim refused to use a condom after they had been intimate for a couple of months and Tim said Jennifer was his "first and only girl." Despite her realistic concerns, Jennifer always gave in to Tim's demands because she was "afraid of losing him" and she needed someone she could feel close to.

Jennifer's family life was a source of stress and little comfort to her. Her parents – both successful professionals – were cold and uncommunicative with each other, and very controlling with all their three children – Jennifer, Corrine, age 12, and Janice, age 9. Sometimes Jennifer felt if she had only been a boy her parents would have been less hard to please. No matter what kind of grades she brought home (usually close to the top), there was always a remark that she could do better. Though Jennifer was by no means overweight, she was always dieting, as her mother let her know in more ways than one that almost anything was better than "getting fat." Jennifer and her two sisters were close and colluded in their complaints against their parents, while Jennifer fought off bouts of depression mostly because she wanted to "be there" for her two sisters. Since both parents seemed so wrapped up in their work, the three girls used to wonder among themselves why they were born in the first place.

During Jennifer's visits with a primary care practitioner at the women's health clinic of the community health center, she learned a great deal about her risk for AIDS and other communicable diseases. She also accepted a recommendation to join an adolescent support group that focused on relationship and self-esteem issues for girls at risk for eating disorders. As a result of these group sessions, Jennifer decided, among other things, that she would refrain from sex until she felt more secure in herself and had better prospects of respect and commitment from her boyfriend.

Meanwhile, at a school dance Jennifer attended with her new boyfriend, Daryl, Tim came by and asked her to dance. Jennifer refused, they got into a loud argument, Daryl came to Jennifer's defense and threatened to "have it out with you [Tim] outside if you don't stay away from Jennifer." Jennifer became very frightened by Daryl's threat of violence, particularly because she had felt much safer with him than with Tim. She asked Daryl to take her home, and at the next week's group session at the health clinic she discussed this incident and what it meant for her. Meanwhile, a teacher chaperone at the dance talked with Tim and persuaded him to see the school counselor. During homeroom periods, this teacher had observed Tim's behavior for some time and sensed a troubled history.

Key concepts and practice implications

This example is replete with suggestions of the psychosociocultural roots of violence and abuse in familial and gender relations in the larger society, including:

- The centrality of family and responsible non-violent parenting in the growth and development process, including self-esteem and firm messages about a child's inherent worth in the human community.
- The process whereby childhood abuse and insecurity in the family lays the foundation for later consequences such as excessive dependency and vulnerability to abuse and violence in an intimate relationship.
- Power and control issues in parent-child and gender relations.
- Learned behavior, including competition and control issues, in familial and community settings.
- The correlation between childhood abuse of boys and later abusive behavior among some; while a history of abuse in childhood does not *determine* future violence, it lays a foundation for learning physical force for problem solving and conflict resolution (Foshee *et al.*, 2004; Molnar *et al.*, 2001; Silverman *et al.*, 2001). An excessive focus on the "intergenerational transmission of violence" can move "victim-blaming" from the individual to the family (see Hoff, 1990, p. 127, and Miller & Challis, 1981, for a 25-year longitudinal study of this issue).
- Cultural messages regarding women's body image ("a woman can never be too thin") which intersect with family dynamics to negatively affect young women's self-acceptance and self-esteem (important buffers to stress and avoiding abuse during conflicted interpersonal situations like Jennifer's).
- The high correlation of "eating disorders" in young women with histories of sexual abuse (Everett, & Gallop, 2001, pp. 44–5).
- The meaning of sexuality and how an adolescent makes informed and healthy life choices about sexual behaviors during the turbulent life cycle phase of adolescence.
- The role of family, couple, and adolescent support groups in alleviating stressors and preventing violence.

Situations related to this example include vulnerability to harassment and violent attack that is exacerbated among adolescents identified as gay, lesbian, bisexual or transgendered (GLBT); the increasing rates of violence by women (especially teens) against each other and/or male partners; and the additional vulnerability to abuse, violence, and self-destructive behaviors among indigenous youth who feel acutely the strains of surviving in two cultures (see Chapter 8).

Power and control manifestations in dating relationships also evoke some deeply embedded values many societies confront which are a source of anxiety for parents wishing the best for their children: the place of corporal punishment in child-rearing patterns; the moral and religious ideals people hold about sexual expression and how these ideals are reconciled with contemporary youth culture and emphasis on individual rights; health issues such as HIV/AIDS and the prevention of unwanted pregnancy; the intersection between self-esteem, gender stereotypes, and "consensual" or "pressured" sex; and the place of sexuality in the total schema of human relationships.

Health professionals are part and parcel of the cultural scene in which these values and conflicts are embedded, and need to acknowledge that traditional claims of "objectivity" and neutrality no longer hold around these issues any more than around violence. Such acknowledgement, of course, does not equate with a "moral lecture" approach to the topic. This example can also serve to help health professionals and their students to examine traditional gender relations within their own ranks as an essential prerequisite to dealing with these issues as they manifest themselves in clinical scenarios. The situation of violence based on bias regarding sexual identity similarly evokes powerful feelings and values that need opportunities for discussion in a non-threatening environment.

Key practice skills needed in this example and related situations among adolescents include:

- The ability of health professionals to teach about the detection and *prevention* of violence as early as possible and in concert with such medical interventions as treatment of communicable diseases.
- The incorporation of psychosocial facets of health into routine medical situations for any family member.
- Teaching young people how to detect and label abusive behavior in dating and other adolescent relationships and the risk of violent attack.
- Networking and inter-agency liaisons with schools and community groups that can assist families with child-rearing and other health-related issues.

Interdisciplinary collaboration includes work with pediatric primary care and dental providers around incorporation of victimization assessment into health assessment protocols and teaching about violence prevention (e.g. when presenting for Chlamydia symptoms or routine dental care). A support group facilitator (any discipline so trained) would explore sexuality, sexual identity, and self-esteem issues, gender relations, violence in dating relationships, and prevention of abuse. Depending on outcomes through primary care channels, mental health providers focusing on family and relationship issues might be engaged. Since undergraduate college students in health and social service programs are so close in age to vulnerable couples in dating relationships, special attention should be directed to students' classroom or clinical site behavior that might suggest their own unresolved issues around this topic (see Chapter 12 for further discussion of this issue).

Case example: neglect and violence in late adolescence – Kendall (the Caribbean) [as told to volunteer counselor Glenda Dubienski]

Kendall, a 21-year-old man from a Caribbean island nation, presents at a community-based health fair with what appears to be a major depressive episode. As Kendall's story unfolds, neglect and violence are the main themes, leaving him with an overwhelming sense of worthlessness.

Kendall's father left his home shortly after the birth of Kendall's younger brother, leaving the boys to be raised solely by their mother. When Kendall was 22 months old, his mother went out on a 4-day drinking binge with her new boyfriend, leaving the boys unattended. Two days after abandoning the boys, a neighbor responded to the children's cries by breaking into the home, taking the children, and placing them in the care of their father. Seven years later, while still in the care of his father, Kendall was raped by his two half-sisters, marking the beginning of 4 years of regular sexual abuse. Unable to share this violation with any family members, marijuana became his consoler.

There was a brief period of hope in Kendall's early pubescent years. Recognizing his enormous talent as a soccer (football) player, a teacher from Kendall's secondary school encouraged him to pursue this extracurricular activity. Realizing the ill effects of marijuana on his ability to play, Kendall gave up the drug and committed fully to the sport. He was so successful playing soccer that there was discussion about the potential of making it a career. This bolstered his self-esteem, granting him the courage to tell his grandparents about the sexual abuse he had endured. Expressing tremendous remorse and empathy towards Kendall and his situation, his grandparents responded by bringing him into their home to live with them. The sexual abuse ended. Shortly thereafter, during a league play-off soccer match, the coach of the opposing team gave specific instructions to one of his team members to take Kendall out of play. The result of this directive was a severe fracture of Kendall's tibia. Improper healing of this injury ended his soccer career, causing him to once again question his sense of self-worth. Choosing not to return to marijuana to dull the pain of worthlessness, alcohol, cigarettes, and risky sexual escapades became his drugs of choice – all of which appear to be acceptable behaviors for men within the island's culture. Whether or not this is the norm for the culture, this legacy of neglect and violence has left Kendall longing for safety, security, respect, and love.

Sociocultural factors contributing to child neglect and abuse

A slave mentality has left its imprint on Kendall's island nation. For example: It is acceptable for men who do physical labor to have "side women" supposedly because their "wife" cannot keep up with them sexually (the strongest men of the plantation were rewarded for their hard work, i.e. given their choice of woman for sexual gratification). Men and women typically are very harsh in dealing with their children; during the slave era, if parents appeared not to care for their children the slave masters would use the children to get back at them, for example, by selling the children to another master.

Children are expected to fend for themselves because their mother works long hours to provide for them, and the father is out of the picture (men were often housed separately from their women and worked long hours in the field). Fatherless homes are therefore even currently more the rule than the exception, while there is little support for single mothers and social services or public assistance are not readily available. Foster care of children is usually left up to extended family members, while the only orphanage on the island has closed down due to poor management and lack of funding. Marijuana is readily available and very inexpensive on this island, while incest and child abuse are rampant. Health statistical estimates are that HIV/AIDS will kill one person in every household on the island.

This scenario of child neglect and abuse on a poor former slave colony has much in common with the risks of poor children in rich nations like the United States and Canada, and their counterparts in ravages suffered by the children of indigenous communities as discussed in Chapter 8.

Hope and growth potential vs. pathologizing wounded and alienated youth

Despite these sad stories of abuse and neglect, there is hope for all children and alienated youth across cultures as this section attests. Health and social service providers collaborating with educators and community workers in programs like these have enormous potential for making a difference in children's lives.

The Circle of Courage

In their classic work, *Reclaiming Youth at Risk*, educators and youth workers Larry Brendtro, Martin Brokenleg, and Steve Van Bockern (Brendtro *et al.*, 1990, pp. 6–7) trace the discouragement and alienation of youth at risk to four ecological hazards:

1 *Destructive relationships*, as experienced by the rejected or unclaimed child, hungry for love but unable to trust, expecting to be hurt again.
2 *Climates of futility*, as encountered by the insecure youngster, crippled by feelings of inadequacy and a fear of failure.
3 *Learned irresponsibility*, as seen in the youth whose sense of powerlessness may be masked by indifference or defiant, rebellious behavior.
4 *Loss of purpose*, as portrayed by a generation of self-centered youth, desperately searching for meaning in a world of confusing values.

In their hope-inspiring book these youth specialists draw on values of a traditional Native society of North America, the Lakota Sioux, as well as spirituality and the ministry, cross-cultural communication, and special education principles in their application of the Medicine Wheel, with its four spokes depicting *belonging, mastery, independence, and generosity*. To many Native peoples, the number four has sacred meaning. They see the person standing in a circle (a symbol of life) surrounded by the four directions – the requisites for a child to feel whole, competent, and cherished as a member of the community. These four spokes of the wheel constitute a powerful "reclaiming" environment for youth facing the aforementioned ecological hazards (Brendtro *et al.*, 1990, pp. 2–3; see also Chapter 8 for application of this principle to work with abusive men):

1 Experiencing *belonging* in a supportive community, rather than being lost in a depersonalized bureaucracy.
2 Meeting one's needs for *mastery*, rather than enduring inflexible systems designed for the convenience of adults.
3 Involving youth in determining their own future [toward *independence*], while recognizing society's need to control harmful behavior.
4 Expecting youth to be care givers [*generous*], not just helpless recipients overly dependent on the care of adults.

Significantly, the ecological hazards placing so many children and youth at risk cross cultural and class boundaries. Some children, as Bobby and Kendall above illustrate, reap the seeds of despair emanating from extreme poverty, substance-abusing parents who themselves are deprived of necessary social supports for responsible parenting, the pain of discrimination, and deprivation based on racial bias and oppression of indigenous peoples over hundreds of years. Some other children whose parents lack nothing by way of material resources and opportunities are over-protected to the point of feeling stifled in their developmental task of achieving independence and generosity, in that little is expected of them except to achieve admission to an elite college. And college admissions officers note that many of the tasks required for college acceptance have in fact been performed by their over-indulgent parents.

While many children of affluent parents nevertheless achieve responsible adult status, statistics on youth suicide and violence toward others often reflect a privileged background (see Chapter 11). For example, the students who carried out the Columbine school shooting that has been imitated across countries were owners of expensive automobiles given by their parents who apparently had little "time" to learn of their children's planned violence; a rich divorced mother living in an expensive neighborhood "rewarded" her out-of-control daughter with a luxury car for her 16th birthday after she spent one year in a Catholic boarding school "without getting in trouble," and continues her financial support with a luxury apartment as the daughter continues her teenage years of deviant behavior and struggles with depression. Thus, while some children are extremely deprived of necessary material and social supports for healthy development, for others nothing significant is expected of them – which can negatively affect a young person's self-esteem in that it suggests a belief in their *inability* to achieve the healthy independence of adulthood.

Brendtro *et al.* (1990, pp. 20–9) refer to such scenarios as "learned irresponsibility," the "tyranny of indulgence," and the "tyranny of obedience" that foster a climate of futility that includes loss of a sense of meaning and purpose in life, and the "misery of unimportance." The Circle of Courage depicting *belonging, mastery, independence,* and *generosity* is compromised further by the rampart practice in mental health circles of pathologizing children's behavior by attaching psychiatric labels that are demeaning and blaming rather than fostering of self-esteem and empathy (Brendtro *et al.*, pp. 13–19; Hoff *et al.*, 2009, Chapter 3). Educators and all health and social service professionals hold key roles in mending the broken circle of injured and alienated youth by focusing *not* on what is *pathological* in children but rather, on what they need to achieve the key features of the Circle of Courage: *belonging, mastery, independence,* and *generosity*.

The ROPE program: Rite Of Passage Experience

This program, developed by psychologist David Blumenkrantz over the course of 30 years doing community-based programs for youth, is currently being expanded to an international arena. It is highly complementary to the Circle of Courage program in its emphasis on young people's potential for growth, rather than their problems or psychopathology. Drawing on van Gennep's (1909) classic work on rites of passage, Blumenkrantz (2008) describes the Initiation of Scholars (IOS) component of the ROPE program as one of the clearest examples for promoting values, ethics and expected behaviors of young people in their climb toward adulthood.

As the vast literature on child neglect, abuse, and youth violence attests, the path toward adulthood is fraught with both danger and opportunity along the way. The ROPE program is based on children's natural predisposition to exploration and learning. However, good students are not born, but must be guided by caring adults to achieve their potential, avoid the pitfalls and dangers that lurk around and tempt them, and develop the intellectual competence, emotional stability, and behavioral attributes necessary for mature and responsible adulthood. A key aspect of the ROPE program is its focus on puberty-age youth not just as individuals, but as members of the whole community. This includes their parents in supportive, non-controlling roles, and teachers who convey to students their respect and hope for the youth committed to their care. Together, these caring adults offer the guidance and support that youth require as they approach various crossroads that can leave them vulnerable to abuse or to joining gangs who afford them a sense of belonging – albeit a very dangerous substitute for what they need.

The IOS component of ROPE is designed to build on a child's understanding of the value that the community places on education and the expectation of a successful academic. This is accomplished by leading children to acknowledge that their "coming of age" requires them to learn certain skills and competently perform certain tasks and behaviors required across a range of areas in their future as adults.

The plight of many youth is visible across cultures. Inner city schools in many US cities see rampant rates of students failing or dropping out altogether, while they and many neighborhood adults fear injury or death from violence-tinged gangs of youth that appeal to them for the connections and support they lack in family and school. Some of these children and teenagers are also highly vulnerable to trafficking (Gozdziak, & MacDonnell, 2007; Chapter 9 in this book). Blumenkrantz suggests that history is not on our side for altering the paradigm of education where schools are not interesting places that encourage attention and enthusiasm (see Chapter 11). He cites Thomas Kuhn's *Structure of Scientific Revolutions* (1970) as a model for the paradigm shift necessary to consider new approaches to education and a promising passage toward adulthood without getting lost to abuse, drugs, or violence – often because of too few healthier options being available to youth from secure and supportive parents, some of whom are unhealed from their own wounds of childhood or domestic violence.

The Circle of Courage and the ROPE program offer hopeful resources and inspiring examples of protecting children, healing those already injured or sexually abused, and nurturing them toward security in supportive communities.

References

Abrahams, N., & Jewkes, R. (2005). Effect of South African men's having witnessed abuse of their mothers during childhood on their levels of violence in adulthood. *American Journal of Public Health*, 95(10), 1811–16.

Blumenkrantz, D. (2008). *The Initiation of Scholars: Bridging the Divide between Playing and Learning.* Hartford, CT: The Center for the Advancement of Youth, Family & Community Services.

Brendtro, L. K., Brokenleg, M., & Van Bockern, S. (1990). *Reclaiming Youth at Risk: Our Hope for the Future.* Bloomington, IN: National Education Service.

De Mause, L. (1975). Our forebears made childhood a nightmare. *Psychology Today*, 8, 85–8.

Eggert, L. L., (1994). *Anger Management for Youth.* Bloomington, IN: National Education Service.

Everett, B., & Gallop, R. (2001). *The Link between Childhood Trauma and Mental Illness: Effective Interventions for Mental Health Professionals.* Thousand Oaks, CA: Sage.

Foshee, V. A., *et al.* (2004). Assessing the long-term effects of the Safe Dates Program and a booster in preventing and reducing adolescent dating violence victimization and perpetration. *American Journal of Public Health*, 94(4), 619–24.

Gozdziak, E. M., & MacDonnell, M. (2007). Closing the gaps: The need to improve identification and services to child victims of trafficking. *Human Organization*, 66(2), 171–84.

Greven, P. (1990). *Spare the Child: The Religious Roots of Punishment and the Psychological Impact of Physical Abuse.* New York: Alfred Knopf.

Havig, K. (2008). The health care experiences of adult survivors of child sexual abuse: A systematic review of evidence on sensitive practice. *Trauma, Violence, Abuse*, 9(1), 19–33.

Hoff, L. A. (1994). *Violence Issues: An Interdisciplinary Curriculum Guide for Health Professionals.* Ottawa: Health Programs and Services Branch.

Hoff, L. A., Hallisey, B. J., & Hoff, M. (2009). *People in Crisis: Clinical and Diversity Perspectives* (6th edn.). New York and London: Routledge.

Kozol, J. (2000). *Ordinary Resurrections: Children in the Years of Hope.* New York: Crown.

Kuhn, T. S. (1970). *The Structure of Scientific Revolutions* (2nd edn.). Chicago: University of Chicago Press.

Miller, D., & Challas, G. (1981). Abused children as adult parents: A twenty-five year longitudinal study. Paper presented at the National Conference for Family Violence Researchers, 21–4 July, Durham, NH: University of New Hampshire.

Molnar, B. E., Buka, S. L., & Kessler, R. C. (2001). Child sexual abuse and subsequent psychopathology: Results from the national comorbidity survey. *American Journal of Public Health*, 91(5), 753–60.

Silverman, J. G., Raj, A., Mucci, L. A., & Hathaway, J. E. (2001). Dating violence against adolescent girls and associated substance use, unhealthy weight control, sexual risk behavior, pregnancy, and suicidality. *American Medical Association*, 286(5), 572–9.

Sonkin, D. (1990). *Wounded Men: Healing Child Abuse.* New York: Harper & Row.

Straus, M. A., Gelles, R. J., & Steinmetz, S. K. (1980). *Behind Closed Doors: Violence in the American Family.* New York: Anchor.

Van Gennep, A. (1960). *Rites of Passage.* Chicago: University of Chicago Press. [French edn. 1909.]

Waring, M. (1990). *If Women Counted: A New Feminist Economics.* San Francisco: Harper San Francisco.

6   Sexual assault of adults

Intimate partner and war victims

- Overview: sexual assault – worldwide prevalence
- Rape as the spoils of war

    - Rape legacy from Rwandan genocide
    - War survivors: Women for Women International

- Rape survivors in Portugal – a qualitative study

    - Participatory study method and collaborators
    - Rape and Portuguese culture
    - Legal definition and types of rape in Portugal
    - The consequences of rape: individual and socioeconomic
    - Myths about rape affecting Portuguese survivors
    - Reporting rape: the police, court, and health systems
    - Study conclusions and implications for service to survivors

- Case example: a lesbian survivor of rape and childhood sexual abuse (Canada)

    - Key issues and concepts
    - Values and diversity issues
    - Related violence and abuse issues

- Clinical practice implications across cultures

    - Interdisciplinary, generalist, specialist, and student roles
    - The SANE program: Sexual Assault Nurse Examiners

- Preventing rape and sexual assault

Rape is a violent crime, not a sexual act. Because of people's attitudes toward the crime of rape, the crisis of rape victims has not received appropriate attention until recently. Feminists and others who have become sensitized to the horrors of this crime are slowly bringing about necessary changes in a legal system that often causes double victimization of the person who has been attacked. The crime of rape is committed against those considered weaker or with less power; women and children are thus the favorite targets, women because they are seen as the "weak gender," children because they are obviously weaker than adults and are dependent on adults for subsistence and protection. Male prisoners are also very vulnerable to rape (Alexander, 1990).

Overview: sexual assault – worldwide prevalence

Among women, the crime of rape crosses ethnic, social, and economic borders, ignoring age, sexual identity, physical appearance, job/occupation, place of living, and so on. The idea that only sexy women are raped is a myth and emphasizes that the woman is to blame – that is, because of her beauty she becomes irresistible.

Although most rape victims are female, male victims of rape are sometimes even more reluctant than women to report the crime and seek help. Until recently, most research and clinical attention has focused on heterosexual female survivors of rape, as they have constituted the majority of victims. But among gay, bisexual, and transgendered men (GLBT), rape is also a serious issue; victims have additional fears of reporting because of homophobia and subsequent bias among some mainstream agency staff.

If a woman is sexually abused or raped by her physician, the chances of successful prosecution are further reduced because (1) the social and political influence of the medical profession is enormous; (2) the average woman thus abused has been seduced into believing the action is part of medical practice; (3) the woman is often afraid to report the incident and cannot imagine that this could happen to anyone but herself; and (4) the woman may have absorbed the message that she invited the rape or did something wrong. This point applies to any professional who violates a position of trust and power (Burgess & Hartman, 1989).

In the US and Canada, rape in marriage is now recognized legally as an offense. However, the cultural notion of woman as the property and appropriate object of man's violence and pleasure still lingers. Fortunately, research findings and public education have changed the attitudes of most American and Canadian physicians, nurses, and police. This is significant when considering the threat to life accompanying many rapes and the great number of acquaintance rapes (mostly female).

In date rape, it is often assumed that if a woman says no she does not mean it and that in some way she invited the attack (Levy, 1991). This issue is complicated when women have drunk too much and are then victimized by a gang of rapists. The woman's intoxication is used as an excuse to exploit her; college women are particularly vulnerable to such attacks. These are reported least often because of the continued tendency to excuse rapists on grounds of their *victims'* behavior. Sometimes even the female friends of raped women make public, victim-blaming statements – for example, "If she hadn't stayed out so late, it probably wouldn't have happened" (students in a college class on sexual assault). One interpretation of such behavior is that it is a potential victim's means of gaining some control and reducing her own vulnerability: "If *I* don't stay out too late or drink too much, I won't get raped." In Warshaw's (1988) study of college students, 50 percent of the men had forced sex on women but did not define it as rape, and only 33 percent said that under no circumstances could they rape a woman. We should not be surprised at these responses in a culture in which women are often considered fair game. Recently, psychiatric and general health personnel have developed rape crisis intervention programs in hospital settings based on principles of equality and a rejection of popular myths about rape.

Perceptions concerning rape situations, rapists and victim/survivors are influenced by a variety of factors related to personal experience, attitudes and prejudice about rape, victims and rapists. These beliefs can even influence mainstream information about this crime. Some investigations reveal that women rarely report the rape to the police. Koss (1993) found that only 8 percent of women who were raped lodged a complaint. Among this 8 percent, 29 percent were raped by strangers, and 3 percent were raped by men they knew.

Cross-culturally, victim-blaming is still alive. Some women victims are advised by clergy that sexual assault is rooted in a women's failure to observe traditional rules that call for their submission to male dominance and limitations on their freedom of movement in society. For example, if women would just "stay at home," and refrain from enticing men, there would be no problem. The fallacy of blaming a woman for her attack because she was "dressed too provocatively" or "out on the street alone" becomes clear in the analogy of a well-dressed man who is robbed of his wallet: no one would say he was robbed because of what he wore. Regarding women who are raped while out at night, we might attend to Golda Meir's response to the curfew proposal for Israeli women at risk of attack: let the men who are raping be curfewed instead.

Another popular myth about rape is that the victim "enjoys rape" and that the average woman entertains fantasies of being raped. This myth was evident at the dawn of the new millennium in the words of a prestigious mental health professional at an international conference when he proclaimed, "There are two kinds of rape – real rape and those who want it." This notion is an echo of Freud's now discredited theory regarding incest, and is reinforced by popular movies, by hardcore and soft-core pornography, and by advertising images in which women are depicted as appropriate objects of male violence. These myths about rape stem from the persistent interpretation of rape as a sexual event (Thornhill, & Palmer, 2000) rather than an act of violence. Societal attitudes, then, play a major part in the outcome of a rape crisis experience. When rape victims are blamed rather than assisted through this crisis, it is not surprising that they blame themselves and fail to express feelings appropriate to the event, such as anger. Such attitudes also impede the process of long-term recovery (Braswell, 1989).

There is still much to be done to change public attitudes, reform institutional responses to sexual-assault victims, and dismantle the widespread belief that women and girls who are raped are "asking for it." Many victims fail to report sexual assault because of fear, their perception that police are ineffective, and the threat of further victimization by authorities (Buzawa, & Buzawa, 1996). Also, some victims do not seek monetary compensation now available through US court-based victim assistance programs because payment was either inadequate or denied altogether (Hoff *et al.*, 2009, Chapter 11).

Rape as the spoils of war

From a human rights perspective, rape as the spoils of war is a gender-based crime, as documented by the United Nations (UN) and by Brownmiller (1975) in her historical account. The crime of rape has continued over centuries and is still a very visible phenomenon during wars worldwide (e.g. Amowitz, 2002), but only now is it being addressed in the International Criminal Court in The Hague.

During the 1990s Bosnian war, at least 20,000 women on all sides were raped. Figures from the conflicts in Rwanda and Darfur are still to be recorded. Over the ages, the alleged rationale was that rape satisfied the sexual needs of men on the battlefield – it reflected the culturally embedded license of men to use and abuse women with few or no legal consequences for their behavior. A woman who testified in the International Criminal Court said that she and scores of other women were raped in classrooms and apartments, while her detained children became ill from unsanitary conditions. This woman's testimony about damage to her health included sexually transmitted disease, insomnia, severe anxiety, and reproductive dysfunction (Socolovsky, 2000). Women survivors of the Rwandan genocide who are raising children begotten when they were raped as teenagers speak of their struggle to reconcile their traumatic memories with a mother's natural love of a child conceived by the rape.

A refugee woman from Cameroon and then Liberia, Canada, and the United States describes a triple trauma – watching her son die at the hands of soldiers, as her hands and feet were tied, she was then beaten to persuade her to talk about her husband, and finally placed in a corner and repeatedly raped (Hartigan, 1999). This woman suffered the additional trauma of social stigma for having been raped, because such women in her culture – as in others – are viewed as unmarriageable. As is true of many survivors of violence, this woman found meaning and healing in telling her story – another small step toward ending the worldwide plague of war in general and violence against women in particular.

Rape legacy from Rwandan genocide

Among the huge number of survivors of sexual assault during the 1994 genocide in Rwanda, the most isolated are women who bore children – estimated at 20,000 – as a result of being raped, in some cases after being forced to witness the murder of their families. In many cases these women not only contracted HIV, but were also rejected by remaining family members. While struggling with ambivalent feelings toward their children conceived through rape, they nevertheless want them to have education and access to other human rights. Here are vignettes from a few of the women who have shared their plight and the bleak post-genocide aftermath they have suffered with their children:

> They took me to a place where they raped me, one after the other – I can't tell you how many .... When I realized I was pregnant, my first thought was that I should abort, but I didn't know where to go for such services. After giving birth, I thought of killing it because I was bitter and didn't know who the father was. It was painful, but eventually I decided not to kill it. I don't know how I am going to live with a boy who has no family. I am physically handicapped because of the beatings .... It is now that I say it is good that I didn't kill that boy, because he fetches water for me. I fail in my duty as a mother ... but it is because of my condition of poverty, not because he is the son of rapists. I am not interested in a family [or love] .... I sometimes look at my situation and compare myself with people who have their families around them, and I regret that I didn't die in genocide.
>
> Survivor, age 28; son, age 12 (Torgovnik, 2008, p. 17)

> I'll never forget that day [my son was born] .... My wish was that he would die immediately after birth .... Why he didn't die, I don't know. My child was almost a skeleton because I didn't have milk in my breasts. But that man, that rapist was with me. He kept raping me again and again. My problem is that boy, my son. When I think about his life, he is like a tree without branches. I am alone. I don't have any surviving relative apart from my old mother. He is my life ... the only life I have. I love him. If I didn't have him, I don't know what I would be. A genocide happened in Rwanda, and we went through torture like no other person has gone through. Tell the world that the legacy of genocide can never be removed. The international community has a debt because they didn't come to the rescue.
>
> Survivor, age 30; son, age 11 (Torgovnik, 2008, p. 18)

> After the war, my father constantly reminded me this kid is bad, her family is bad, her family killed my relatives, that there was no reason for me whatsoever to love that girl. When I see her, she reminds me of the rape. ... The first rape, the second rape, all the rapes that followed, I relate them to her. I can't say I love her, but I can't say I hate her either. Now she lives with my aunt, where I went through the horror. Every step of that hill, every grass, every tree,

every stone, every house reminds me of 1994. I don't want to go there.

Survivor, age 26; daughter, age 13 (Torgovnik, 2008, p. 19)

Similar stories could be told about sex abuse by military personnel in the Democratic Republic of Congo, Sierra Leone and the Sudan, where perpetrators and civilian authorities largely go unaccountable for the crimes (Amowitz, 2002). Thousands of women have had surgeries performed on mutilations carried out by militia groups in the Congo. In the Sudan the longest war in recent times continues with mass murders and rapes of women and entire Darfur villages burned to the ground. The light in this dark tunnel is that the International Criminal Court in The Hague and the UN Security Council emergency relief branch are making charges of crimes against humanity for prosecution in the International Criminal Court. The hope is that every person of goodwill and the international community at large will find ways to not only stop these crimes, but also look to the larger picture of preventing violence and its horrendous cost to innocent victims through social and political action supporting the rights of all to safety and security.

War survivors: Women for Women International

Among all the works attempting to deal with the age-old and worldwide scar of treating women as the "spoils of war," one of the most searing and promising examples of what can be done about these crimes is the work of Zainab Salbi (2006), documented in her *The Other Side of War: Women's Stories of Survival and Hope*. In 1993, Salbi, originally from Iraq and a war survivor herself, founded Women for Women International, a non-governmental activist group whose mission is empowering marginalized women survivors of war and assisting them in rebuilding their lives through job skills, human rights awareness, and education (see the online resources in Part IV). Her 2006 book, a collaboration with award-winning photographers and with a preface by prolific author, Alice Walker, features narratives and stunning photos from the war-torn nations of Afghanistan, Bosnia, Rwanda, Congo, Sudan, and Columbia.

The women describe not just the atrocities of rape, mutilation, infection with HIV, death, sexual enslavement, incredible losses and cruelty, but also and equally incredibly, how the women endured and rose above their plight with courage and creativity. Together, Salbi and Walker show that gender inequality was deeply ingrained in these societies and that once war undoes a society's social fabric, the major burden of cleaning up the mess and restoring the torn fabric falls on women. And as if that were not enough, Salbi points out this example of insult added to injury: when a man is injured in war, he is declared a hero. But when a woman is raped or mutilated, because of rape being seen as a male entitlement and the spoils of war, she is more likely hidden and set aside as an object of shame. Awareness of such atrocities and injustice might leave many feeling helpless or hopeless, but this book is a powerful example of what one person, Zainab Salbi, can do: she and the courageous women who feature, have made visible around the world (through the National Geographic Society) the possibility of moving beyond victim identity despite what they have suffered.

Rape survivors in Portugal – a qualitative study[1]

The purpose of this qualitative study was to ascertain from the women's stories what had happened during and after the crime of rape up to the time they sought advice or assistance from two organizations that collaborated in the study: The Portuguese Association of Support to Victims (APAV) and the Women's Association against Violence (AMCV). A convenience sample of 10 women victim/survivors of rape agreed to collaborate in this research through in-depth interviews conducted over a period of two months. The study also included interviews with judges, lawyers, police agents, and health professionals of the crisis centers offering aid to rape victims (Maria, 2004).

Participatory study method and collaborators

The feminist participatory model used for this exploratory study coincides with the research principles recently adopted in Portugal. Early studies of sexual and other violence against women had contributed to victim-blaming and attributions of the women's purported psychopathology (Mawby, & Walklate, 1994). Practitioners working with victim/survivors therefore need to examine study methods and possible bias of researchers for their implications on service outcomes. In contrast to some researchers' claims to "objectivity," feminist researchers make no such claims, but rather make explicit the fact that factors such as gender and race might influence research outcomes (Hoff, 1990; Renzetti, 1997; Reinharz, 1992). See the online resources in Part IV for feminist research models.

The women who collaborated in this study revealed a variety of sociodemographic features: ethnic, social and economic, professional, and educational. Their ages ranged between 22 and 49; three were single; five were married or living with a mate; two were in process of divorce. The number of children ranged as follows: one woman had three; one had two; four had only one child; and four had no children. Seven of the women were Portuguese; one was Portuguese but born in Angola; one was Cape Verdean; and one was German/Portuguese. Occupations included teacher (2); clerical and sales (3); hairdresser (1); factory and housekeeper (3); unemployed (1). Income per month ranged from 67 to 450 euros. Education level ranged from 6th grade and primary school (3); secondary school (4); university level (3).

Rape and Portuguese culture

These demographic factors even in this small sample reveal the incidence of rape across social roles and other boundaries (Costa, & Alves, 1999) Beyond the family, schools in Portugal have helped to reproduce gender roles and social differences taught by the family; for example, students' books show the mother in the kitchen and the father at work (Liñares, 1989). Public advertising (on radio, television or press) is another factor leading to stereotypes, because the images highlight the idea of the sexually appealing woman as an object of admiration under a man's control, a housewife and mother, as well as the idea of a successful man, the one who is the leader, gentleman and so on (Silva, 1995)

For example, during the Portuguese expansion, in the Iberian Peninsula the letter M (woman in Portuguese is *mulher*) was used with three words that are correlated: Maria (a very common name for a woman); *mulher* (woman) and *mãe* (mother). The name Maria is linked to Christianity's roots, while the other nouns mean the two unquestionable roles for women in most societies: wife and mother (Magalhães, 1994, p. 705). Until the beginning of the twentieth century, Portuguese women were still totally submitted to their husband's control (Silva, 1995).

It was only in the 1960s that the relationship between women and men in Portugal changed as part of the "third wave of feminism" that emerged in Western societies (Silva, 1995). In a feminist framework, rape was defined *not* as a sexual act, but as a crime, an act of humiliation and abuse of power. Accordingly, while rape may appear at first sight as an individual problem, it is actually a structural problem of unequal power distribution between the sexes (Sousa, Mateus, & Lopes,

1993). The result of the domination and exploitation of women by men makes clear that rape is not defined as a sexual act but as a crime.

Today in Portugal, despite some reform of the institutional responses to rape, and integration of other perspectives, the patriarchal ideal and limited actions to hold perpetrators accountable persist. The victim-blaming phenomenon is more pronounced when women are raped by people they know. On the one hand, people in general believe that, in some way, the women must have known the men's intentions. On the other hand, in trying to answer the question "Why?" the tendency is to blame somebody, and unfortunately the person blamed in the majority of the cases is the survivor (Allison, & Wrightsman, 1993).

Legal definition and types of rape in Portugal

Rape is, in fact, both a personal crisis and a political phenomenon. Being so, some believe that one result of the victim-blaming phenomenon is that women become more alert and develop, as it were, a "sixth sense" in detecting risk of rape. Rape is a kind of social control, in the sense that it restricts both the rights and behaviors of women. Each country defines what is meant by rape, what is acceptable to count as rape, and which punishment would be fair. However, beyond these formal written definitions, there are the informal ones, and these are the established practices based on the myths about rape that over centuries have not yet disappeared from people's minds (Waldron, 1990).

According to the Portuguese Punishment Law[2], rape crime is in the chapter entitled "Crimes against the freedom of sexual self determination." Article 164° – "Violation of the law" – states:

1   Anyone who, by means of violence, serious threats or having rendered a person unconscious for this purpose, or having made it impossible for that person to resist, forces another person to be subjected to or perform with him or her or with a third party, copulation or anal or oral coitus shall be liable to 3 to 10 years' imprisonment.
2   Anyone who, abusing a relationship of authority in the context of a hierachical relationship or one of financial dependancy or, in the workplace forces another person, by means of orders or threats not included in the previous paragraph, to be subjected to or perform, with him or her or with a third party, copulation or anal or oral coitus shall be liable to a term of imprisonment of up to 3 years.

A major reason why rape is misunderstood is the assumption that rape is committed by strangers. In fact, many rapes occur in other contexts, especially marriage and dating relationships, in which the victim knows the rapist. Although this is a real crime, in Portugal it is not seen as a crime in a majority of such situations. Even if predicated in law, it rarely exists in the plurality of people's consciousness.

In this study, 50 percent of the women were raped by their husbands. Conceição Brito Lopes, (a well-known Portuguese lawyer who specializes in the area of women's rights) notes that married women who were frequently raped by their husbands and forced to endure sexual acts against their will were in most cases unaware that they were victims of the crime of rape or sexual abuse. They were uncomfortable, revolted, but, as the aggressors were their husbands, they didn't refer to the situations as rapes. Their husbands used to beat them in order to have sexual relations but they presented the general idea that as the husband "he had the right." They defined rape or a sexual crime as an act done with *another* person, not their husband.

It is thus not surprising that some of the women in this study are still living with their rapists, as found in the Layman *et al.* (1996) study in which significant numbers of raped women keep on living with their rapist, and forced sex continues. The truth is that a woman who is raped by her husband might not show the same type of resistance as one raped by a stranger. But even though women survivors of rape by men they know tend to avoid regarding the experience as rape, that doesn't mean the experience is less traumatic. This affirms the need to inform women that rape is never their responsibility, and that rape committed by a person they know is still a crime. Banning rape within marriage requires changing the social structure that has created and perpetuated inequality between men and women, between husbands and wives, as the crime of rape is an abuse of male power, either in society or at home.

The consequences of rape: individual and socioeconomic

Researchers Norris and Feldman-Summers (1981) found these factors influencing the psychological impact of rape: (1) lodging a complaint; (2) assuming responsibility for the rape; (3) lack of understanding from others; and (4) the harshness of rape. The authors concluded that except for the first factor, all the other ones are significantly correlated with the damaging psychological impact of rape. That is, the harshness of rape correlates strongly with the frequency of psychosomatic symptoms, blaming oneself, lack of understanding from others, the victim's level of seclusion (e.g. no longer able "to go alone to pubs, concerts and cinema").

The effects of rape on survivors' physical, emotional, personal and spiritual health – as well as ramifications on work and family life – are almost always deep (Koss *et al.* 1996). Here are some of the psychological and physical health consequences expressed by the Portuguese participants in this study:

> I lost a great amount of weight ... became very thin, because I didn't want to do anything .... Apart from losing weight I also lost blood due to nerves.

> I have a urinary incontinence [problem].

> I lost the will [to] be myself ... [and] the pleasure of dressing up, of washing up .... I have nightmares ... I was afraid of falling asleep ... that smell of his. There was a time that I thought I was going mad, I couldn't sleep, I couldn't eat, I didn't want to go out, all I wanted was to stay alone without hearing noise. I couldn't help thinking "Why did that happen to me?"

> Having the abortion was a big trauma, because I wanted to have the baby because it was mine, but I didn't want to have it because of him .... It was very hard.

> I have depressions, I am always crying.

Similar to the economic consequences of domestic violence cited by Fátima Monteiro (2000), the expenses of court, hospitals and other services relative to rape are added to these psychological and physical health problems rape survivors suffer. Raped women also reported a decrease of sexual activity immediately after the rape, and over time, had thoughts of suicide and homicide and acknowledged using psychiatric drugs or alcohol to calm down:

> I felt very down and tried suicide twice with pills [the first time on the day it happened] .... I felt very bad and fainted three or four times in the bathroom. I took [the pills] to forget everything .... I felt dirty [wells up with emotion] .... I washed myself with bleach. ... If I had

a gun at that time, God forgive me, I would already have killed him. He has no right to do such an evil thing to a person.

I take Xanax [an anti-anxiety drug] but I don't get the expected result.

One woman thought of killing her husband by poisoning his food. Another said about suicide:

I even got into the car and thought about crashing against a wall and afterwards I thought "Who is going to up bring my children?" so I changed my mind. I opened the window and I thought "I'll jump." I was really sure about that, but my daughter came to me with a glass of water and that idea was gone.

Rape trauma also affected the women's relationships with other people in general – their mates, relatives, and children. For example:

When I am with my friends I feel more insecure, I became distant .... I know they are not to blame, but nowadays one can't rely on anyone. In the beginning, it affected [her relationship with her son]. I was not patient ... but at those times I felt rage, I fed him and told him to watch television so that he was quiet, not to bother me.

I am more aggressive, I feel dirty. ... I am more mistrustful.

It strongly affected my relationship with my relatives ... now I don't even trust my own family. The word family has now another meaning ... it is not the paradise I used to think it was.

Here is how rape affected the women's professional life and daily life in general:

I made a lot of mistakes [in job performance evaluation] and knew that my job depended on that evaluation .... I spoiled everything.

I left the company .... I couldn't work. It really affected me .... I stayed at home during two or three months because I wasn't able to work.

Now I don't go out. I don't go to discos, I don't go out at night.

I was a person who used to laugh a lot, I was very cheerful. People who know me have asked me what was wrong with me because I didn't laugh anymore. I don't go to a café to drink a coffee, I can't go out alone [she cries, and a deep silence follows].

These testimonials show that women survivors of rape experience huge problems resulting from rape over a long period of time. They have quite high levels of stress, they don't enjoy their daily routines, they show that they feel tired and stressed and have more problems in socializing.

Myths about rape affecting Portuguese survivors

The study also revealed that the survivors had internalized common myths about rape, with the end result of feeling responsible for what had happened. Responses included:

To avoid being raped you have to stop going to unsafe places.

But there are also women who like to excite men, who are not made of iron.

He told me that he was my husband and he had the right to do it.

Maybe he is insane ... I guess he has an emotional instability.

Women's acceptance of myths about rape leaves them feeling guilty or responsible which can be harmful to their recovery:

... and then I think about what I should avoid ... because my window wasn't shut ...

I felt guilty. I thought that I shouldn't have been in the street at that time. I am a woman, why was I out here alone at that time?

I supposed I was the worse woman in the world ... there is no solution, maybe he did it because of me. It was hard for me to believe that I didn't influence him.

I was so silly ... I shouldn't have entered the car of a person I didn't know.

Several women said they felt "angry ... dirty ... guilty."

Many victims/survivors of rape present high levels of responsibility for the rape (Meyer & Taylor, 1986). And when the victim's family or others also believe in these myths, the victim's feelings of responsibility for the rape increase, as attested in these remarks:

My mother says that I have to be patient with him.

They tried to find excuses for what has happened, for example, my aunt says that the cause of it might have been the fact that I wore a black mini-skirt.

They say "You shouldn't have entered that car ever in your life."

There are still people who think we are married and we must do that [submit to unwanted sex] ... or suppose we had what we deserved because we might have excited the man.

Crisis and other service providers must be careful not to reinforce these unhealthy self-blame responses. For example, they might say: "No matter what you did or did not do, you are not responsible for the criminal behavior of another person .... Perhaps it was unwise to accept a ride home, but that is not an excuse for someone to attack you." A public statement like this can help in changing the widespread culture of "victim blaming."

Reporting rape: the police, court, and health systems

Ascribing responsibility for rape to the victim rather than the perpetrator is a major factor contributing to victims' reluctance to report the crime. She is thus victimized again in a system that should help her, not add to her trauma (Sousa *et al.* 1993).

Alexander and Waldron (1990) cite the following reasons for the rare reporting of rape: fear of revenge; fear of the police, medical and court procedures; in the case of teenagers, they are afraid of their parents; they are afraid people don't believe in them; they feel shameful and guilty; they fear their husband's, mate's, boyfriend's reactions; they are afraid reporting can bring more problems; they don't trust police because of past unsuccessful experiences, or believe they don't have enough evidence, especially if raped by men who are close to them.

Some may question the report of a rape crime for a variety of reasons, such as, lack of proof, but this doesn't mean that the crime has not happened. In fact, stories of rape victims who were treated badly by authorities influence other victims to lose motivation to lodge a complaint. Da Cruz (1990) notes that a woman may give up on a complaint if she becomes emotionally upset from harsh and repeated questioning, or if police assume she is lying about the rape, or is looking for money compensation.

The police are still the most important key in the criminal justice system concerning rape. The importance of police agents lies in their powerful role in the process of lodging complaints about rape crimes; typically, police agents are the first people the victim meets when turning for aid to the justice system. The interaction between police and victim will influence the victim's feelings in either a positive or negative way. For some victims the first point of contact post-rape is the health system, primarily hospital emergency departments. If either police agents or medical professionals have doubts about survivors' stories and they convey their beliefs about victim "responsibility" (implicitly or explicitly) to the victim, rape survivors will feel guilty and most likely their recovery process will be negatively affected (Norris, & Feldman-Summers, 1981).

Persons representing the court system presented similar thoughts about rape, while the beliefs of the crisis center professionals were significantly different and lacked the "victim-blaming" tone of the other entities. The whole process of survivors' recovery is touched by the responses of every professional met by raped women. Thus, if responses from society to survivors are cued to their needs, not on myths and stereotypes, further harm is avoided and the recovery process will be easier. It is necessary, therefore, to demystify the crime of rape in order to ban from society the reason why so many women suffer in silence (due to feelings of guilt, fear, and lack of aid, etc.) when they lack assurances that the rapists who are to blame will be identified and punished.

Norris and Feldman-Summers (1981), among others, have written about the insensitive welcome from the elements of court systems that may underline rape victims' feelings of shame, guilt, and impotence. Since the mid-1970s many countries have been changing their laws on rape, but it is important to know how these changes have affected legal practice. Since police agents are the "entry" point to the court system, they need to understand and respond to these changes.

Portuguese agents in the "Police Superior School" who were interviewed for this study affirmed that their training regarding sex crimes focused only on the legal side, with no attention addressed to the psychological needs of victims. However, the police have made efforts to find a policewoman to be in charge of the raped woman's case, noting that while the policewomen aren't specialists, they are able to get closer to the victim; they assume that the raped woman would feel more comfortable or at ease with another woman.

Victim/survivors in this study cited five reasons for why they did not lodge a complaint: (1) fear; (2) mistrust of police; (3) feeling that they were going to be blamed or that nobody would believe them; (4) shame; (5) desire to avoid more suffering and fear of disappointing people they love. Only four of the ten women had lodged a formal complaint to police, but all ended up discussing it with the researchers because of the suffering they had endured.

Among these women, seven had gone to the police, and three did so immediately after the rape, but one of them declared only that she had been robbed, and two others went to the police some months after the rape. Four of them went to the police because not only were they rape victim/survivors but also domestic violence victims. We also learned that the Portuguese police have some projects that aim to call the attention of professionals to meeting service standards for raped women, for example the project INOVAR, which belongs to the Internal Management Ministry, with two counterparts: the police and GNR (Republican National Guard). Its goal is to increase rape victims' trust of the police forces through an adequate response as soon as a raped woman lodges a complaint.

   While there are many references in Portugal regarding the correct treatment of rape survivors by doctors, an exploratory interview of a doctor revealed the following:

> There isn't any specialized service to attend raped victims. Neither do I know a hospital that has such a service.

The same doctor states that she still feels that it is hard to deal with rape situations:

> I don't feel it is hard when I am treating physical wounds, but when it has to do with advice or information about behavior in the future, I find it very difficult.

Concerning graduation and medical studies this doctor says:

> I have learned how to deal with hard situations in general, for example to tell bad news or to listen to more complex situations, but not specifically rape situations. I think it would be very important if our studies included specific training on the rape issue, because we are not ready, we don't feel comfortable when we have to face a situation like this, and sometimes we don't do the right procedures .... The community has omissions at different levels. There is so much that is missing. But in the case of rape, immediate support is the most important thing. ... If women have that support and need it often or later on they come for help, if [she doesn't get that help], there will be more problems later.

Here are comments on the women's appeals to Portuguese health services:

> I think that here in Portugal they are not trained. I know that in foreign countries they do "body delict" [a term from Brazilian Portuguese meaning collection of physical evidence] ... here, in Portugal, they don't do it.

> In the 'Legal Medicine Institute' I was attended by a foreign doctor who told me that, in Portugal, there was little information on rape, at the hospital they should have taken photos, do every exam, but they haven't done so. At that moment I should have been supported by the police, right there at the hospital, but they didn't follow any of these procedures; I left hospital and went to the police to lodge a complaint. In the Legal Medicine Institute I did the exams that should have been done at the hospital, but it was too late, [it was] after the doctor did other exams and asked me all those questions about how did it happen.

> At the hospital when I said that my husband had mistreated me, they didn't even tell me to go to the police; neither did they write anything on paper ... they just told me to go home.

> Later on I was scared so I did some analysis [tests to ascertain whether she had a sexually transmitted infection] and everything was fine. I did them on my own.

Study conclusions and implications for service to survivors

The data from this study have led to the following conclusions:

- The raped women who appealed to APAV and to AMCV all experienced deep negative consequences of rape, and they are so serious that the process of recovering for them has been very slow and difficult.
- Rapes in the context of marital relationships are a reality, and some of the survivors were also victim/survivors of domestic violence.
- Prevailing myths about rape, believed in our communities, make many women feel guilty or responsible for their rapes, and impede the process of recovering. When women realize they are not to blame, it is important for their recovery.
- Support institutions play a very important role in the recovery process of these women. However, they had difficulties obtaining help (for example, from "Crisis Support Services," having an advocate present when the victim goes to hospital or other services, support for others significantly related to the victim, information/advertising campaigns). It is important to underline that the raped women who were interviewed in this study made a great effort to recover from the situation. Most of these women identify themselves with the word "survivor."
- The data reveal that rapes are not reported to the police or other services because of fear, mistrust on justice, fear of being blamed or that others won't believe them. Some raped women still think that if they keep their silence they won't suffer so much and won't make significant others suffer either.
- Justice and laws in Portugal don't readily fit to rape situations. While there has been reform of the laws in Portugal regarding rape, the women we interviewed did not seem to benefit from these reforms. There is no strong victim advocacy program in the courts.
- Another significant finding is that the women in this study and Portuguese society in general are not well informed about rape as a crime situation, which weakens responses to the needs of sexual assault victims.
- The services to which these Portuguese women appealed for help presented difficulties in dealing with rape situations efficiently. The lack of unity and inter-agency collaboration, and of specialized techniques to provide necessary support, is quite obvious. What is more, there appeared to be no communication between the services to which raped women appeal (police, health services, the "Legal Medicine Institute," support institutions).

Case example: a lesbian survivor of rape and childhood sexual abuse (Canada)

Susan is a 35-year-old woman with two children, currently working as an advocate in a rape crisis center. As a child, from age 6–11 she was sexually abused by an uncle who assisted her mother with child care, especially while her father was away for week-long stints on his job as a traveling salesperson. Not only was Susan unable to tell her mother about the abuse, but she also was emotionally abused by her mother and physically abused by her father. On one of those occasions her teeth were knocked loose, but Susan's mother told the dentist a story to cover up what really happened. To escape her miserable home life she left at age 16, worked as a waitress while finishing high school, and married her boyfriend at age 18. Susan is now aware that she married for financial security and to escape her abusive background. Her marriage was never on solid ground; in response to her disinterest in sex, her husband "forced it on me" several times, but "I didn't think of it then as rape." After coming out as a lesbian, Susan finished college, divorced her husband, and now shares joint custody of the children with him, saying their relationship is "friendly." She describes him as a "good man, a good father" and understanding of her lesbian identity. Susan lives alone, has a supportive group of friends, and is now drug-free and successfully employed.

Before reaching this point, however, for several years Susan was frequently depressed, dependent on tranquilizers and anti-depressant drugs, and in emotional turmoil, primarily, she says, as a survivor of childhood sexual abuse, the effects of which she dealt with through repression and dissociation:

> I really repressed my memories and had all the symptoms that now I recognize ... I had nightmares, I had eating disorders, I had this, I had that, and then I had a breakdown .... I find it very interesting that looking back [in the psychiatric hospital] I was never asked any questions about what my marriage was like, and what my childhood was like or if I had been abused. No one ever asked those questions. I'd sit there through those OT sessions trying to paint or whatever was going on for the day, and most of the time I just couldn't concentrate. But no one would help me make a connection with my past. They looked at the symptoms and treated me for depression, including shock treatments and drug therapy. And so I walked out of there after six weeks, discharged myself against this doctor's orders and I stopped all my medications.

A few months later Susan met some counselors who had dealt with sexual abuse:

> They were able to start putting the puzzle pieces of my life together .... In therapy my nightmares got worse, I got to be a real mess, and during the next five years I attempted suicide several times.

One of those attempts (an overdose of anti-depressants) was nearly fatal, requiring intensive care and a heart monitor:

> I don't think I really wanted to die, I wanted the pain to end ... I just wanted out. I didn't see any other avenue .... I really do think that therapy is necessary but I also think that it's a re-abuse experience because you have to re-live it all. I think it's the only way but it's horrible.

After her divorce, and the successful therapy dealing with the abuse history, Susan went on to finish a degree in human services administration, developed a very solid relationship with her lesbian partner, a professional in government service, and was doing very well in her class work. In college, one of Susan's classmates became interested in her romantically:

> He kept coming on to me and I finally said to him, "You know, I'm not interested and I'm a lesbian but you know we could be friends." So he said that was fine, no problem, and we'd just be friends. And months went on in class and I got quite comfortable with him and we were working on a project together at my apartment and it ended up in sexual assault. And afterwards, even though I know better, I went through all the typical things that rape survivors do .... All these emotions and all the myths that were given all our life really do come into play. So I thought, why did I let him in my house, maybe I was asking for it, maybe I gave him mixed messages, I knew he was interested in me. But then I thought I had given him a very straight message about who I was. And I always thought previous

to this experience that if a man ever tried to assault me I would just about kill him. But what in fact happened was when the assault started, I went right back into my child. My childhood abuse just overwhelmed me and I became like a little child and I just whimpered and cried and begged him not to, instead of being able to be an assertive strong woman. So for a while I blamed myself. He left and phoned me the next day, wanting to see me again. And I said: "You raped me." And he said, "Oh, I don't see it that way." And I said, "Well, that's what you did. That was sexual assault. That was rape. And I could report you and have you charged." And he said, "Well, I don't think you should do that, because I know your partner's name, and that wouldn't look good for her if it hit the press, would it?" So I hung up the phone and never went back to my classes.

I couldn't tell my professors the real reason when I started to fail my classes. I did see my gynecologist and arranged for an AIDS test, but couldn't tell her what happened ... I just said I was careless about sex. But I did persuade her to give me a prescription for a tranquilizer. It took me a couple weeks even to tell my partner. She was very supportive, but there was just too much to deal with, so we ended up splitting up because I was so traumatized I started running away from her, from my apartment. Finally I started talking to my friends and was really pressured to take this man to court. But you know the fact that I'm a lesbian and my partner was a public official all had big repercussions on my choice. I felt limited in my choices, but then I felt guilty because this man is still at large. And I felt angry at myself for not handling it well. You know I think actually my lesbianism probably was a factor in this man because you know there is this real myth and lie out there that lesbians just need a good lay and they'll never be lesbian again. That's all they need.

Key issues and concepts

Susan's response to rape as an adult intersects with her history of sexual abuse by relatives during childhood. It reveals several concepts to be addressed in mitigating the interrelated outcomes of rape, while underscoring the fact that regardless of earlier neglect, it is never too late to support survivors in moving on from the damaging effects of sexual assault. Here are the key concepts that must be understood in offering services to survivors like Susan:

- Non-violent parenting roles, including protection from abuse by others (relatives/neighbors/strangers).
- The traumatic aftermath of childhood sexual abuse: nightmares, eating disorders, depression.
- Psychosexual development and sexual identity.
- The *non*-equivalence of childhood sexual abuse with sexual orientation: many women have been sexually abused as children – most are heterosexual; some are lesbian.
- Labeling theory, "spoiled identity," and homophobia.
- The interrelationship between victim-blaming, self-blame, and self-destructive behaviors.
- The relationship between repressed emotion and various physical ailments.
- The rape trauma syndrome.
- Additional trauma from risk of AIDS and other communicable diseases following sexual assault.
- Resilience following trauma, mastery, and the healing role of social support and non-judgmental therapy.
- Social isolation and its mental health impact.

- Risks of unhealthy coping through drug dependence in the absence of more appropriate supports.
- The particular stress on a lesbian relationship (exacerbating violence potential) when heterosexist bias limits community sources of support.
- The limits of legal restitution in a cultural milieu of victim-blaming, homophobia, and prejudice against those perceived as "different."

Values and diversity issues

Susan's situation dramatically illustrates the process of multiple victimizations that can be traced to several deeply embedded values in mainstream culture:

- Abusive parenting and simultaneous failure to protect a child from abuse outside the family; the unavailability of parents as a support following such abuse.
- Collusion by health and mental health professionals in the cultural tradition of defining abuse as a private matter, as illustrated by non-attention to Susan's history of abuse and failure of a gynecologist to elicit current sexual assault incident.
- The "medicalization" of sociocultural problems: i.e. professionals' apparent unawareness of how traditional treatment such as psychotropic medication and electroshock therapy can compound a victimized woman's problem.
- Heterosexism and stereotypes regarding gay, lesbian, bisexual or transgendered (GLBT) persons which increase their vulnerability to sexual assault.
- Assumptions about the legal/court system and its equal availability to a disadvantaged population such as GLBT persons.

Related violence and abuse issues

Susan's experience suggests attention to the related issues involving violence and abuse: sexual abuse by psychotherapists; abuse of women with developmental, physical or mental disabilities; lesbian and gay teens whose suicide risk originates from identity crisis combined with verbal abuse and threats of violence motivated by homophobia; child custody disputes and visitation access following the divorce of a battered woman concerned with the safety and protection of children; the exacerbation of custody disputes experienced by lesbian women; the particular challenges of confronting accountability for rape in marriage, which until recently was not included in legal definitions of rape. In regard to lesbian and gay male battering, it is important to note factors such as bias and the social isolation faced by many of these couples which constitute additional stressors in their relationship and may leave them more vulnerable to intimate partner violence than is the case with heterosexual couples (Renzetti, 1992).

Clinical practice implications across cultures

Susan's situation and the plight of the Portuguese women who were raped illustrate multifaceted practice skills as well as primary, secondary, and tertiary prevention:

1 Victimization assessment and crisis intervention skills immediately following Susan's childhood sexual abuse and the rape as an adult might have prevented some of the most damaging traumatic aftermath she experienced. The failure of such primary and secondary preventive efforts demands victimization assessment skill and tertiary prevention efforts

– albeit delayed – which correctly identify the primary problem as victimization. Had such assessment been conducted, some of the psychological trauma Susan and the Portuguese women suffered (depression, self-destructive behaviors, suicidal ideation, eating disorders, etc.) might have been avoided or been less severe.

2   Linkage of rape survivors to peer support and community-based (and perhaps college-based) sexual assault services.

3   In Susan's case: consultation with lesbian groups and legal resources regarding the particular needs of lesbian women around disclosure, custody issues, etc.

Interdisciplinary, generalist, specialist, and students roles

At intersecting professional roles and levels, several points of early identification were possible for Susan: a school *nurse* might have identified her childhood abuse; Susan's *dentist* would have recognized the mother's cover-up "story" for what it was and would have communicated explicitly about the nature of dental damage and patterns of abuse while providing resource information and an appropriate referral along with active encouragement to follow through. Later, in psychiatric settings, any member of the *mental health team* might have identified the primary problem as prior victimization; while in the community, the *pharmacist* would have observed Susan's mood (and physical evidence such as black eyes) when filling her prescription of psychoactive drugs, particularly repeated refills. Routine victimization assessment by *all* professionals might have averted the series of self-destructive episodes. *Specialists* in this case include a psychotherapist (any mental health discipline) or group sensitive to gender, sexual abuse, and diversity issues, including peer support groups for survivors of sexual abuse.

Students of any discipline in a psychosocial or psychiatric course would participate in identifying the primary problem of victimization regardless of where someone like Susan is seen in the total health system. The student who observes that such identification has not been made by the interdisciplinary medical or psychiatric team should confer with the clinical instructor or preceptor regarding strategies to make this primary issue visible in the treatment planning process in psychiatric settings. Routine victimization assessment could have assisted health and mental health staff to focus on Susan's primary problem much earlier. As Warshaw (1988) documented, college women are prime targets of sexual assault – their vulnerability exacerbated by transition from home-based parental oversight and binge drinking on college campuses. Therefore, seminar discussions on transition state stress, alcohol abuse, homophobia, and rape might help students avoid crises around sexual assault (see the teaching/learning strategies in the online resources in Part IV).

The SANE program: Sexual Assault Nurse Examiners

Some of the problems rape survivors cite about services after reporting and seeking evaluation and treatment in the health sector could be alleviated by institution of the Sexual Assault Nurse Examiners (SANE) program. This program is now available to rape survivors in numerous sites across the United States and Canada. It was developed in response to the piecemeal and unsatisfactory responses cited by survivors seeking emergency medical treatment following rape.

SANE's primary function is to provide objective forensic evaluation of sexual assault victims after the patient's immediate medical condition is stabilized. Typically, a SANE is an advanced practice emergency or psychiatric nurse who receives additional training and certification in the basics of forensic medicine which, in practice, is integrated with the holistic perspective of nursing in its focus on the *whole* person – in this case the emotional and social sequelae of rape – in addition to obtaining objective forensic evidence that a victim may use if choosing to pursue legal action against the alleged perpetrator.

Because SANE programs follow cases from the initial evidence collection in emergency medical settings on to possible prosecution, they often gather data such as finding sperm and the likelihood of a sexual assault victim's injuries being traceable to the assault. SANEs can also help build a more accurate picture of victimization, such as drug-facilitated assaults, the victim's healthcare needs, and reasons why victims do or do not report the assault to law enforcement. SANE program operations may differ depending on factors such as a community's Sexual Assault Response Team (SART) protocol. Basically, however, SANE programs use a pool of SANEs who are on call 24 hours a day, and who are available to respond in emergency medical centers within 30 to 60 minutes.

Successful SANE programs do not operate in isolation, but work closely with SARTs, the police, prosecutors, judges, forensic laboratory staff, victim/witness specialists, and child protective services. Their aim is to meet the multiple needs of victims and to hold offenders accountable for their crimes. Community-based sexual assault victim advocate programs (often called rape crisis centers) have laid the groundwork for improving the quality of emergency medical and forensic evaluation of sexual assault victims. These groups are now promoting the SANE model to promote a comprehensive and victim-centered community response to sexual assault. The operation of one such program, the Avalon Centre in Halifax, Nova Scotia, is illustrated with an example in Chapter 13, which also includes medical and psychological follow-up services after emergency medical treatment (for further information, visit http://www.sane.com).

Preventing rape and sexual assault

Long-range strategies to prevent rape include dismantling the myths and centuries-old norms that promote the double victimization of women. Such a campaign should cover education, health, social service, and criminal justice systems worldwide, as well as the public at large – in short, the Social-Ecological Model of Prevention.

At the individual level, a woman whose life is threatened can do little or nothing to prevent sexual assault. In some cases, however, women can lessen their chances of attack by training themselves to be street-smart – alert at all times to their surroundings when outside. Potential victims should remember that even though crime may appear to be random, the would-be criminal has a plan. That plan includes attacking a person who appears to present the greatest chance of success at the crime with the least amount of trouble. Women and children on the street who are alert and make this evident therefore have, to some extent, equalized the criminal-victim relationship. Signals of an escape plan may be as simple as looking around frequently or carrying a pencil flashlight – cues that alert a would-be attacker that you are not an easy target. The attacker does not know what else you may possess – perhaps mace or karate expertise – and generally will not take unnecessary chances with people who appear prepared to resist. Alertness at home is also important. For example, a 56-year-old woman was raped in her home by a man posing as a delivery man, in spite of a highly organized neighborhood patrol on her street.

Self-defense training is also useful as an immediate protection strategy. It provides physical resistance ability as well as the psychological protection of greater self-confidence and less vulnerability. However, women should not rely on self-defense excessively because (1) it may lead to a false sense of security and neglect of planning and alertness, and (2) some attackers are so fast and overpower the victim so completely that there may be no opportunity to put self-defense strategies to work.

Preventing the sexual assault of children includes not leaving children unattended, instructing them about not accepting favors – including car rides – from strangers, and keeping communication open, so that a child will feel free to confide in parents about a threat or attack. Just as important is public education about the dangers from those closest to us, a grim reality that is difficult for many to acknowledge (Hoff *et al.*, 2009, Chapter 11).

References

Alexander, K., & Waldron, C. (1985). The realities of rape. In E. Crespo, & C. Waldron (eds.), *Reclaiming Our Lives*, pp. 15–31. Massachusetts: Department of Public Health.

Alexander, K. O. (1990). Profile of the rapist. In E. Crespo, & C. Waldron (eds.), *Reclaiming Our Lives*, pp. 33–44. Massachusetts: Department of Public Health.

Allison, J. A., & Wrightsman, L. S. (1993). The rapist. In J. A. Allison, & L. S. Wrightsman (eds.), *Rape: The Misunderstood Crime*, pp. 20–45. Newbury Park: SAGE Publications.

Amowitz, L. L. (2002). Prevalence of war-related sexual violence and other human rights abuses among internally displaced persons in Sierra Leone. *Journal of the America Medical Association*, 2887(4), 513–21.

Bart, P. B. & O'Brien, P. H. (1985). *Stopping Rape: Successful Survival Strategies*. UK: Pergamon Press, Inc.

Braswell, L. (1989). *Quest for Respect: A Healing Guide for Survivors of Rape*. London: Pathfinder Press.

Brownmiller, S. (1975). *Against Our Will*. New York: Simon & Shuster.

Burgess, A. W., & Hartman (eds.) (1989). *Sexual Exploitation of Patients by Health Professionals*. New York: Praeger.

Buzawa, E. S., & Buzawa, C. G. (1996). *Domestic Violence: The Criminal Justice Response*. Thousand Oaks, CA: Sage.

Costa, J. M., & Alves, L. B. (1999). Perspectivas teóricas e Investigação no domínio da delinquência sexual em Portugal. *Revista Portuguesa de Ciência Criminal*, 9(2), 281–312.

Da Cruz, A. M. (1990). Violação. Comunicação apresentada no colóquio Internacional sobre Criminalidade e Cultura, Centro de estudos Judiciários, Lisboa.

Ellis, E. M., Atkeson, B. M., & Calhoun, K. S. (1981). An assessment of long-term reaction to rape. *Journal of Abnormal Psychology*, 90(3), 263–6.

Hartigan, P. (1999). "It's like I had this war in me." *Boston Globe*, 16 June, pp. E1, E4.

Hoff, L. A. (1994). *Violence Issues: An Interdisciplinary Curriculum Guide for Health Professionals*. Ottawa: Health Programs and Services Branch.

Hoff, L. A., Hallisey, B. J., & Hoff, M. (2009). *People in Crisis: Clinical and Diversity Perspectives* (6th edn.). New York and London: Routledge.

Koss, M., *et al.* (1996). Traumatic memory characteristics: A cross-validated mediational model of response to rape among employed women. *Journal of Abnormal Psychology*, 105(3), 421–32.

Layman, M. J., Gidycz, C. A., & Lynn, S. J. (1996). Unacknowledged versus acknowledged rape victims: Situational factors and posttraumatic stress. *Journal of Abnormal Psychology*, 105(1), 124–31.

Levy, B. (1991). *Dating Violence: Young Women in Danger*. Seattle: Seal Press.

Liñares, E. (1989). Disparidades ao nível do casal. In Direcção Geral da Família (ed.), *Tempo para o Trabalho, Tempo para a Família* (pp. 175–90). Lisboa: Ministério do Emprego e Segurança Social.

Magalhães, M. I. M. (1994). Maria: um corpo de duas faces. In M. Reynolds de Souza, *et al.* (eds.), *O Rosto Feminino da Expansão Portuguesa*, pp. 705–13. Lisboa: Comissão para a Igualdade e para os Direitos das Mulheres.

Maia, G. (1999). *Código Penal Português Anotado (13ªedição)*, Lisboa: Almedina.

Maria, S. (2004). *Mulheres Sobreviventes de Violação*. Lisboa: Livros Horizontes.

Meyer; C. B., & Taylor, S. E. (1986). Adjustment to rape. *Journal of Personality and Social Psychology*, 50(6), 1226–34.

Monteiro, F. J. (2000) *Mulheres Agredidas Pelos Maridos: De Vítimas a Sobreviventes*. Lisboa: Comissão para a Igualdade e para os Direitos das Mulheres.

Norris, J., & Feldman-Summers, S. (1981). Factors related to the psychological impacts of rape on the victim. *Journal of Abnormal Psychology*, 90(6), 562–7.

Reinharz, S. (1992). *Feminist Methods in Social Research*. New York & Oxford: Oxford University Press.

Renzetti, C. M. (1992). *Violent Betrayal: Partner Abuse in Lesbian Relationships*. Thousand Oaks, CA: Sage.

Renzetti, C. M. (1997). Confessions of a reformed positivist: Feminist participatory research as good social science. In M. D. Schwartz (ed.), *Researching Sexual Violence, Against Women: Methodological and Personal Perspectives*, pp. 131–43. London: Sage Publications.

Russell, D. E. H. (1986). *Secret Trauma: Incest in the Lives of Girls and Women*. New York: Basic Books.

Silva, L. F. (1995). *Entre Marido e Mulher Alguém Meta a Colher*. Celorico de Basto: À Bolina.

Socolovsky, J. (2000, April 26). Rape victim testifies against Serb soldiers. *Boston Globe*, p. A17.

Sousa, E., Mateus, F., & Lopes, P. (1993). Decisões em matéria penal: o caso da violação e o peso de variáveis extralegais. *Sociologia, Problemas e Prática*, 14, 141–57.

Thornhill, R., & Palmer, C. (2000). *A Natural History of Rape*. Cambridge, MA: MIT Press.

Torgovnik, J. (2008). Intended consequences: Rwanda's living legacy of violence. *Amnesty International*, Spring, 2008, 16–20.

Waldron, C. (1990). The sociological and political implications of rape. In E. Crespo, & C. Waldron (eds.), *Reclaiming Our Lives*, pp. 8–13. Massachusetts: Department of Public Health.

Warshaw, D. (1988). *I Never Called it Rape*. New York: HarperCollins.

Notes

1 Excerpted from Maria (2004), translated from the Portuguese by Maria João Ramos and edited by Lee Ann Hoff.

2 The Portuguese Punishment Law of 1995, with changes in 1998 by the Act 65/98 of September 2. In this revision, the number 1 of the Article 164° changes to be constituted by the numbers 1 and 2 of the previous version and the number 2 is added. This means that, before this revision, the law did not foresee that men in authority could be guilty of rape. The Punishment Law is noted by Gonçalves Maia (1999).

7   Abuse and neglect of older adults

Bonnie Joyce Hallisey

- Elder abuse: overview
    - Elder abuse, family situations, and violence
    - Caregiver issues
    - Self-neglect and coercive intervention
- War as violence and abuse
- Risk factors for elder abuse
- Protective factors against elder abuse
    - Society's services
- Case example: a Haitian immigrant
    - Key issues and concepts
    - Attitudes and values
    - Clinical practice skills

The population of the world is aging, with the exception of areas devastated by war, disease and natural disasters. More people are living longer than ever before in history. Declining birth rates, immigration to lands of greater economic prosperity and civil order, surges of population growth such as the "baby boom" after World War II, medical advances, and public health successes have all contributed to this rising "Age Wave" (Dychtwald, 1990) which has the force to change the landscape of societies worldwide. There is both opportunity and danger in this demographic revolution. Increased longevity in richer countries with government benefits may allow a standard of living later in life that is unsurpassed in modern times. However, even in these countries, not all share equally in the bounty. In poorer countries with no income for elders after they stop working, families may become more impoverished, leading to an even greater disparity between rich and poor nations in the future (Ayres, 2005).

Where there is greater need than the social environment can meet, older persons are at risk. When we consider protective and vulnerability factors later in the chapter, we will understand that it is the discrepancy between resources available (finances, housing, family) and needs/ environmental demands which makes an elder vulnerable. Risk can result in abuse and neglect when vulnerability is high, stress or environmental demands are great, and protective forces are not enough to buffer the danger.

Elder abuse: overview

Elder abuse can be physical, sexual, verbal, emotional, financial, or involve the neglect of basic necessities. Between 1 and 2 million Americans age 65 or older have been injured, exploited, or otherwise mistreated by someone on whom they depended for care or protection (National Research Council, 2003). The American Psychological Association (APA, 2005) estimated that 2.1 million incidents of neglect or abuse of elders occur yearly. Almost half of elder maltreatment is neglect, with psychological abuse comprising about 35 percent, financial exploitation 30 percent and physical abuse 25 percent (National Center on Elder Abuse, 1998). Current estimates put the overall reporting of financial exploitation at only 1 in 25 cases, suggesting that there may be at least 5 million financial abuse victims each year (Wasik, 2000). It is estimated that for every one case of elder abuse, neglect, exploitation, or self-neglect reported to authorities, about five more go unreported (NCEA, 1998).

Ninety percent of abuse allegations involve family members and take place at home (US AoA, 2005). Two thirds of victims are women. Most states have laws requiring mandatory reporting of elder (60 years and older) abuse, neglect and financial exploitation. Mandated reporters are typically health and public safety providers. The US Department of Justice reports only 1 in 14 cases are reported, usually by medical professionals, to authorities.

Elder abuse happens in our midst, not just on the fringes of life nor in nursing homes, but in the homes of neighborhoods across all segments of society. Often it is subtle and the distinction between a bad, stressful time and abuse may not be easy to determine. Like other forms of violence, abuse of elders is never acceptable no matter how difficult the situation might be. Sometimes older adults harm themselves by not eating, failing to seek medical care or take medications, etc. resulting in the most frequent type of elder abuse reported which is self-neglect or abuse. Awareness and intervention by health and social service professionals may prevent or limit real harm.

Elder abuse, family situations, and violence

Many situations contribute to violence in the family. There can be a history of intergenerational violence that takes different forms throughout the life cycle. Marital violence can persist into old age, with some spouses even being grateful if abuse is "only" verbal/ emotional at this point, although physical abuse can persist as well. If a mistreated partner or child becomes an overly stressed caregiver for the spouse or parent who victimized them for much of their life, there can even be a changing of roles from victim to abuser/neglecter, "turning the tables," so to speak. However, most who were treated unfairly do not dole out the same punishment and try their best at care-giving. Changes to lifestyle, such as the financial, social and physical accommodations necessary with care-giving, complicate relationships within the whole family. Resulting stress can take a toll on even the most resourceful families.

Generally when people think about intimate partner abuse, they picture a young woman with children, not a white-haired woman in her 70s (Brewer, 2007). Research in the 1980s and 1990s debunked the myth that most elder abuse was caused by caregiver stress. Instead the research showed that the elder abuse was occurring within a spousal relationship with a long history of domestic violence (*Wisconsin Lawyer*, 2000). As the general population grows older, estimates of domestic violence among the elderly are expected to increase dramatically – putting additional pressure on service providers (Hurme, 2002).

There are several patterns of domestic violence among the elderly: "Spouse abuse grown old" in which victims have been abused most of their adult life; "late onset" beginning in later years of an ongoing, mature relationship; or in the new relationship of older persons (Nerenberg, 1996). The National Center of Elder Abuse (NCEA, 2006) reports that the majority of elder abuse victims are female, and abusers are most frequently adult children, family members and spouses. Abuse occurs in all social classes, in heterosexual and same-sex relationships, across all races, ethnicities and religions. Researchers Mouton *et al.* (2004) studied the prevalence and incidence of abuse among postmenopausal women. In addition to the usual stigma associated with domestic violence situations, older victims are further disadvantaged by services being geared toward younger victims; fear of institutionalization (being sent to a nursing home); possible changes in memory; and the shame of perceived failure of parenting when it is one's own child who is abusing.

Harris (1996) found that physical and sexual abuse decreases with age, whereas psychological abuse remains. Psychological abuse is also most likely to co-occur with other, more severe forms of abuse, as in this case from my own clinical experience:

> My husband has always been abusive. I am thankful now that it is "just words" and not being hit. He no longer has the strength since his stroke. He doesn't have the mobility either. Our son brings him three cans of beer a day, that's all. He can't get drunk on that, yet it satisfies him. What can I do? We've been married for 55 years. I am Catholic and also believe in fate. This is my fate. I have 8 children who are all good to me. They are my reward and the reason I say my marriage was worth it.

This Vietnamese woman has obviously suffered many decades of abuse and has chosen to stay with her husband for family, faith and cultural beliefs, as well as perhaps lack of alternatives in her community.

Questions for consideration:

· While her son is offering his own version of tertiary prevention, are there services that a health provider could offer even at this late juncture that may support her resilience?
· Is the expression "just words" as innocuous as she makes it sound? Can providers confirm the dignity/right of every human being to non-violence while empathetically honoring her survival ability?
· If she were still being beaten, what would be the responsibility of healthcare providers?

Abuse takes a negative toll on the quality of life for older persons, affecting both physical and mental health. Older women who are abused are more likely to experience:

· depression
· anxiety
· digestive problems
· chronic pain

These are red flags to health providers to screen for possible mistreatment.

A few minutes alone with the elder is crucial for such screening because abuse is generally perpetrated by people routinely involved in the victim's life (Fisher & Regan, 2006). Older people who suffer abuse or mistreatment experience a much higher incidence of depression (Pillemer, & Finkelhor, 1988; Pillemer, & Prescott, 1989). Experiencing such abuse is a risk factor for nursing home placement (Lachs *et al.*, 2002).

Cross training is advised among domestic violence workers for them to become more aware of resources available on aging and also for elder protective service workers for them to become more aware of domestic violence resources. For further information on domestic violence, see Chapters 4 and 8.

Caregiver issues

Most caregivers are females, the majority of whom are wives and daughters. The gender imbalance is improving slightly as males are stepping into the role and the void created by divorce and both men and women working outside the home. Males tend to provide instrumental, less personal care and report less guilt and more pride in their role while women tend to be involved in all aspects of care-giving, including hands-on personal care, and feel more guilt and stress.

Most caregivers find themselves in the role without having appropriate training, information or resources. The needs of the dependent elder can overwhelm their own needs, resulting in an imbalance that threatens to throw the family system out of balance. The following example illustrates the near despair and danger of a murder-suicide when a caregiver lacks professional resources and support (Hoff, 1994, pp. 42–3):

> Catherine is 64, a former teacher, and now the home caregiver for John, her 69-year-old husband. John has been cognitively impaired since his early 60s, and has been a wheelchair user for the last 10 years due to knee and other injuries from a car accident. In addition, John has various cardiovascular ailments and sometimes becomes very irritable and physically resistant to care, though he recognizes Catherine and seems to take comfort in her continued presence. Catherine is very active as an advocate on behalf of the needs of caregivers who increasingly are left to pick up the pieces when public services are terminated.
>
> Catherine says regarding termination of professional nursing services: "I don't think I can go it alone." Asked if she's ever been abusive to her husband, Catherine says: "No, no ... you have to be careful of yourself even if you know better ... One of the real feelings you live with is guilt. When I lose my temper it's over the silliest thing. Well, it really isn't silly ... It's an awful lot of work ... I would never hit him, you can be sure of that. But, my brother phoned me at Christmas and it had just been a terrible time and he asked 'What are you going to do?' And I said, 'I'm looking for two plastic bags, two pieces of rope and somebody to pull them both.' And he said, 'Well, I better come in.' And I said, 'No, don't come near me' ... Things like that are very stressful ... Christmas and those things are really bad ... usually, though, I just take an extra tranquillizer."

The older person being cared for may become abusive to the caregiver, especially if dementia results in aggressive behavior. Without skills for managing difficult behaviors or resources to replenish the system, caregiver stress can lead to neglect and abuse. In addition to caregiver stress being a risk factor for abuse, dependency contributes greatly to this risk. Sometimes the caregiver is impaired by physical or mental illness or addiction, or is financially dependent upon the elder. Such conditions are likely to worsen under the burden of caretaking (APA, 2005). Consider the following case from my own clinical experience:

> Her son never heard her calls for help to get out of the shower. He had passed out on the couch drinking, with the TV blaring. When she tried to shut off the faucet herself, she mistakenly turned off the cold water, leaving only hot water which scalded her. While attempting to escape the steaming onslaught, she slipped and fell into the scorching water. She remembers seeing murky patches in the water and thinking how dirty she must have

been. Her skin had sloughed off from the burning. Like a beached whale, the stroke-disabled mother desperately tried to fling herself to safety. She made it over the side of the tub, falling on the bathroom floor, screaming. A neighbor called 911. After months of hospitalization and rehabilitation, she was admitted to a nursing home. Her only child was not a fit caretaker so she could no longer live in her own home. Her son would be evicted and proceeds of the house sale would be put towards the expenses of her long-term care.

Questions for consideration:

- Is there anything that a health provider could have done which might have foreseen or prevented this outcome?
- Would adding in-home services, such as a personal care assistant, have enhanced the safety of the patient?
- What if the client refused such services out of fear of angering her son and being sent to a nursing home?
- Is our focus as health providers strictly on the patient or does it also include the patient's home environment/family?
- If the alcoholic son smoked in the house and his mother was on oxygen, would this change the right to self-determination/safety equation?

Self-neglect and coercive intervention

One of the most difficult problems facing modern society is the balance between respecting the autonomy and independence of older persons in the community, offering supportive services with the least restriction to their living situation yet intervening before it becomes too dangerous. When independence becomes the enemy is a particularly salient concern among those working with older people. The following are the ethical principles of the National Center on Elder Abuse (NCEA):

- Adults have the right to be safe.
- Adults retain all their civil and constitutional rights unless some of these rights have been restricted by court action.
- Adults have the right to make decisions that do not conform with societal norms as long as these decisions do not harm others.
- Adults are presumed to have decision-making capacity unless a court adjudicates otherwise.
- Adults have the right to accept or refuse services.

Self-neglect/abuse typically includes failure to take necessary medications or seek medical care for life-threatening conditions; poor nutrition; misuse of alcohol or drugs; fire hazards such as leaving the stove on; being easy prey for financial exploitation; having inadequate protection from extremes of temperature whether lack of warmth in winter or excessive heat in summer; wandering in unsafe ways such as walking into busy roadways without regard for traffic; driving which endangers self or others; getting lost/stranded repeatedly, etc. Such matters must be evaluated qualitatively and quantitatively. As a bottom line, independence is curtailed when responsibility for self and to others threatens life.

Suicide is the ultimate self-abuse by most societies' standards. The segment of the population in the USA that has the highest suicide rate is older white males living alone. Most of these individuals have seen a doctor within the last 30 days. This underscores the vital opportunity for intervention by healthcare professionals. Older people may experience emotional distress as physical symptoms, so being pro-active and empathetic in inquiring about the concerns and total well-being of patients may yield a more accurate assessment.

War as violence and abuse

War is State-sponsored violence that affects people in profound and varied ways relevant to their role/experience. Whether one was a soldier in combat duty, a provider of medical care to the wounded, a civilian whose country was at war or a family member of a war casualty, the experience of war dramatically alters people, as in the following cases from my own clinical experience:

> "They wouldn't open the box. I couldn't even see my own son, my first born," laments Joseph an 86-year-old immigrant from Jamaica. Forty years after the death of his son in the US-Vietnam War, he is like a stuck record playing the same refrain over and over again. His unresolved grief in not being able to see his son's remains, not knowing if it was really him in the box they were burying. Feeling in his gut that there was some subterfuge leaves Joseph in a story without an ending, in desperate search of resolution, retelling his saga to anyone and everyone who lends a kind ear.

Questions for consideration:

- Joseph clearly has not been able to move beyond this tragedy of war. How might this affect his health?
- Does this place him at greater risk for depression/suicide?
- How would this be assessed?
- Could Joseph benefit from mental health counseling, a grief support group or services from a veterans' agency?

In a senior center, the metal-legged chairs are dragged across the linoleum tiles to ready for an event. The noise enters her ears like a flock of screeching seagulls vying for the same food. The sound reverberates in her head until it consumes and transports her back in time and place:

> In my village the bombs came screeching down, blew up the house next door to me. I grabbed my baby and ran, didn't have time to find my parents and grandmother and never saw them alive again.

This is when her headache comes, exploding in the center of her temple. It immobilizes her. She cannot talk, be near other people or tolerate light until the pain leaves her, usually hours later, when she is spent and diminished:

> They wanted us young, pretty and single to work with the soldiers. I was good at my job, supported my whole family not only by working as a chef but by selling handmade items the soldiers could send back home and purchasing from the PX what my people needed. When I got pregnant it was a big shame for my family. When the Americans left Vietnam, Amerasians were the scum of the earth. My son wasn't allowed to go to school. He was beaten up by other kids. He's a good boy, doesn't eat meat, won't kill living things, is attentive to his mother.

Questions for consideration:

- What is a country's responsibility to the victims of war?
- Do providers have any responsibility to advocate for needed services for veterans and refugees?

Children who are born in war as offspring of the military's liaisons with local population, whether forced as spoils of war, an economic necessity by mothers trying to support their families, or a result of love relationships, suffer as half-breeds with terrible consequences for themselves and their families (Nguyen, 2001). Many Amerasians conceived during the Vietnam War were ostracized in their villages, suffered severe discrimination and grew up without education and sometimes even without parental support (Hanes,1992; see also Chapter 5).

Those who survive war but are physically and psychologically injured are also casualties of war, as are their families. An estimated 10,000 recent veterans of Iraq and Afghanistan are returning from war with injuries that would have been fatal in other wars (Wounded Warrior Project, 2008; Military Family Network, 2008; Coalition to Salute America's Heroes, 2008). "This is a war of disability, not a war of deaths," says Army physician Ronald Glasser, MD, author of *Wounded: Vietnam to Iraq* (2006). "Its legacy is the orthopedics and neurology wards, not the cemetery." "As more troops than ever are surviving the fearsome injuries of war, parents are increasingly being thrust into the role of long-term caregivers" (Yeoman, 2008). Most of the wounded are young and single, returning to their parents who quit jobs, shelve retirement plans, and step into the daunting role of primary caretaker for an adult child with long-term, debilitating injuries.

Questions for consideration:

- What happens when these aging parents need care themselves and their adult child is disabled?
- Are the risk factors for violence higher for survivors of war?
- What protective factors can be built in to reduce the long-term disabling effects of such trauma?

Risk factors for elder abuse

Age is a complex phenomenon comprising chronological years, biological health, physical characteristics, social role, psychological attitude, etc. Those 75 and older are most likely to be dealing with chronic illness, decreased physical and mental capability, deaths of spouse, partner, friends, be less mobile and need help with daily activities. This is not to say that a 55-year-old would not be challenged by these same conditions or that an 85-year-old wouldn't be working independently – just that it is more likely in advanced age to encounter these stressors. It is also important to note that it is the oldest old who are the fastest growing segment of the population in industrialized countries.

Isolation is a key risk factor, not only geographic separateness from others but social separateness as well. Anonymity within a high rise apartment building in the middle of a city can be as deadly as rural inaccessibility. Elders who live alone without the support of family or close friends are the most vulnerable.

Disability/dependence of elder: Being dependent upon others is trying even under the best of circumstances. To need others for very survival generates profound feelings in both the person needing care and those who are providing care, with resulting psychological and social consequences (Berman-Rossi, 2001). The dependence can be from loss of sight or limb, acute or chronic illness such as cancer, diabetes, AIDS, developmental disability. Mental illnesses, addictions, and dementias can exist apart from and in addition to other conditions. Whenever capacities and resources are limited, stress is inevitable.

Disability/dependence of adult children/family members: When an adult child/family member is disabled and/or dependent, this adds exponential stress on the resources of the family system. The dependent adult child may be frightened and upset that their needs are no longer being met by the older parent. An older person not only must deal with his/her own aging concerns but may feel tremendous anxiety about being able to provide for their dependent kin, as in this case from my clinical experience:

> I thought about sitting in my car in the garage with the motor running. If I checked out, he would have to go with me. I've cared for him my whole life. No one cares for him like I do, that's a parent's job. I couldn't leave him alone in this world, to be institutionalized at the mercy of strangers.

So said the mother of a Down syndrome middle-aged son, himself showing symptoms of early dementia. Only when the mother became disabled and had to directly face her own mortality was she able to break the symbiosis and allow her son to go to a group home. Visits home had to be stopped because either son or mother would end up in an emergency room by the end of the weekend as the excruciating psychic pain of separation was reactivated. Unalleviated stress in such dire situations can lead to abuse or even a tragic murder/suicide response.

Questions for consideration:

- Is it predictable that both the aging parent and the Down syndrome adult child would need increasing assistance?
- What services could be added to increase the coping ability and reduce the hazardous nature of this family situation?
- How would you assess both the suicide and homicide risk inherent in this mother's conversation?

Abuse in childhood can cause individuals to grow up to be wounded adults who partner and parent with their capacity for attachment deeply scarred, as in this case from my clinical experience:

> They took something from me that I can never get back. They amputated my trust, cut the core right out of me. I can't even hug my grandchildren without having to have a conversation with myself in order to get out of my own way and let my precious little grandbabies snuggle up to me. My family doesn't get the full me; I don't get the full me. I am an emotional amputee.

This 90-year-old still hides her face in revealing what "stained her soul" in childhood, carrying an unearned shame through eight decades of life. She marvels at the illogic of it but cannot help herself feeling this way, even well into old age. Consider this description of the psychic conflict caused by such unspeakable acts from Joy Kogawa's novel *Obasan*:

> If I speak I will split open and spill out. To be whole and safe I must hide in the foliage. ... But already the lie grows like a horn, an unfurled fiddlehead fist, through the soft fontanelle of my four-year-old mind.
>
> (Kogawa, 1981, p. 63)

Post-traumatic stress disorder (PTSD): Older age can inflame the symptoms of PTSD. The shift from doing to thinking, from long-range planning to reminiscing, from preoccupation with the busyness of everyday life to unstructured leisure creates the space where earlier trauma comes flooding back. The coping strategy of activity may no longer be effective in the relative stillness of aging. Erik Erikson postulated that integration is a major task of senescence (Krystal 1981, 1988). When there is incredible quantity and quality of loss, people may have used excessive repression, denial, psychic splitting and externalization just to go on. However, the life review thought to be common in older years makes it even harder to manage the guilt, rage and shame of trauma.

The losses normative in older years revive earlier traumas. Children grow up, may leave home and live farther away. Spouses and friends die. Older persons may feel abandoned all over again. In hospitals, rehabilitation facilities or nursing homes, people are uprooted and confined. They may be told what to do for their own good and feel humiliated at being helpless. The dehumanizing experience of institutionalization may recapitulate previous trauma. For victims of trauma, time may not heal, rather it may intensify their response to subsequent ordeals. As the narrator of Elie Wiesel's novel *The Accident* puts it:

> You must look at them carefully. Their appearance is deceptive. They look like the others. They eat, they laugh, they love .... But it isn't true. Anyone who has seen what they have seen cannot be like the others ... The thing that they have seen will come to the surface again sooner or later.
>
> (Wiesel, 1970, pp. 79–80)

As survivors age, those who have been the most successful in life may paradoxically be in greatest danger. Working hard may have been a very effective coping strategy. Without the protective buffer of constructive activity, they may be at the mercy of traumatic memories. Survivor guilt may be too difficult to bear. Work can be a protective shield against memories. It offers routine, structure and purpose as well as relationships. Consider what it may mean to survivors of concentration or "re-education" camps when the inability to work meant death. For some older persons, it may not be advisable to stop working if they are so able. At the very least, having a constructive role, a way to contribute and be involved, may be a lifeline (Danieli, 1995, pp. 9–22).

Poverty, gender, minority, and immigrant status can exacerbate other risk factors for abuse or neglect of older people. Consider the following poem by Barbara Bolz, entitled "Social Security":

> She knows a cashier who
> blushes and lets her use
> food stamps to buy tulip
> bulbs and rose bushes.
> We smile each morning as I
> pass her – her hand always
> married to some stick
> or hoe, or rake.
> One morning I shout
> "I'm not skinny like
> you so I've gotta run
> two miles each day."
> She begs me closer, whispers

to my flesh, "All you need
honey, is to be on welfare
and love roses."

(Bolz, 1987, p. 127)

Even this can be a rosy (no pun intended) picture of being poor in the USA. The stereotypic image of the poor elderly buying cat food in supermarkets for their own meals may have wider applicability today as costs for essentials such as heat and food rise along with co-pays for medication. Even lower- and middle-income older persons are at risk of impoverishment due to prohibitive costs of long-term care (Freeman, 1997).

Social Security-like programs in industrialized countries have lifted many elders out of poverty, yet the likelihood of being poor increases with age (Porter *et al.* 1999). Older persons, especially women over 75 years of age who are living alone, whether single, divorced or widowed, are more likely to be poor, near poverty or in a lower income range than other adults (Wu, 2003). The poverty threshold in the USA for those over 65 years of age (US$9,944/year) is lower than that for those under 65 years of age (US$10,787/year) (Institute for Research on Government, 2009) due to the index established in 1964 by the Social Security Administration based on the premise that older people have lower nutritional requirements. The poverty rate for females is greater than for males due to lifelong disparities in wages and years absent from employment due to child bearing/rearing, homemaking and caretaking. It is greater still for minorities. Blacks have a 24.4 percent poverty rate, Hispanics 22.5 percent and Whites just 8.2 percent (Bishaw and Iceland, 2003).

African American and Native American women are at greater risk for extreme impoverishment. Recent immigrants, who have not worked in this country long enough to accrue benefits, may live under particular hardship. If there is a language barrier with mainstream culture, they are often trapped by the inability to communicate and access needed services. Those who do not fit the mainstream categories of heterosexuality, or polarized male-female gender identity, are frequently targets of societies' prejudices. There are serious consequences of increased health problems and decreased longevity for those not favorably sanctioned by society. Over a lifetime, there can be an accumulation of disadvantage that results in a "pileup of hardship" and chronic stress (Berman-Rossi, 2001, pp. 715–38).

If one adds together multiple disparities of age, gender, marital status, minority and immigrant conditions, sexual preference and gender identity, the vulnerability increases exponentially. Given the fact that women, people of color, immigrants and the oldest old are the fastest growing segment of the US and other societies, we are facing an increasingly vulnerable elderly population. Protections against potential violence such as by installment of security systems or moving to a safer neighborhood are less affordable for the poor and many immigrant groups.

Protective factors against elder abuse

Despite risk factors, there can also be an accumulation of *advantage* that better positions a person to weather the storms of aging. In the body there is such a thing as "organ reserve," referring to the extra capacity available to meet greater challenges. The "reserves" that are often born of privilege from a certain class, gender, race, nationality, etc. may allow a person greater power to manage the demands of life. Such advantage may also bestow optimism and perceived control to direct one's life. This is amply born out in the "psychological reserves" and strength gained through successfully weathering various crisis episodes over a lifetime (Hoff *et al.*, 2009). One who has ample reserves and a relatively predictable, ordered world can afford to take risks (financial or otherwise) whereas one who is at chronic disadvantage and under others' control may need to conserve (Hobfoll, & Wells, 1998).

Society can provide buffering forces to its members. The "poor houses" of yesteryear were society's way of providing for those needy and dependent. The fact that these were often not available to minorities may have, of necessity, maximized the self-reliance and kinship patterns of Blacks in the United States (Martin, & Martin, 1985). While Whites outlive Blacks until the age of 75, there is a "Black-White crossover" that occurs around 75–85 years of age wherein the minority elders' health risks actually decline (George, 1996). Hardship can build resilience and privilege may provide little incentive for fortitude, although one would not trade categories to garner this possible byproduct.

Society's services

In the United States, formal services to elders typically follow the medical model which favors institutional care. While only a very small percentage – approximately 4 percent of people over 65 in the USA – live in nursing homes, a high percentage of Medicare and Medicaid funds go to "for profit" long-term care facilities (Meiners, 1996).

The vast majority of older people live in the community with families providing most of the care informally. Most care needed by frail elders is of a personal, hands-on, functional level rather than medical (Brody, & Brody 1987). Families struggle to do their best to take care of older family members, each "rediscovering the wheel" as they navigate the maze of eligibility standards and government programs. Those with sufficient funds may hire geriatric care mangers to help them manage the complex and time-consuming avenues of care. Poor elders in institutions or programs may benefit from the expertise of case managers. Community and home-based services offer some continuum of care but such services are fragmented, not equitably distributed and often difficult to access.

In 1965, the Older Americans' Act (OAA) established a national network of services to older Americans including senior centers, nutrition advice, homemakers, home healthcare, information and referral, and legal assistance. Due to insufficient funding to provide programs for all older Americans, services are targeted to at-risk groups such as those who are poor, those at risk of nursing home placement, and those who are rural and/or a minority (Markson, 2003). The Adult Day Health program, respite care, multipurpose community centers, nutrition programs and home care have lessened the need for institutionalization and enhanced the quality of life for elders in the community. Initiatives such as the Boston Partnership for Older Adults (2003) seek to develop a "consumer-focused and culturally competent long-term care system for vulnerable older adults." Such a system would assist elders and their families to be resilient in their aging by building in such protective factors as:

- senior centers;
- nutrition programs;
- information and referral;
- easy access to crisis services if in immediate or suspected danger;
- in-home services such as a homemaker, home health aid, personal care assistant, respite care, etc.;
- caregiver education and support;
- geriatric care/case managers.

In addition, healthcare providers can become more skillful in addressing the needs of elders by being culturally sensitive, viewing the patient in context of their environment, being alert to risks factors for violence, and utilizing services which can moderate the risk and reinforce resilience. Consider the following case from my clinical experience that highlights some of these factors and their relevance in *cultural context*.

Case example: a Haitian immigrant

Renald is a 78-year-old newly arrived Haitian immigrant whose uncontrolled diabetes is of great concern to his doctor. Although he is overweight, Renald reports that his daughter doesn't feed him, leaves him alone all day "in a prison of a home" until she finally returns from work in the evening.

To fully attend to their patients, health providers must be sensitive to how culture permeates behavior. Communication style is shaped by culture. A specific question by a provider will typically be answered by a Haitian with a story. The time-pressed Western healthcare system can be frustrated by this method. Haitians tend to be polite and agree with whatever the provider says. A medical professional is an authority. They would not want to ask a question or say no to any question posed by an authority.

Therefore, taking Renald's statement that his daughter doesn't feed him as a fact evidencing abuse/neglect would be an unfortunate starting point. It is a beginning point of inquiry and the family needs to be considered in the problem solving.

When the social worker contacted the daughter she explained that she brought her parents over from Haiti to be with her because her mother was gravely ill and needed care. The mother died a month ago. Her father is grief stricken, bereft of his lifetime companion and his homeland. The daughter is having a difficult time managing the demands of her job and her father. Before she leaves for work, she gives her father his breakfast then prepares his mid-day meal but he won't heat it up nor take it out of the refrigerator for himself. In Haiti the young orphan girl who lived with them served every meal. His wife used to do much for him. Now he is expected to fend for himself for the first time in his life.

In the new world of the United States, Renald expected to "have it in the shade ... because God comes down every Friday" when you get your check. However, Renald doesn't know the language of this new land nor how to find his way around. It is freezing here in winter, too icy to go out. None of his friends are here. He is a disjointed person, a self divided between two cultures, in shock at the juncture of two worlds. He cannot return to Haiti because it is a political and economic nightmare. The years of violence and insecurity plague him.

Key issues and concepts

Cultural knowledge

The Haitian population is growing in the USA and the need for services for Haitian elderly is significant. Waves of migration began in the early twentieth century and continue to present times due to political upheaval, violence and economic hardship. Through migration, Haitians have experienced racial discrimination unknown in their country of origin – the first Black sovereign nation, Haiti was established in 1804 and is the second oldest republic in the Americas. In Haiti, patriarchy and age are respected. In the modernized lands to which many immigrant elders come, they are often marginalized and disempowered by the mainstream culture and eventually within their own family system.

Great emphasis is placed on family in Haitian culture. Three generations often live together with little intergenerational conflict. Children are the parents' survival hope. Authority rests with father and is to be respected and accepted without question. The will of the parent is law. Children are brought into existence not to follow their own inclinations but to look to their parents for guidance, not to govern but to be governed. Discipline and obedience is required. Conformity is encouraged. A mother's responsibility is to identify the problem and the father's is to decide what to do. Control of children by parents often extends into adulthood, even including choice of career (HAPHI, 2006). In Haiti, the current literacy rate is 65 percent. Most Haitian elders have little or no formal education, although many of them have been hard working parents who pushed their children to higher education. Their literacy issue is compounded by lack of English-speaking abilities in the US. They may pretend to understand a question when it is, in fact, not understood. The language barrier, the bureaucracy of the US healthcare system, and the difficulty of adult children to take time off from their jobs to tend to their parents often cause the elders to feel overwhelmed and abandoned.

Culture impacts one's concept of pain, health, illness and avenues for healing. In Haiti they say "*Sante se riches*," meaning health is wealth. In Haitian culture, disease is often understood in terms of hot versus cold. A "cold" for instance would be treated with a hot, herbal remedy. Infection with fever would be treated with cold compresses, a cool bath. A mental disorder is often understood as a spell or bad spirit cast on the individual as a punishment from another or from God. Congenital deformity is often understood as a supernatural problem. For Haitians, there is a continuum from not feeling well, to being sick, to very sick, to dying: "*Kom pa bon*" (I don't feel well) to "*Moin mald*" (I am sick) to "*Moin malad anpil*" (I am very sick) to "*Moin paprefe*" (I am dying). The gradations of illness implied here are essential to understanding the extent of their health complaints. Haitians often have a strong belief in God and spirits and prefer these avenues for cure. Home remedies are usually tried first, followed by a traditional healer. Disease may be treated by biomedical means only when complications set in or traditional resources yield no positive result. Medical intervention is often the last resort. Haitians may expect an expedient cure and tend to stop medication as soon as they feel relieved. Their diet tends to be rich in spices, salt and sugar. Being big is perceived as being healthy. To be fat is healthy; to be skinny is bad, meaning you don't eat meat (HAPHI, 2006).

Knowledge of violence and victimology

Awareness of how violence occurs can result from the imbalance between the needs of the person and the discrepancy between resources available (finances, housing, family). Risk can result in abuse and neglect when vulnerability is high, stress or environmental demands are great, and when protective forces are not enough to buffer the danger. If providers are cognizant of the statistics and demographic data which alert us to higher risk populations and combine this with empathetic inquiry and skillful intervention, the incidence of violence could be reduced.

Medical professionals in Renald's case would be well aware of the health risks associated with diabetes and poor nutrition. Physical and mental health professionals would also know that depression often accompanies diabetes. Someone who spoke the same language would probably elicit a fuller response from Renald, allowing a culturally sensitive understanding of his felt problems. Renald may share that his wife recently died and that they had just come from Haiti a short time ago to live with their daughter, who is loving but too busy at work to take care of him. The loss of a spouse and new immigrant status are risk factors for depression and suicide. Protective factors could be added to minimize risk, relieve stress and maximize resilience. An ethnically sensitive Adult Day Health program with daily structure, meals, medication monitoring, etc., or lunch and activities at a culturally appropriate community center may offer Renald a home away from home. These would supplement the caring but limited family support of his adult child caretaker.

Attitudes and values

While this case illustrates Haitian culture, we could be speaking about many other cultures as well. It is vital to recognize other world views and realize the far reaching impact of culture. It helps to have a sense of history and acquaintance with people and places around the globe. There is both a value and a caution with generalizations. Broad-spectrum knowledge offers a background but should not be considered expertise nor used to stereotype. No cultural group is homogeneous and every group contains diversity.

While literacy, education, religion, family structure, gender roles and values may differ according to culture, our common humanity unites us. We are all members of the human race sharing basic needs for physical survival, love and belonging, and meaningful activity in life. Immigrants share similarities with the mainstream culture of their adopted land while differing significantly at the same time.

The immigrant experience is a profound adjustment. People are torn between cultures, feeling shock at the juncture of two differing worlds which necessitates a double consciousness which can even be a divided self. As one Vietnamese refugee said, "Tears are the water of a new life." Many immigrants are glad to be in a land with greater opportunity for themselves and their children and yet miss their native land and people they left behind. Not all immigrants come to their adopted land by choice. The unique migration of Africans brought against their will as slaves for cheap labor in North, Central, and South America, the Caribbean islands, etc. bespeaks a continuing legacy of discrimination that impacts the health and very longevity of current descendants. Countless others have been forced to leave their homelands due to wars, political violence and natural disasters over the generations (see Chapters 8 and 9).

While empathy and compassion are called for in working with people, it is also vital to not take on the mantle of a rescuer. To do so means we are not working with, but for – that we are taking over instead of empowering, that we have the answers instead of helping others find their own answers.

Clinical practice skills

Broaden the context – from individual to system, from current to history. It is wise to bear in mind that we are all part of a system; that no individual is an island unto him/herself. We all are limited by our own perspective and cannot have a totally objective, complete picture. No single event is isolated in time and stays out of the context of one's life. Even if an event is solitary and traumatic, it becomes part of the fabric of that person's tapestry. The elders we serve have a lifetime of experiences. They are not only the person we see before us but a rich compilation of who they have been and what has gone on at all previous times in their life.

Pro-active and non-judgmental asking of questions about physical and psychological safety can open the door for more frank discussions. Making sure that providers are able to speak with elders alone may give the space necessary to talk about concerns within the family. Most elders are in contact with health providers at numerous points in their victimization. The earlier one can identify the problem and offer support, the less might be the exposure to violence and its devastating aftermath.

Just as important as the clinical skills of risk assessment and intervention is that providers also have a responsibility to *advocate* for public policy which does not victimize segments of the population and provides needed services. Visiting community centers for older persons in your geographic area and finding out about services available to enhance and maintain people in their homes enhances one's repertoire of practice skills. A growing number of programs are emerging, especially in urban areas, which are culturally relevant and attempt to be more comprehensive. Enhancing services in the community builds protective factors and reduces the risk of violence. See the online resources in Part IV for examples of such programs.

Speaking with elders from different cultures to learn about their rich history is an illuminating endeavor. Exploring cultural events and resources and participating in ethnic festivals, celebrations of food, music, art, etc. brightens the colors of our universal tapestry.

Suggested readings/viewings

Anderson, J., Coolidge, M, & Heche, A. (dirs.) (2000). *If These Walls Could Talk 2*. Home Box Office.

Gruen, S. (2001). *Water for Elephants: A Novel*. North Carolina: Algonquin Books of Chapel Hill.

Martz, S. H. (ed.) (1987). *When I Am An Old Woman I Shall Wear Purple*. CA: Papier-Mache Press.

References

APA – American Psychological Association (2005). *Elder Abuse and Neglect: In Search of Solutions*. APA Online: American Psychological Association. Retrieved March 10, 2009 from www.apa.org/pi/aging/eldabuse.html

Ayres, R. (August 1, 2005). *The Economic Conundrum of an Aging Population*. Worldwatch Institute.

Berman-Rossi, T. (2001). Older persons in need of long term care. In A. Gitterman (ed.), *Handbook of Vulnerable and Resilient Populations*; New York: Columbia University.

Bishaw, A. and Iceland, J. (2003). Poverty: 1999. *Census 2000 Brief*. Retrieved March, 2009 from http://www.census.gov/prod/2003pubs/c2kbr-19.pdf

Bolz, B. (1987). Social Security. In Martz, S. H. (ed.), *When I Am An Old Woman I Shall Wear Purple*. CA: Papier-Mache.

Boston Partnership for Older Adults (2003). Website: http://www.bostonolderadults.org/

Brewer, J. (2007). Boston-based collaborative works to improve the response to older victims of intimate partner abuse. *The FJC Monthly*, Family Justice Center of Boston, 1(3), April 2007, retrieved March 10, 2009 from http://www.cityofboston.gov/fjc/pdfs/FJCNews_April07.pdf

Brody, E. M., & Brody, S. J. (1987). Aged: Services. In R. L. Edwards (ed.), *Encyclopedia of Social Work*, pp. 106–26. Silver Springs, MD: National Association of Social Workers.

Coalition to Salute America's Heroes (2008). Website: http://www.saluteheroes.org/

Danieli, Y. (1995). As survivors age: An overview. *Journal of Geriatric Psychiatry* 30(1), 9–26.

Dychtwald, K. (1990). *Age Wave*. New York: Bantam Books.

Fisher, B. S., & Regan, S. L. (2006). The extent and frequency of abuse in the lives of older women and their relationship with health outcome. *Gerontologist*, 46, 200–9.

Freeman, I. C. (1997). Nursing home reform: Fait accompli or frontier. *Journal of Aging and Social Policy* 9(2), 7–18.

George, L. K. (1996) Social factors and illness. In R. H. Binstock, & L. K. George (eds.), *Handbook of Aging and Social Sciences* (4th edn.), pp. 229–52. New York: Academic Press.

Glasser, R. (2006). *Wounded: Vietnam to Iraq*. New York: George Braziller.

HAPHI – Haitian-American Public Health Initiatives, Inc. (2006): Website: http://maacoalition.org/?q=HAPHI

Hanes, P. J. (1992). *The Vietnamese Experience in America*. Bloomington, IN: Indiana University.

Harris, S. (1996). For better or for worse: Spouse abuse grown old. *Journal of Elder Abuse & Neglect*, 8(1), 1–33.

Hobfoll, S. E., & Wells, J. D. (1998) Conservation of resources, stress, and aging: Why do some slide and some spring? In J. Lomranz (ed.), *Handbook of Aging and Mental Health: An Integrative Approach*, pp. 121–43. New York: Plenum.

Hoff, L. A. (1994). *Violence Issues: Interdisciplinary Curriculum Guide for Health Professionals*. Ottawa: Health Canada.

Hoff, L. A., Hallisey, B. J., & Hoff, M. (2009). *People in Crisis: Clinical and Diversity Perspectives* (6th edn.). New York and London: Routledge.

Hurme, S. (2002). Perspectives on elder abuse. *Abuse Against Older Persons: Report of the United Nations Secretary-General*. Retrieved March 10, 2009 from http://assets.aarp.org/www.aarp.org_/articles/international/revisedabusepaper1.pdf

Institute for Research on Government (2009). *What are Poverty Thresholds and Poverty Guidelines?* University of Wisconsin: Madison. Retrieved March 10, 2009 from www.irp.wisc.edu/faqs/faq1.htm

Kogawa, J. (1981). *Obasan*. Massachusetts: Godine.

Krystal, H. (1981). Integration and self-healing in posttraumatic states. *Journal of Geriatric Psychiatry*, 14(2), 165–89.

Krystal, H. (1988), *Integration and Self-Healing*. Hillsdale, NJ: Analytic Press.

Lachs, M., Williams, C., O'Brien, S., & Pillemer, K. (2002). Adult protective service use and nursing home placement. *The Gerontologist*, 42, 734–9.

Markson, E. W. (2003). *Social Gerontology Today*. CA: Roxbury.

Martin, J. M., & Martin, E. P. (1985). *The Helping Tradition in the Black Family and Community*. Silver Spring, MD: National Association of Social Workers.

Meiners, M. R. (1996). The financing and organization of long-term care. In R. H. Binstock, L. E. Cluff, & O. Von Mering (eds.), *The Future of Long-Term Care*, pp. 191–214. Baltimore: Johns Hopkins University.

Military Family Network (2008). Website: http://www.emilitary.org

Mouton, C. P., *et al.* (2004). Prevalence and 3-year incidence of abuse among postmenopausal women. *American Journal of Public Health*, 94(4), 605–12.

NCEA – National Center on Elder Abuse (1998). *National Elder Abuse Incidence Study: Final Report*. Washington, DC: Department of Health and Human Services, Administration for Children and Families and Administration on Aging. Retrieved March 10, 2009 from http://www.ojp.usdoj.gov/ovc/ncvrw/2001/stat_over_7.htm

NCEA (2006). *Survey of Adult Protective Services*. Washington, DC: US Administration on Aging. Available online at: http://www.ncea.aoa.gov/

NCEA (2007). *Ethical Principles and Best Practice Guidelines*. Available online at: http://www.ncea.aoa.gov/NCEAroot/Main_Site/Find_Help/APS/Principles_Guidelines.aspx

National Research Council. (2003) *Elder Mistreatment: Abuse, Neglect and Exploitation in an Aging America*. Panel to Review Risk and Prevalence of Elder Abuse and Neglect. Washington, DC: National Academies Press.

Nerenberg, L. (1996). *Older Battered Women: Integrating Aging and Domestic Violence Services*. San Francisco Consortium for Elder Abuse Prevention.

Nguyen, K., & Andrews, F. (2001). *The Unwanted: A Memoir of Childhood*. Boston: Little Brown and Company.

Pillemer, K., & Finkelhor, D. (1988). The prevalence of elder abuse: A random sample survey *Gerontologist*, 28, 51–7.

Pillemer, K., & Prescott, D. (1989). Psychological effects of elder abuse: A research note. *Journal of Elder Abuse & Neglect*, 1(1), 65–74.

Porter, K. H., Larin, K., & Primus, W. (1999). *Social Security and Poverty among the Elderly: A National and State Perspective*. Washington, DC: Center on Budget and Policy Priorities.

Ryff C. D., Singer, B., Love, G. D., & Essex, M. J. (1998). Resilience in adulthood and later life. In J. Lomranz (ed.), *Handbook of Aging and Mental Health: An Integrative Approach*, pp. 69–96. New York: Plenum.

US AoA – United States Administration on Aging (2005). *Older Women*, United States Administration on Aging. Retrieved March 10, 2009 from http://www.aoa.gov/naic/may2000/factsheets/olderwomen.html

Wasik, J. F. (March/April, 2000). The fleecing of America's elderly. *Consumers Digest*.

Wiesel, E. (1970), *The Accident*. New York: Avon.

Wisconsin Lawyer (2000, September). 73, 9.

Wounded Warrior Project (2008). Website: http://www.woundedwarriorproject.org

Wu, K. (2003, March). *Poverty Experience of Older Persons, A poverty study from a long-term perspective*, AARP Public Policy Institute. Retrieved March 10, 2009 from http://assets.aarp.org/rgcenter/econ/2003_02_poverty.pdf

Yeoman, B. (July–August, 2008). When wounded vets come home. *AARP Magazine*, 60–4, 80.

8 Oppression, abuse, and enslavement of indigenous people across continents

- Overview: violence, destruction of indigenous cultures, and its consequences
  - The historical power of Native women
  - Female and male sex roles
- Cross-cultural examples
  - Australia
  - The Caribbean
  - Canada
  - The United States
- Key concepts and commonalities across cultures
- Survivors' responses in rebuilding their cultures
  - Cangleska, Inc.: serving the Oglala Lakota people
  - Lakota Sioux values regarding sex roles and violence
  - The Older Native Women's Health Project – Canada
  - Internalized oppression
  - Unnatural power and control vs. natural life-supporting power
  - Cangleska Healing Program for Offenders
  - The Indigenous Wellness Institute
- Practice implications for non-indigenous professionals and students

History is replete with examples of wars – tribe against tribe, nation against nation, and the winner subduing and imposing cultural, economic, and other rules on the conquered, often with the tragic consequences observable today in indigenous cultures. The contemporary scene of these conquests – aided and abetted by missionaries over decades, even hundreds of years – includes the imposition of values and beliefs about women together with the introduction of alcohol to colonized people. *Colonization* is the term representing this process across continents. Significantly, the United States – once "colonies" themselves subject to the British Crown – waged war against the indigenous people who welcomed them, and developed the "reservation" system where these Native Americans comprise some of the poorest and most isolated of the country's population of 300 million. All this was done while building the newly independent nation's wealth on the backs of African slave labor, the remnants of which still linger. Similar conditions exist among other indigenous groups across continents.

The rates of intimate partner violence and sexual assault among indigenous women exceed national averages across population groups (Evans-Campbell *et al.*, 2006; Harris *et al.*, 1997).

In the United States, the National Violence against Women Survey revealed that the highest rates of all forms of violence occur among American Indian/Alaska Native (AIAN) women: 34 percent reporting rape, 61.4 percent physical assault, and 17 percent reporting stalking (Tjaden, & Thoennes, 2000). Evans-Campbell *et al.* (2006, p. 1416) cite other research suggesting that AIAN women have higher rates of victimization by violent crime, domestic violence homicides, witnessing traumatic events, and psychological trauma related to victimization (Manson *et al.*, 2005). Seventy percent of violent victimizations experienced by Native women are more likely to occur from other races, mostly Black and White men, a difference from other populations of women most at risk of assault from members of their own race, which is intertwined with tribal jurisdiction issues (Artichoker, 2007).

This chapter connects these themes to the serious problems of interpersonal violence and abuse among indigenous peoples worldwide, with examples from Australia, Canada, the Caribbean, and the United States. The term "indigenous" is used generically throughout, while recognizing different usage across countries: in Australia, the most common term is "Aboriginal;" in Canada it is "First Nations;" in the United States it is "American Indian and Alaska Native – AIAN." The examples are followed by discussion of rural and urban programs illustrating how survivors of cultural suppression are rebuilding their lives through a combination of traditional values and adoption of contemporary education and research approaches. While the focus is on indigenous populations, many of the issues apply as well to the African American population suffering the intergenerational effects of slavery and challenges that many still face in a society where – over centuries – purported democratic principles and civil rights were constitutionally and by cultural acceptance denied to slaves and their descendants. For example, "Black-on-Black" violence must be understood in a context similar to Native American "Indian-upon-Indian" violence – not as excusable under the law, but as one manifestation of "oppressed group behavior."

Two programs are featured:

1   The Sacred Circle National Resource Center to End Violence against Women, a project of Cangleska, Inc., serving the Oglala Lakota people in South Dakota. Funding is from the Administration for Children and Families, Family and Youth Services Bureau, US Department of Health and Human Services. It is headquartered on the Pine Ridge Reservation in western South Dakota, and serves both rural and urban dwellers.

2   The Indigenous Wellness Research Institute in the Department of Social Work at the University of Washington in Seattle, Washington. Through its university affiliation, Native scholars have bridged some of the gaps in violence research discovery among urban and reservation-based American Indian and Alaska Native groups (Evans-Campbell *et al.*, 2006). While originally confined by force to reservations with bleak prospects for livelihood, today about 60 percent of AIAN members live in urban areas in search of more opportunity, while they confront and struggle with another set of challenges common among all marginalized groups in cities – e.g. street crime, the drug trade. Together, these programs capture an underlying theme of this book – *knowledge is power*:

    •   a victim/survivor's knowledge that the violence and abuse suffered "is not my fault" – often because health and social service providers have assured their clients that the *perpetrator*, not the victim, is accountable for the violence;
    •   professional practitioners' and educators' knowledge of *how to help* without further disempowerment of survivors;
    •   the powerful governmental institutions' *enactment of public policies from what we know*

about the serious consequences of violence for individuals, families, and all of society with a goal of preventing violence.

Newton Cummings, the Chair of the Board of Trustees of Oglala Lakota College on the Pine Ridge Reservation, presents this sage comment about knowledge in reference to the great buffalo herds that once provided his ancestors with all of life's necessities (food, shelter, clothing, medicine, art, etc.): "Today I consider higher education to be the new buffalo. For it offers our people everything we need to break free from a century of oppression and poverty and take control of our own future" (Cummings, 2008).

Overview: violence, destruction of indigenous cultures, and its consequences

Sadly, the contemporary scene for many indigenous people reveals how powerless people (across Africa, North and South America, and other former colonies) may turn upon one another in violence and abuse, not only because their traditions have been suppressed, but out of extreme economic deprivation and despair – this from having absorbed the conquering culture's value of "power and control" *over* others in contrast to harmonious living *with* one another and "mother earth." It is noteworthy and gratifying that mainstream societies are beginning to emulate worldwide some of the traditional values and rituals prized by indigenous people. For example, the increasing development of "green" programs to save an endangered planet from the effects of industrialization resembles the Lakota Sioux's "love of mother earth," a central tenet of their belief system.

On the other hand, violence against and within members of tribal groups and accountability for it is compounded by the challenge indigenous people face in adapting their lives to two cultures – their traditional one and that of the dominant group, including unresolved issues regarding jurisdiction over crimes committed. That is, Indian tribes in the United States are "limited sovereign nations" within the US boundaries, with Congress exercising plenary power over Indian affairs – in essence a unique relationship similar to that of ward and guardian (Hobson, 2006, p. 28). Attorney Hobson notes the root of this "trust relationship" in the doctrine of discovery and the way the US was settled. As is well known, violation of this trust relationship across continents is also basic to the loss, sorrow, and suffering of indigenous people. This is discussed further in connection with the Cangleska program for domestic violence offenders among the Lakota Sioux below.

The historical power of Native women

The sovereignty of Indian tribes is an inherent right and is rooted in the unique historical, political, and legal relationship between the tribes and the United States government. Before confinement of Native Americans to reservations, tribal justice systems and cultural supports were in place to ensure the safety and protection of tribal women (Artichoker, 2007). In pre-reservation societies both men and women held an honored place in society. The hero archetype for Native American women is a female. Among the Hopi, it is the "Corn Mother;" the Navajo, the "Change Woman;" the Taos, the "Deer Mother;" and Lakota Black Elk (2000) cites the "White Buffalo Calf Woman" from whom one learns how to be a truly integrated person through teachings brought to men, women and children. As Karen Artichoker (2007, p. 2) notes:

Prior to colonization, Native women were property owners, legislators, diplomats, and policy makers. The oral history and customary practices of tribal kinship networks and Indian nations describe women as full participants in all aspects of tribal life. Teachings about respect for women were brought by feminine, supernatural powers that held women as sacred and counseled the people that women were to be treated accordingly.

Pre-reservation society is also captured in author Barry Unsworth's fictional account of the slave trade in his Booker Prize-winning book, *Sacred Hunger*. Besides depicting the degradation experienced alike by slaves and poor British men recruited to keep the Africans under control before delivering them to the colonies, we learn of the secret "utopian" colony that the abused sailors, an ethical British doctor, and freed slaves set up in Florida with Native Americans after a mutiny on the high seas from Africa to Liverpool. Noteworthy in this story is the tender love relationship between the British doctor and an African woman – untouched by later laws forbidding interracial marriage. When the colony is found and done in by the son of the ship's owner wreaking revenge on his cousin, the doctor, the stage is set, so to speak, for later wars against Native peoples and their cultural traditions.

Female and male sex roles

In Lakota Sioux creation stories, women – as creators of life and the lodge owner along with its furnishings – were created first and men were made compatible to women. They were traditionally acknowledged as spiritually powerful, and offered leadership in decisions regarding the household and the *tiyospaye* – roles non-existent in the reservation system imposed on the Lakota Sioux. In this pre-reservation system, the union of man and woman married to each other was not a family, but was called the *tiyospaye* (relatives living together). The partners could choose a spiritual ceremony to bless their union, but divorce was not viewed as breaking a religious code or "sinful" as in Christianity. Basically, marriage was part of a household (*tiyospaye*) in which a woman ranked her brothers first, then her sons, her cousins, and her husband last.

Oral histories describe the balance between the male and female with feminine power honored and recognized. Tribal worldview was circular, not hierarchical. Every nation and all the elements had a place and function within the circle. Natural law afforded Native women the safety and protection of her kinship network and tribe (Artichoker, 2007, p. 2). The Medicine Wheel (see Figure 8.1) depicts this worldview application to ending violence against women.

In pre-reservation society, men held definite roles as providers and protectors. In this they are not unlike men in other traditional societies. The difference lies in the Lakota philosophy of equality between men and women, in contrast to "patriarchal" Western societies in which women, children, servants, and the entire estate were under the control of – and therefore subservient to – the "patriarch," who owned all. Thus, for example, if an aggrieved wife desired a divorce, it was understood by societal law that custody of any children automatically was accorded to the "patriarch." Modern mainstream society divorce laws (perhaps as an over-correction in some cases) most often award custody to mothers, sometimes irrespective of the mother's fitness, but sometimes custody is awarded to the father because of his economic advantage (not his primary caretaker role).

For traditional male leadership in Lakota society, men had to demonstrate valor, bravery, wisdom, and dignity that meant respectful self-conduct and non-violent, compassionate behavior – along with other behaviors like putting the needs of the people first and contributing to consensus decision making for the good of the people. "Men were taught that women were to be respected, even in thought. The man who was unable to recognize her sacredness was reduced to a pile of bones" (Artichoker, 2007, p. 2). When genocide failed and a military presence was no longer needed, the prisoner of war camps evolved into the present day reservation system which has exacted an enormous and tragic toll on traditional female and male roles and the natural laws ensuring the proper behavior of individuals.

Anthropologist Eleanor Leacock describes how the open, friendly, warm tribal people met by early White travelers also left them vulnerable and easy to exploit. The analog to conquest by soldiers was the conquest and degradation of Native women by men, Indian and otherwise. The plan to Christianize Native people included introduction of the European family structure emphasizing male authority, female submission and fidelity, and eliminating the right to divorce – thus enabling the shift from an egalitarian, gynocratic social structure to a patriarchal hierarchical one (Leacock, 1980).

Artichoker (2007, p. 3) similarly describes the resulting dissolution of female power and its impact on traditional relations between Native men and women:

> The civilizing of Native people became synonymous with Christianizing. Federal government policy was to remove Indian children from their families and place them in residential Christian missions or government boarding schools. This tactic destroyed or distorted traditional parenting abilities predicated on the worldview that children are sacred beings and replaced it with experiences of corporal punishment that reflected the teachings of the church. Similarly, Indian boys and girls were immersed in an environment that reflected male domination/female subservience.

> Mission and boarding school experiences reinforced earlier role modeling of cavalry and government officials. Women were obviously devalued and not allowed to participate in earlier treaty-making and negotiations between sovereign tribal governments and a fledgling U.S. government. Treaties between Indian nations and the United States government, made in exchange for promises of tribal sovereignty, have not been honored and, in combination with subsequent congressional policy and legal decisions, culminate today in a sorry lack of protection and safety for Native women.

The examples that follow offer a glimpse into indigenous peoples' contemporary struggles. For the Oglala Sioux, Nicholas Black Elk (2000, pp. 199–201) recounts the history of this struggle that culminated at Wounded Knee Creek on December 29, 1890 at Pine Ridge Reservation:

> Dead and wounded women and children and little babies were scattered all along there where they had been trying to run away. The soldiers had followed along the gulch, as they ran, and murdered them .... I saw a little baby trying to suck its mother, but she was bloody and dead .... Men and women and children were heaped and scattered all over the flat at the bottom of the little hill where the soldiers had their wagon-guns .... It was a good winter day when all this happened. The sun was shining. But after the soldiers marched away from their dirty work, a heavy snow began to fall .... There was a big blizzard .... The snow drifted deep in the crooked gulch, and it was one long grave of butchered women and children and babies, who had never done any harm and were only trying to run away.

Black Elk's book is a classic among all who wish to learn about the religious beliefs of the Plains Indian, and has become a North American bible of all tribes. These beliefs included the warrior's role to protect and defend women and children, not harm them – a tradition that Oglala Sioux men today are trying to recapture in their program for fellow men who abuse women. In the massacre at Wounded Knee, Oglala Sioux warriors were defeated in their protective role by the US soldiers' wanton murders of all in their sight.

Cross-cultural examples

Australia [recounted from the consultation and clinical experience of Joy Adams-Jackson, 2008]

Example 1

The Aboriginal health worker, Grace, made a home visit to a 32-year-old Aboriginal mother of three children following a call from the local school principal who expressed his concerns about the children's ongoing absenteeism. Grace was alarmed to see the state of the woman's home; it was putrid, and the children were filthy and full of head-lice. Grace asked what was going on. The woman responded that the black bastard of a boyfriend had beaten her up and then taken off with her money. Grace arranged for the woman to see the Aboriginal police liaison officer and insisted that she take out an AVO [a protection order] against her ex-partner. The woman refused because she claimed she was fearful of reprisals from the ex-partner, his mates, and other members of the local Aboriginal community. Grace felt frustrated and annoyed; all she could do was to try and impress upon the woman how important it was for the children to attend school. She also informed the woman of the consequences to her if the children continued to remain absent from school.

Example 2

Grace received a visit from Mona, the local Women's Health Nurse Consultant. Mona had seen a young Aboriginal woman earlier that morning and was concerned that her partner was emotionally and sexually abusing her. Mona had performed the necessary evaluation, but wanted Grace to have a word with her client. She thought it best that an Aboriginal woman deal with anything potentially culturally sensitive. Grace agreed to talk to the woman and suggested a home visit. Grace went to the woman's home and after a lengthy conversation the woman confirmed that she was being abused. Grace put forward a list of options for the woman and stressed her concerns about the woman's safety. Despite acknowledging her abusive situation, the woman refused any outside help and declined any offer of police assistance. When Grace asked why she was refusing any help, she replied "If he don't beat ya, he don't love ya." She also believed that other people in the Aboriginal community would further abuse her.

The Caribbean [recounted from community service work by Glenda Dubienski, 2008]

Laura, a 35-year-old devoted mother of 4, has been considering leaving her abusive and un-faithful husband of 19 years. With the extremely high risk of AIDS in this island nation, Laura is confronted with the reality that his philandering ways could very likely bring this plague upon her. Professing a strong Christian faith and subscribing to the teachings of the local church, Laura is torn as to what to do about her situation. Her church has taught her that divorce is wrong and that remarriage is adulterous. Fearful that she will disappoint God, she is choosing to separate from her husband and not ask for financial support. Her church community has been her primary support throughout the most difficult times of her married life.

Laura seriously questions whether or not the community will shun her if she does divorce her husband. Certainly, divorcing him and suing him for a portion of his assets seems out of the question, despite the fact that she started and maintained their business, which has made them wealthy by island standards.

Typically the church in this former colony is patriarchal and legalistic, and not egalitarian. However, the island's current legal system highly favors women who have proven grounds for divorce. They are often granted all their ex-husband's assets. Presently, Laura is not financially self-sufficient and does not feel she is capable of providing for her children. Lax in his attempts to hide the details of his affairs, Laura's husband was recently witnessed by their eldest daughter dining with his current "side woman" (i.e. "mistress" in Western terms). Uncertain as to how to approach this sighting, their daughter collected more information about the relationship and confronted him with it in their home. In front of the entire family, a heated argument ensued. Feeling trapped by the confrontation, the father attempted to knock his daughter to the ground. Adrenaline won out and the young lady was able to overpower her father. This altercation left Laura with the harsh realization that her children are not immune to the violence she has withstood for so many years. She now has the resolve to remove herself and her children from her husband's house. However, the logistics of such are difficult.

Canada [excerpted with permission and edited from Hoff, 1994]

Clara, age 40, is the daughter of Joseph and Magdalene who spent most of their childhood and adolescence in one of the residential church schools to which most Indian children were sent until the 1970s. Clara's parents died in their 50s from injuries incurred from a car crash which occurred while driving under the influence of alcohol. The oldest of five children, Clara divides her time working as a social services administrator, as a peer counselor for adolescents on a reserve in Ontario, and as caretaker of her three children. She and her husband also have assumed responsibility temporarily for the care of one niece, age 10, and two nephews, ages 12 and 15, children of her sister who is studying dental hygiene at a local community college after escaping from an abusive marriage.

Clara poignantly describes the intergenerational odyssey of First Nations people struggling to deal with their rage and the human misery wrought by subjugation of a whole people through colonization and the destruction of Native culture. Her parents' memories of life in the residential school included the dramatic image of "a Bible in one hand, and a zipper in the other" to describe the widespread sexual abuse of children in these schools. With only abusive authoritarian "caretakers" as role models, no formal preparation for the preservative tasks of parenting, and easy availability of alcohol as an escape from despair, Clara readily understands why her parents did not know how to parent her and her siblings. Though now closed, the cycle of abuse set in motion by these schools as agents of the mainstream culture's colonizers has been visited upon generations to come. Clara says that it has left "blood memories" which some elders want desperately to unlock so that they can heal from their rage. And how do they heal? "Maybe someone is just kind to them," Clara declares. But most important is getting in a circle with their own people and listening to elders who know, who remember and cherish their own culture.

As a result of the residential school system's damage to her parents, Clara lived for a time with her grandparents, but at age 9 was taken away from them and placed in a foster home sponsored by Children's Aid. There she was sexually abused by both the foster father and one of his sons. When the social worker made supervisory visits, she made it clear that she did not want to talk with Clara about the abuse; instead, the focus was on how clean the house was. After leaving the abusive foster home at age 15 and attempting reconciliation with her family, Clara finally began to understand her rage, and has been able to grieve for herself, her extended family, and her people by attending the healing circles conducted in her community. The support and process of self-healing she experiences there have also given her the insight and strength to facilitate the healing of her nephew, Jason, now in her care, and attending an adolescents' healing group sponsored by the school and health center on the reserve. Jason, age 15, was arrested when he was caught trying to steal a car, and while in jail, was raped by an inmate – all this while his mother seemed locked in a violent marriage.

Clara emphasizes the importance of providing a safe place among their own people for First Nations members where they are allowed to feel and to grieve their losses. These healing circles are pivotal, no matter how many years may have passed since victimized persons buried their wounds and the rage they have directed toward themselves instead of the people and the unjust institutions that victimized them. Clara says that some women in these circles are already in their 60s and 70s when they disclose for the first time the assaults they have suffered.

The United States

Patricia, age 29, is the mother of three children, two boys and a girl – ages 12, 8, and 6. Her ethnic and racial heritage is mixed – her mother is Lakota Sioux and her father Caucasian. Her mother began college in a New England state, but dropped out during the first year after becoming pregnant with Patricia. When she was age 4, Patricia's parents divorced primarily because of her father's drug abuse for which he would not follow through with treatment. Patricia's mother then moved back to the reservation in North Dakota. At age 18, Patricia married Allesandro (Alex) a man of mixed Latino and Caucasian heritage who worked on the reservation as a mechanic. Alex had always been controlling of Patricia, but after the birth of their second child, he began beating Patricia and threatened to kill the boy when he was still an infant. He also struck the older boy, Dennis, and accused Patricia of infidelity – denying he was the father of Dennis.

Key concepts and commonalities across cultures

What can we learn from these four women? The situations of these women and their families illustrate the toll taken on the human spirit and on physical and mental health by colonial policies calculated to eliminate entire cultures.

Central to colonial subjugation are the multiple losses and unresolved grief felt by entire communities who lost their children to a foreign education system, their culture, and their homeland. The *individual* pain, grief, and disproportionate frequency of self-destructive or violent behaviors among indigenous people must be situated in the *sociocultural* context of their oppression as an *entire society*. Without such an historical perspective, the tenacity of the victim-blaming tendency may surface in work with individual victims who need help – not judgment – as they strive among their own people to rebuild their lives beyond victimhood.

Facilitating the grief work and continued healing of these survivors and their families, and other indigenous people, demands attention to several key factors:

The systematic disempowerment of Native people by *others* must be replaced by the people *themselves* assuming responsibility for dealing with the destructive effects of colonization, especially through Healing Circles and communication with elders. This does not exclude whatever services are available and appropriate from *other* outside sources. Significantly, some of the women in these examples had little awareness of the connections between their individual victim/survivor status and how it both resembled that of women from mainstream cultures and was linked to the disadvantaged status of entire indigenous communities; for example, the Aboriginal woman visited by health worker Grace revealed that she had absorbed the Western acceptance of battering as part of the marital relationship when she said "If he don't beat ya, he don't love ya" – which could pass as a page from Erin Pizzey's (1974) book that launched the activist "battered women's movement" in the UK and other Western countries. This cultural acceptance of wife abuse also surfaced in mainstream research, as in "the marriage license as a hitting license" uncovered in the first national survey on violence in the American family (Straus *et al.*, 1980).

Indigenous women fear the implications of reporting partner violence and the impact it could have on their communities given the disproportionate rates of aboriginal men in prison and the high rate of aboriginal deaths in custody. Some aboriginal women prefer not to criminalize a violent partner. This has profound consequences with aboriginal women placed at greater risk of death from violent assault than non-indigenous women. Non-members of the indigenous community must also control paternalistic or rescue impulses, some of which may be rooted in "White guilt" for what their own ancestors wrought against indigenous people in decades and hundreds of years past.

- Social support must replace social isolation as a prerequisite for unlocking the "blood memories" and discharging rage away from self and family members into non-violent channels.
- Grief counseling includes forgiveness of self as well as others, for example, a parent like Clara's who did not provide a safe environment due to alcoholism or one's own grief.
- Spirituality and traditional teachings have key roles in the stabilization of individuals, the family, and the community.
- Traditional family roles and communal responsibility need integration with contemporary child-rearing, discipline, and non-violent resolution of female/male conflict situations.
- Young people, in attempting to reconcile values from traditional and mainstream cultures, need special support, many may try to "pass" as a way to survive in the dominant culture (see Chapter 5 for the Circle of Courage).

The implications of these key concepts for practice with indigenous victim/survivors are addressed in this chapter's last section in relation to the programs featured in the next two sections.

Survivors' responses in rebuilding their cultures

The efforts by indigenous people to revive their traditions and rebuild their cultures have very promising results for individual survivors of interpersonal violence. Central to this process is rekindling among both victim/survivors and offenders their own values before subjugation to the values and behavior of the colonizers – in this case the contrasting approaches to intimate partner abuse. Education toward prevention and service programs for survivors and offenders are key to this rebuilding process.

Cangleska, Inc.: serving the Oglala Lakota people (excerpted and edited from "Women are Sacred – Violence is not a Lakota Tradition" and the Cangleska website (http://www.cangleska.org))

Before the founding of Cangleska (which translates as "Medicine Wheel"), formerly known as Project Medicine Wheel, Native women abused by their intimate partners had been jailed at a shelter to protect them from their batterers or were left to find refuge wherever they could. Cangleska was incorporated and chartered in 1994 by the Oglala Sioux tribe during the same period that the Violence Against Women Act (VAWA) was passed in the United States Congress. Cangleska's founders, Karen Artichoker and Marlin Mousseau, envisioned incorporating the Lakota Sioux people's traditional values of respect, bravery, generosity, and wisdom into responses to end violence against Native women and their children.

Embedded in the programs of Cangleska is the concept of "sovereign women within a sovereign nation," whose safety is paramount. With the Lakota principle of "we are all related" infused in all its programs, Cangleska offers a comprehensive and collaborative approach to domestic violence on the local, state, and national levels. Its model programs, policies, and practice protocols for service to survivors and law enforcement for perpetrators are replicable across Indian country because they are grounded in the values of Native culture and respect for tribal sovereignty. Key features of Cangleska's philosophy and programs for survivors and offenders are summarized here for consideration by indigenous people across cultures with whom the Lakota Sioux share similar consequences of colonization and confinement on reservations or their equivalent on other continents. The introduction of alcohol to Native peoples has compounded the plight and confinement of indigenous people to oppressed reservation life.

Lakota Sioux values regarding sex roles and violence

Before confinement to reservations, *tiyospaye* (relatives living together) social laws were based on the Lakota values that ensured the central goal of safety, harmony and continuity of the *tiyospaye*. There was no "battle of the sexes" because in the deeply enmeshed pre-reservation philosophy was the belief in equality between adult men and women, with their defined roles of equal importance to the nation, as discussed above.

Wife battering was considered a violation of respect and the nation's social law which disrupted the camp's harmony. It was therefore a rare occurrence and was treated very seriously. As Artichoker (2007, p. 2) notes:

> The oral histories of many tribes describe the harsh and severe nature of punishment in the event a husband abused his wife. Mental self-discipline was highly valued and those unable to adhere to customary practices of respectful behavior experienced consequences from kinship networks and social societies with the power to physically punish, shun, banish or even kill an abuser of women.

The Lakota believe that today's reality of wife battering can be traced to the disintegration of Native peoples' freedom, their life-ways, and beliefs resulting from colonization and the reservation system. Development of this system was carried out by the US government cavalry who guarded the reservation. The Lakota were appalled at the behavior of these soldiers – drinking, gambling, cursing, and being disrespectful toward women. In that system, it was not uncommon for US government cavalry soldiers to take and hold Lakota women against their will, repeatedly rape them, impregnate them and return them to their families, only to repeat the crimes

THE MEDICINE WHEEL

*The Medicine Wheel is said to be a mirror from which
anything can be reflected, a mirror in which to look so that
we can see how we got to be who we are and where we can be.
This **Figure focuses** on the dynamics
of abuse from the philosophy of the Medicine Wheel.*

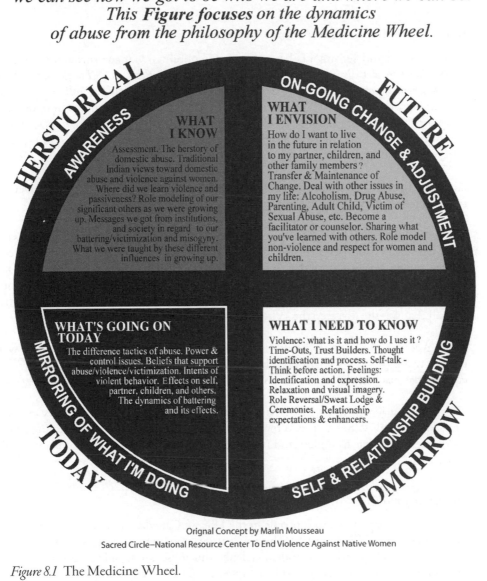

HERSTORICAL

AWARENESS

**WHAT
I KNOW**

Assessment. The herstory of
domestic abuse. Traditional
Indian views toward domestic
abuse and violence against women.
Where did we learn violence and
passiveness? Role modeling of our
significant others as we were growing
up. Messages we got from institutions,
and society in regard to our
battering/victimization and misogyny.
What we were taught by these different
influences in growing up.

ON-GOING CHANGE & ADJUSTMENT

FUTURE

**WHAT
I ENVISION**

How do I want to live
in the future in relation
to my partner, children, and
other family members?
Transfer & Maintenance of
Change. Deal with other issues in
my life: Alcoholism, Drug Abuse,
Parenting, Adult Child, Victim of
Sexual Abuse, etc. Become a
facilitator or counselor. Sharing what
you've learned with others. Role model
non-violence and respect for women and
children.

**WHAT'S GOING ON
TODAY**

The difference tactics of abuse. Power &
control issues. Beliefs that support
abuse/violence/victimization. Intents of
violent behavior. Effects on self,
partner, children, and others.
The dynamics of battering
and its effects.

WHAT I NEED TO KNOW

Violence: what is it and how do I use it?
Time-Outs, Trust Builders. Thought
identification and process. Self-talk -
Think before action. Feelings:
Identification and expression.
Relaxation and visual imagery.
Role Reversal/Sweat Lodge &
Ceremonies. Relationship
expectations & enhancers.

MIRRORING OF WHAT I'M DOING

TODAY

SELF & RELATIONSHIP BUILDING

TOMORROW

Orignal Concept by Marlin Mousseau
Sacred Circle–National Resource Center To End Violence Against Native Women

Figure 8.1 The Medicine Wheel.

against other women. As with the Australian Aboriginal woman visited by health worker Grace who seemed unaware of the political and cultural origins of her battering, some Lakota men today treat women the same way the US cavalry did, in effect, taking on the "same appalling characteristics of the very men that were sent here to kill us off" – often unaware of the impact of colonization and not realizing that they are behaving just like the men their ancestors fought and despised (adapted from Sacred Circle, 2008).

The Older Native Women's Health Project – Canada

Similar oppression and sentiments have been made public in Canada through the Older Native Women's Health Project's 1995 report, *Sharing Our Health Circle: The Grandmothers' Health Assessment Report.* The Healing Circle of this multicultural interdisciplinary team in Saskatchewan province features these four interrelated elements: (1) strengths in our traditions; (2) disruptions, influences; (3) concerns of today; and (4) teachings, solutions, hopes, vision. Here are some of the individual voices within their collective report that reflect these four elements:

> Aboriginal people had a balanced, holistic view of health which included spiritual, emotional, intellectual, and physical health all in harmony (p. 2).

> Those of us who are Treaty were "put in pastures (reserves) and couldn't eat the grass on the other side." People never owned anything, Indian Affairs did .... Then they introduced welfare and we were worse off than before. There was no incentive to work in exchange for welfare so as to retain our precious pride and dignity .... From the time I could walk until I was 6 years old I lived in moccasins. When I got my first pair of shoes [in the residential school] that was the first step the White society took to rob me of my heritage (p. 3).

> Many Aboriginals are left with bitterness and an inferiority complex because of the way they are treated by others. Many take alcohol and drugs to compensate .... Balancing the two cultures has made my life miserable. I did not connect to my Indianness (p. 7, 8).

> My auntie ... made me understand that I had to connect with my Indian identity in order to move forward. When I started to learn about my traditions, then the healing began .... White society has to understand Native culture and it's time to speak up about this (pp. 11, 13).

Internalized oppression

These scenarios among indigenous people in the US and Canada evoke the concept of "oppressed group behavior" (Friere, 1989). This concept is central in the Lakota Sacred Circle and central to understanding Indian-to-Indian violence and abuse: an outside group's power and authority imposed over another group's belief system and values (*external oppression*) results in *internalized oppression.* This occurs when the controlled group comes to behave according to the external group's values and life-ways and to believe in them as a reality to adopt. The results are "self-hate," shame, "internalized racism," and the disowning of one's own cultural reality.

Thus, fighting and disrespect for women were "foreign" behaviors modeled by the US cavalry which worked their way into Native communities so that external pressure is no longer needed because "we now do it to ourselves and each other." This "divide and conquer" tactic is observed throughout the world, not just in Native communities – for example, in Black-on-Black violence and the lateral or "horizontal" violence and abuse among nurses (see Chapter 11 for a discussion of this topic regarding workplace violence). A common manifestation of the widespread evidence of oppressed group behavior among marginalized groups includes "women are their own worst enemies."

In the Lakota Sacred Circle philosophy, people learn how to live harmoniously together without violence. Doing so requires bringing internalized oppression to *conscious* awareness as a *first step* toward preventing battering and atoning for violence. Group support and a healing atmosphere are essential to this process – as in the Healing Circles already noted. Significantly, few of the women interviewed for this book, and from the clinical experience of authors and contributors, revealed awareness of the connection between their current plight from abuse and its historical underpinnings – a point noted in Chapter 2 (see Figure 2.1) – illustrating self-destructive and other negative effects on *individuals* when the *sociocultural roots* of violence and its prevention hold only back-burner attention.

Unnatural power and control vs. natural life-supporting power

The Sacred Circle-Cangleska program offers an adaptation of the Power and Control Wheel developed at the Domestic Abuse Intervention Project in Duluth, Minnesota, USA. This powerful depiction of the key dynamics (power over women) operating in intimate partner violence is also widely used in mainstream violence prevention programs. In the Cangleska programs, trainers use it to contrast power and control tactics with a *natural non-violent life-supportive power and values*. The *unnatural* tactics of physical and sexual abuse that treat women as objects include:

- *Male privilege*, e.g. acting like "king of the castle."
- *Isolation*, e.g. by controlling all her activities.
- *Intimidation*, e.g. instilling fear through smashing things or showing weapons.
- *Emotional abuse*, e.g. putting her down, calling her names, etc.
- *Minimize, lie, and blame*, e.g. shifting blame to her for his abusive behavior.
- *Using children*, e.g. threatening to take them away.
- *Economic abuse*, e.g. taking her money, or making her ask for money.
- *Coercion and threats*, e.g. making or carrying out threats to leave her or commit suicide.
- *Cultural abuse*, e.g. competing for "Indianness" or misinterpreting culture to prove male superiority.
- *Ritual abuse*, e.g. using religion as a threat, or "God doesn't allow divorce."

See Figure 8.2 for full description of these tactics used in battering situations.

In stark contrast, the Natural Life-Supporting Power Wheel builds on the traditional Lakota Sioux values of respect, bravery, generosity and wisdom, and includes the beliefs of humility, compassion, hard work, fortitude, love, courage, and mutual sharing. *Natural life-supporting power* is built on indigenous people's reclaiming the values, belief systems, and life-ways demonstrated in one's behavior and relationships with others and all things in the non-violence power wheel emanating from belief in *equality*:

- *Spiritual reflection* on walking your own path and on your relationship with the Creator.
- *Economic partnership* by making decisions together and assuring mutual financial benefits.
- *Negotiation and fairness* through satisfying conflict resolution and willingness to compromise.

BATTERING

Along the left edge of the triangle: PUNCHING - KICKING - CHOKING - PHYSICAL VIOLENCE PUSHING - SLAPPING - PULLING HAIR

Along the right edge of the triangle: PHYSICALLY ATTACKING THE SEXUAL PARTS OF HER BODY SEXUAL VIOLENCE TREATING HER LIKE A SEX OBJECT

MALE PRIVILEGE
Treats her like a servant. Makes all the big decisions. Acts like the "king of the castle." Defines men's and women's roles.

ISOLATION
Controls what she does, who she sees and talks to, what she reads. Limits her outside involvement. Uses jealousy to justify actions.

INTIMIDATION
Makes her afraid by using looks, actions, gestures. Smashes things. Destroys her property. Abuses pets. Displays weapons.

EMOTIONAL ABUSE
Puts her down. Makes her feel bad about herself. Calls her names. Makes her think she's crazy. Plays mind games. Humiliates her. Makes her feel guilty.

MINIMIZE, LIE AND BLAME
Makes light of the abuse and doesn't take her concerns seriously. Says the abuse didn't happen. Shifts responsibility for abusive behavior. Says she caused it.

USING CHILDREN
Makes her feel guilty about the children. Uses the children to relay messages. Uses visitation to harass her. Threatens to take away the children.

ECONOMIC ABUSE
Prevents her from working. Makes her ask for money. Gives her an allowance. Takes her money. Doesn't let her know about or access family income.

COERCION AND THREATS
Makes and/or carries out threats to do something to hurt her. Threatens to leave her, to commit suicide, to report her to welfare. Makes her drop charges. Makes her do illegal things.

CULTURAL ABUSE
Competes over "Indianness." Misinterprets culture to prove male superiority/female submission. Uses relatives to beat her up. Buys into "blood quantum" competitions.

RITUAL ABUSE
Prays against her. Defines spirituality as masculine. Stops her from practicing her ways. Uses religion as a threat. "God doesn't allow divorce." Says her period makes her "dirty."

UNNATURAL POWER & CONTROL

Battering= the purposeful use of a system of multiple, continuous tactics to maintain power and control over another. This intentional violence results from, and is supported by an unnatural, misogynistic, sexist societal and cultural belief system. Battering is a crime against individuals, families, and communities.

Produced by Sacred Circle - National Resource Center to End Violence Against Native Women

Figure 8.2 Unnatural power and control.

- *Non-threatening behavior*, e.g. talking and acting so she feels safe.
- *Respect*, e.g. listening non-judgmentally and valuing opinions.
- *Trust and support*, e.g. of her life goals and right to her own feelings, etc.
- *Honesty and accountability*, e.g. acknowledge past use of violence and admit being wrong.
- *Responsible parenting*, e.g. sharing parental responsibility and presenting non-violent role models.
- *Shared responsibility*, e.g. agreeing on a fair distribution of work and making decisions together.
- *Sexual respect*, e.g. understanding the difference between love, sex, and intimacy, and right to control her own body.
- *Partnership*, e.g. listen with your heart and treat your partner as an equal human being.
- *Cultural respect*, e.g. understanding your relationship to others and all things in Creation, and respecting that people have their own path.

Cangleska Healing Program for Offenders

The Sacred Circle Medicine Wheel approach is pivotal in Cangleska programs for victim/ survivors as well as perpetrators. Lakota Gene Thin Elk in the "Red Road Approach" compliments the "natural life-supporting power wheel" in his description of traditional Lakota healing concepts and ceremonies dedicated to keeping in balance the four basic essences of personhood and wellness: Spirit, Mind, Body, and Emotion (Thin Elk, 1995, p. 159). As Thin Elk notes about this holistic and timeless principle applicable well beyond the indigenous community: "We are more the same than different." Or, as the father of Western medicine, Hippocrates, said of holism: "It is better to know the man who has the disease, than the disease the man has."

Another aspect of the Cangleska Healing Program for Offenders draws on the "Seven Philosophies for a Native American Man" (Deucheneaux, 2008; see the online resources in Part IV for other training resources). The "Seven Philosophies" are briefly summarized here, and are widely applicable across cultures regarding men who abuse women:

1 *To the Women.* The cycle of life for the woman is the baby, girl, woman and grandmother ... the four directions of life. She has been given by natural laws the ability to reproduce life. The most sacred of all things is life. Therefore, all men should treat her with dignity and respect. Never was it our way to harm her mentally or physically. Indian men were never abusers. We always treated our women with respect and understanding. So from now on, I will treat women in a sacred manner.

2 *To the Children.* As an eagle prepares its young to leave the nest with all the skills and knowledge it needs to participate in life, in the same manner so will I guide my children. I will use the culture to prepare them for life.

3 *To the Family.* The Creator gave to us the family ... where all teachings are handed down .... to the child .... I realize the importance for each Indian man to be responsible to the family .... By doing this, I will break the cycle of hurt and ensure the positive mental health of the children .... For example, I must never give up and leave my family only to the mother.

4 *To the Community.* The Indian community provides many things for the family ... to belong to "the people," and to have a place to go. Our Indian communities need to be restored to health so the future generation will be guaranteed a place to go for culture, language, and Indian socializing. For example, as an Indian man, I will care about those in my community so that the mind changes, alcohol and drugs will vanish, and our communities will forever be free of violence.

5   *To the Earth*. Our Mother Earth is the source of all life ... the two-legged, four-legged, winged
    ones or human beings. The Mother Earth is the greatest Teacher, if we listen, observe and
    respect her .... Just as I would protect my own mother, so will I protect the Earth.
6   *To the Creator*. As an Indian man, I realize we make no gains without the Great Spirit ...
    Being Indian and being spiritual has the same meaning .... This day, I vow to walk the Red
    Road [Thin Elk, 1995].
7   *To Myself*. I will think about what kind of person I want to be when I am an Elder [and]
    start developing myself now to be this person .... I will seek out the guiding principles which
    guided my ancestors. I will walk in dignity, honor and humility, conducting myself as a
    warrior. I choose to do all these things myself, because no one else can do them for me.

As an aid for translating these philosophies to individual probation and violence prevention
action, offenders brought before the tribal court for assault, abuse, threats, or terrorizing an
intimate partner are provided a handbook outlining the meaning of probation and all the conditions, rules, and procedures of the Cangleska Probation Department and the Oglala Sioux Tribal
Court. The handbook provides a place for personal notes, special conditions, and ready access
for recording important information like the name and phone number of the Probation Officer.
Broadly, these rules and consequences for those who do not abide by them correspond to the
nationwide Emerge program in the US described in Chapter 10 – the first of its kind directed
at all offenders regardless of race or ethnicity (Adams, & Cayouette, 2002).

The Oglala Sioux offender program is also comparable to the model developed in the Quincy,
Massachusetts District Court. The basic principle in this program emulates the Oglala Sioux
"Seven Philosophies" and puts emphasis on accountability of offenders for their violent behavior,
and their personal responsibility to not re-offend if they are to avoid jail or prison. This view is
supported by Klein's (1994) study of 664 men who were issued civil restraining orders by the
Quincy, Massachusetts District Court. Reliance on such orders alone did not prevent more
abuse, especially among younger, unmarried abusers with prior criminal records who also
abused alcohol. Klein, chief probation officer of the Quincy Court, asserted, "These male batterers look like criminals, act like criminals, and re-abuse like criminals" (Klein 1994, p. 111). The
majority of men in this study who re-abused were not arrested and if arrested were not sentenced
to jail or probation supervision. Another finding of this study with particular relevance for those
who ask, "Why doesn't she leave?" was that many of the victims had either divorced or physically
separated from their abusers – suggesting how little control women have in preventing re-abuse
(p. 113). Klein's study supports earlier critiques of the criminal justice system that has failed to
treat domestic violence as criminal behavior.

For tribal courts and the success of programs such as Cangleska's, additional constraints in
holding offenders accountable are intertwined with the byzantine complexities and intertwining
of tribal, federal and state jurisdictions, some of which date back to the mid-1800s and the
succeeding decades of colonization and enactment of the reservation system. Attorney Traci
Hobson (2006) notes, for example, that tribal courts do not under any circumstances have
jurisdiction over non-Indians (p. 28). This constraint, however, seems to muddy the intent of
the US Federal Violence Against Women Act (US Congress 1994a, 1994b) in its various forms.
This public law provided US$1.6 billion to enhance investigation and prosecution of violent
crimes against women, including pre-trial detention of the accused and imposition of mandatory
restitution by those convicted. In practical terms, it complicates the prospects of a program like
Cangleska in holding offenders accountable, for example, in border towns where non-Indian
men assault Indian women, but in effect, fall between the cracks of accountability – given the
unclear lines of tribal, state, and federal jurisdiction for various crimes (Hobson, pp. 29–31).

The Indigenous Wellness Research Institute

Given that *knowledge* of the past is essential to healing wounds and building peace and promoting health among individuals and nations, the interdisciplinary Indigenous Wellness Research Institute (IWRI) at the University of Washington in Seattle underscores the critical role of collaborative work toward that end. The faculty and staff of IWRI, housed in the School of Social Work, are comprised entirely of American Indians and Alaska Natives. It collaborates with various tribal groups to conduct community-based participatory research focusing on health and wellness among indigenous people (see also Bird *et al.*, 2002).

The IWRI's scholarly publications include, for example, the groundbreaking research of Tessa Evans-Campbell (2006) on interpersonal violence suffered by urban American Indian and Alaska Native women (AIAN) in the largest AIAN population in the United States – 98, 922 in metropolitan New York City. It works with other indigenous groups across the nation, for example, the Indian County Child Trauma Center at the University of Oklahoma, and across continents, such as the International Network of Indigenous Health Knowledge and Development among the Maori in New Zealand. The IWRI also provides a supportive environment for Native students who can feel social isolation among thousands of predominantly White students in a large university. Imbued with the Medicine Wheel philosophy and collaborative principles, this research and learning center offers great promise for supporting the "natural life-supporting power" and healing of indigenous people from the consequences of systematic oppression and abuse by State-sponsored conquerors.

Practice implications for non-indigenous professionals and students

While many practice skills are applicable across various cultural groups, particular issues are paramount in healing work with persons whose trauma from violence and abuse is deeply intertwined with race-based oppression of indigenous people. These include:

- Recognition by mainstream professionals of the importance of facilitating health provision within the Native community itself whenever possible.
- Because Native people may be reluctant to disclose interpersonal abuse or sexual assault to a non-Native professional, assessment of victimization trauma and its sequelae needs to be done at various entry points to the health service system.
- Since alcohol is so prominent as a coping device – minus ready access to health and social services – substance abuse and its intersection with suicidal danger must be prominent in assessment of suicide and assault potential (Bohn, 2003)
- Grief counseling, particularly in Healing Circles facilitated by Native people themselves, should play a prominent role in comprehensive mental health service.
- Advocacy and political action (by mainstream and Native groups) to redress the historic injury done to indigenous people, and the connecting of such action to the counseling process as an aid to moving beyond self-blame and violence (see the Crisis Paradigm in Chapter 13 (Figure 13.1), and US Commission on Civil Rights, 2003).
- Community mobilization for appropriate housing, healthcare, and other primary prevention resources for those at particular risk of abuse and violence.

The communal values characterizing traditional peoples suggest that many of the services provided to indigenous people will emphasize teamwork and collaborative roles, regardless of particular professional identity (see Fong *et al.*, 2006; McGoldrick, & Hardy, 2008). Physicians, nurses, physical therapists, and dental practitioners have pivotal collaborative roles in assessment and treatment of the immediate injuries and chronic pain sustained by violence and accidents often related to substance abuse, while also seeking opportunities for supporting the Native community's role in taking charge of their own healing. The most important specialists for Native survivors are elders, spiritual healers, and others prepared by the Native community to assume primary responsibility in the healing process special to their people. Students of all professions from the Native community can observe and assist as directed by the particular discipline, elder, or spiritual healer; mainstream students from all disciplines can observe and/ or assist as invited or needed on behalf of various survivors.

Learning and student practice situations include:

* Introduction of cross-cultural concepts and values of indigenous cultures early in the curriculum for all students.
* Attendance of community events celebrating Native values and culture.
* Invitation to an elder or Native health professional to address a class.
* A mini-field experience and writing assignment followed by seminar discussion focusing on cross-cultural differences, ethnocentrism, and the health status implications for individual victim/survivors of colonial oppression.
* Required reading of literature citing the particular needs of this group inasmuch as indigenous survivors will be seen in mainstream as well as Native health service agencies.

References

Adams, D., & Cayouette, S. (2002). Emerge: A group education model for abusers. In E. Aldarondo, & F. Mederos (eds.), *Programs for Men Who Batter: Intervention and Prevention Strategies in a Diverse Society*, pp. 4-1–4-23. New York: Civic Research, Inc.

Artichoker, K. (2007). Tribal issues. Unpublished.

Artichoker, K. (2009). Discussion with Lee Ann Hoff, Cangleska, Pine Ridge Reservation.

Bird, M., Bowekaty, M., Burhansstipanov, L., Cochran, P. L., Everingham, P. J., & Suina, M. (2002). *Eliminating Health Disparities*. Santa Cruz, CA: ETR Associates.

Black Elk, N. (2000). *Black Elk Speaks: Being the Life Story of a Holy Man of the Oglala Sioux* (twenty-first-century edn.). Lincoln and London: University of Nebraska Press. (Originally published in 1932 by the John G. Neihardt Trust.)

Bohn, D. K. (2003). Lifetime physical and sexual abuse, substance abuse, depression and suicide attempts among Native American women. *Issues in Mental Health Nursing*, 24, 333–52.

Cummings, N. (2008). Letter to donors: Oglala Kakota College. Kyle, SD.

Deucheneaux, H. (2008). Discussion with Lee Ann Hoff, Cangleska, Pine Ridge Reservation.

Evans-Campbell, T., Lindhorst, T., Huang, B., & Walters, K. L. (2006). Interpersonal violence in the lives of urban American Indian and Alaska Native women: Implications for health, mental health, and help-seeking. *American Journal of Public Health*, 96(8), 1416–22.

Fong, R., McRoy, R., & Ortiz Hendricks, C. (eds.) (2006). *Intersecting Child Welfare, Substance Abuse, and Family Violence: Culturally Competent Approaches*. Alexandria, VA: CSWE Press.

Freire, P. (1989). *Pedagogy of the Oppressed*. New York: Continuum.

Harris, M., *et al.* (1997). The road to freedom: Ending violence against women. *Women's Health Issues*, 7(2), 99–107.

Hobson, T. L. (2006). Criminal jurisdiction in United States Indian country: A practical guide. *Practicing Anthropology*, 28(1), 28–31.

Klein, A (1994). Re-abuse in a population of court-restrained male batterers after two years. Development of a predictive model. Unpublished doctoral dissertation, Northeastern University, Boston.

Leacock, E. (1980). Montagnais women and the Jesuit program for colonization. In M. Etienne, & E. Leacock (eds.), *Women and Colonization*, pp. 25–42. New York: Praeger.

Manson, S., Beals, J., Klein, S., Croy, C., & the AI-SUPERPFP Team (2005). Social epidemiology of trauma among 2 American Indian reservation populations. *American Journal of Public Health*, 95, 851–9.

McGoldrick, M., & Hardy, K. V. (2008). *Re-Visioning Family Therapy: Race, Culture, and Gender in Clinical Practice* (2nd edn.). New York: Guilford.

Older Native Women's Health Project. *Sharing Our Health Circle: The Grandmothers' Health Assessment Report* (1995). Saskatoon, Saskatchewan: Older Native Women's Health Project.

Pizzey, E. (1974). *Scream Quietly or the Neighbors Will Hear You*. Harmondsworth, England: Penguin.

Sacred Circle – Sacred Circle National Resource Center to End Violence Against Native Women (2008). Kyle, SD: Pine Ridge Reservation.

Straus, M. A., Gelles, R. J., & Steinmetz, S. K. (1980). *Behind Closed Doors: Violence in the American Family*. Garden City, NY: Anchor Books.

Thin Elk, Gene. The Red Road Approach. In D. Arbogast (ed.), *Wounded Warriors: A Time for Healing*. Minneapolis: Little Turtle Publications, 1995.

Tjaden, P., & Thoennes, N. (2000). *Full Report on the Prevalence, Incidence and Consequences of Violence against Women*. Washington, DC: National Institutes of Justice Publication NCJ 183781.

US Commission on Civil Rights (2003). *A Quiet Crisis: Federal Funding and Unmet Needs in Indian Country*. Washington, DC: US Commission on Civil Rights.

US Congress (1994a). Violence against Women Act (VAWA). Title IV, secs. 40001–40703. Washington, DC: US Congress.

US Congress (1994b). Violent Crime Control and Law Enforcement Act. HR 3355, Public Law 103–322. Washington, DC: US Congress.

York, G. (1990). *The Dispossessed: Life and Death in Native Canada*. London, UK: Vintage.

9 Torture and trafficking survivors, and abuse of immigrants

Studies of stressful and traumatic life events and experience with anyone who faces a move from secure residence – whether by choice or by force – reveal how migration can threaten physical and mental health, economic security, and our basic human right to shelter and safety from natural events or violent threats to survival. In the case of torture during political strife, and the systematic trafficking of women and adolescents in the sex trade, deprivation of basic needs and fears for survival greatly magnify the stress of ordinary moves from one residence or geographic region to another.

This chapter addresses the extraordinary trauma faced by survivors of torture and human trafficking, and the further abuse endured by migrants displaced during war after arriving in what they presumed was a safe place. It also captures what we have known for sometime about the intersection between gender, race, and class issues as context for this facet of violence and abuse: poor women and girls of color are the predominant victims of trafficking; whole families are displaced by war; men of means (mostly white) are the primary traffickers as well as the clients of women held in sexual and economic bondage to the sex trade. There women suffer cruelty and a combination of crimes that should signal outrage and systematic international attention to stopping these crimes and enforcing human rights standards.

Among abused and exploited immigrants, a similar combination of gender, race, and class status is central to understanding and responding to the degrees of injury inflicted. For example, poor women of color escaping domestic violence and femicide at border crossings between Mexico and the United States try to eke out a living for themselves and their children in a presumed "safe" society, only to encounter abuse, fear of deportation, and financial exploitation in the "host" country to which they fled. Migrants from African countries seeking refuge from political strife find themselves in camps where many are subjected to rape, and most suffer deprivation of the most basic human rights (see Chapter 10).

Interrelated factors affecting immigrants and survivors of torture and trafficking

Even under the best of circumstances, moves to a strange country or continent entail the loss of familiar surroundings, extended family and friends, and fear around confronting many unknowns. But in the case of a forced move, many other questions arise: Will I be safe? How will those foreigners accept me? Will I be able to learn the language so I can get along? Who will help me if things go wrong? What if I want to come back and don't have the money? What if I can't get the right papers and they send me back?

Even if not a survivor of torture or trafficking, these questions are more urgent for some immigrants, as nations tighten their borders and entry rules for people who intend no harm and who are only seeking a job and better life for themselves and their children. Immigrants trying to escape grinding poverty in their own country often face grueling and dangerous hazards at work, while fearing deportation if they complain or report (see Chapter 11). And immigrants to the United States, with its easy access to guns, confront dangers on the streets intermingled with ethnic conflict and stereotypes about immigrants that can quickly dash their dreams of peace and economic security.

In the past few decades, universities and major medical centers in Europe, Canada and the United States have established special service programs for such refugees, and have also conducted studies revealing the serious physical, psychological and social consequences suffered by survivors of torture, genocide, and trafficking (Gozdziak, & MacDonnell, 2007; Jaranson *et al.*, 2004; Marshall *et al.*, 2005; Robertson *et al.*, 2006; Vulliamy, 2005). A study of the mental health status of Cambodian refugees two decades after fleeing the brutal Khmer Rouge regime of the mid-1970s, in which more than two million of their countrymen were killed, revealed evidence of continued post-traumatic stress and that time does not heal all wounds (Hausman, 2007). The United Nations (UN), the World Health Organization (WHO), Amnesty International, the International Criminal Court, and Human Rights Watch are other groups seriously engaged in exposing and stopping these crimes against humanity, and in sponsoring criminal justice and other interventions on behalf of survivors.

Complicating the traumatic consequences of torture and trafficking is that survivors have suffered a combination of physical, sexual, and psychological abuse, as well as economic losses and separation from their families and the supports of everyday life that most immigrants face. The potential for crisis and prolonged suffering is even greater for the following uprooted groups:

- Parents who are forced to leave their children behind.
- Older people – dislocated because of war or disaster and forced out of housing where they have lived all their lives.
- Mentally ill patients with impaired cognitive, social, and economic capacities to take care of themselves.

- Abused women and their children who are forced to leave their homes and even their country to avoid beatings or death.
- Migrant farm workers earning minimum wages and living in sub-standard housing who must move each year in the hope of earning a marginal subsistence.

Globally, many refugees not only have lost family members and property but also face dramatic cultural differences, tripled social burdens, and social isolation. Thousands of teenagers and young people – even in affluent societies – either have no home "safety net," run away from home, or are simply "on the move." Many young people who run away do so because they are physically or sexually abused, or because they have come out as gay, lesbian, bisexual, or transgendered and are wholly rejected by their families. Often they lack housing, food, and money; many are further exploited sexually or feel forced into prostitution for survival; still others succumb to substance abuse (Greene *et al.*, 1997); in extreme cases they are killed by police for petty stealing and vagrancy. In shanty towns of sprawling cities this frightful scene of abandoned and sexually exploited children is multiplied many times over across continents.

War refugees who are crowded into camps in neighboring countries face similar hazards – unsanitary conditions, indifference, brutality, and even rape by soldiers and officials. As if these prices of civil and ethnic strife were not enough, some refugees face grim prospects for immigration, depending on the racial and political biases of a prospective host country. In the United States, for example, because of immigration quotas negotiated between Congress and the Immigration and Naturalization Service, far fewer African refugees are admitted than are admitted from Asia, Latin America, and Europe. International debates and advocacy continue in an effort to protect refugees who are the most vulnerable and are fleeing from war or persecution (Amnesty International, 2000, p. 21).

There are also groups of people who have been relocated by their own governments. Dramatic historic examples include the 1953 dispatching of 85 Inuit people from northern Quebec to the High Arctic, where their families were wrenched apart and they endured extreme hardship and deprivation (Aubry, 1994) and the creation of racially segregated communities in South Africa (Sparks, 1990). As a result of these government actions, the Inuit and South African Black majority are still seeking justice.

A European study: trafficking of women and adolescents

The London School of Hygiene & Tropical Medicine, with several collaborating European institutions, led a two-year 18-country study of the multiple injuries suffered by women and adolescents trafficked to the European Union (Zimmerman *et al.*, 2003). Seven of the countries (mostly Eastern European) were the origin of trafficking, while 11 were the destination (in Eastern and Western Europe, the Middle East, and Southeast Asia). Of the 23 respondents, all were under age 30, a third of them were under 21, and five were under 18. The consequences of trafficking are similar to those experienced by other victimized groups whose plight is illustrated throughout this book.

This study's aim was focused on damage to the trafficked women's physical, reproductive, and mental health from a combination of abuse cited by women interviewed for the study:

- physical, sexual, and psychological abuse;
- the forced use of drugs and alcohol;
- social restrictions and manipulation;
- economic exploitation and debt bondage;

- legal insecurity;
- abusive working conditions;
- the range of risks confronted by any migrant or marginalized group.

The health needs of the trafficked women were addressed as they occurred during five stages of the trafficking process:

1 *Pre-departure*: factors that influenced the women's decision to migrate and which left them vulnerable to trafficking and exploitation included poverty, single parenthood, membership in a disrupted household, and a history of interpersonal violence.
2 *Travel and transit*: during this stage the women faced risk of arrest, illness, and death from dangerous modes of travel and high risk border crossings, while half of those interviewed had been confined, raped or beaten in transit. The initial trauma they experienced triggered survival responses including extreme anxiety that can inhibit memory and recall for providing later criminal investigation. Trafficked women may blame themselves for not having recognized early on the deceptive and violent recruitment tactics used on them by traffickers, and for failing to escape – all affecting their self-esteem and ability to trust others.
3 *Destination*: this is the stage during which the women experienced the most extreme violence and psychological stress. The violence was pervasive and affected every aspect of the person's life:
   - *Physical health impact*: the women reported broken bones, high fevers, gastrointestinal problems, pelvic pain, complications of abortions, deprivation of food and human contact.
   - *Sexual and reproductive health*: all the interviewed women reported sexual abuse, including forced anal, oral, and unprotected sex, and gang rape; had no knowledge of where to receive medical care; and were forced to be sex workers with most having 10–25 clients per night, and some as many as 40 or 50 per night.
   - *Mental health*: the traffickers used psychological control tactics such as threats, lies, and deception to keep the women intimidated, dependent, and uncertain of their future if they did not obey the traffickers' demands. The most common mental health symptoms were crying more than usual, feeling tired, unhappy and sad, and permanently damaged – a sense of "spoiled identity."
   - *Substance abuse and misuse*: the women were forced to use drugs and alcohol with a goal of taking on more clients or performing acts they would otherwise find too risky. Some women used drugs, alcohol, and cigarettes as a coping device.
   - *Social well-being*: some of women were physically confined and under regular surveillance, while all were restricted in their movement, time, and activities, and the majority had no contact with family.
   - *Economic and legal security*: women were subjected to financial arrangements that involved serving more clients and more risk, while keeping very little of their earnings and thus severely limiting their capacity for maintaining hygiene and basic health measures. Few of the women had possession of their identity papers, and all felt insecure about their immigration status and legal rights, thus leaving them hesitant to seek out and use health and other services.
   - *Occupational and environmental health*: nearly all the women described their seven-day-a-week working conditions as "bad" or "terrible" including being forced to perform acts dangerous to their health and sleeping in the same place they worked.

Together, these damaging experiences in the destination stage of trafficking presented the extreme limitations of the women's access to needed health services (discussed further in the "Specialized services" section below).

4   *Detention, deportation, and criminal evidence*: findings from this stage of the trafficking process are based primarily on interviews with law enforcement officials and several service providers. Only one of the women viewed herself as the victim of a crime, while most trafficked women do not view law enforcement officials as a source of assistance. And indeed, these officials in the UK, Italy, and Ukraine noted their lack of victim-sensitive procedures on behalf of trafficked women – not unlike findings in the Portugal study of sexual assault (Maria, 2004; see Chapter 6). Service providers and police suggested a "reflection period" to precede criminal investigations of trafficking in order to foster victims' participation in the proceedings, and avert the significant toll on physical and mental health exacted by the experience of testifying.

5   *Integration and re-integration*: the positive or negative effects on trafficked women during this stage were found to be directly related to the amount and quality of support received. Study findings revealed that only the smallest minority of trafficked women received the physical and psychological support needed. Also, while many suffered serious and enduring physical and mental health complications, they do not fit the image of a "destroyed victim" – underscoring a major finding of work with traumatized victims of all sorts: a human capacity for resilience, the centrality of support and needed services, holding perpetrators accountable, and the ability to move beyond a life-time identity as "victim" as illustrated in Figure 2.1, the Downward Spiral (see Chapter 2).

Case example: a torture victim seeking asylum

Rose, age 30, is a refugee in the United States from an African country rife with internal political strife. She was married, had two children, ages 5 and 8, and was pregnant with a third child when the first of several violent episodes ensued. Rose worked as an elementary school teacher, while her husband Joseph, age 34, held a mid-level administrative position in the government office of social services. They lived in a modest home that they shared with Rose's widowed father.

Without notice, Joseph was fired from his job. He and Rose concluded that the firing occurred because he was on the "wrong side" of the current ruling political establishment. One evening three thugs forced their way into their house, brutally beat Joseph, and demanded that Rose have sex with her father. Upon refusal to do so, she was also beaten up and put in jail. Both children were witnesses to this brutality. In jail, Rose was gang raped and suffered a miscarriage of her child. Upon release from jail she learned that her husband had died of bleeding from his wounds. She went with her children to live with her in-laws. The same team of thugs found her there and raped her 65-year-old mother-in-law in the presence of her children. Through a friend of her murdered husband, Rose reached the US Embassy where she was granted a visa and political asylum status for travel to the United States. She was not allowed, however, to bring her children with her.

Her plan was to stay with a friend of her husband's friend who had helped her obtain the visa. Upon arrival in the large American city she directed the taxi driver to take her to the house of the friend's friend. Instead of doing so, the driver took her to his own house where he raped her. Rose finally found help in an agency specializing in settlement and services for refugees and asylum seekers. There she received counseling and legal assistance in processing her papers for political asylum in the United States. She is very concerned to keep her identity and address secret, as she believes the political "enemies" and thugs responsible for her husband's death and the other brutal crimes against her and her extended family will try to find her in the US and wreak still more harm. She also fears for the safety of her children, although she trusts her extended family members to care for and protect them insofar as they are able.

Key concepts and practice implications

Most survivors of torture and trafficking require specialized services by sensitive and informed providers. But just as often they may appear in ordinary health and social service agencies without divulging the truth of their situation; or providers caring for them may not be prepared to deal with medical needs originating from their torture experience and therefore complexly related to sociopolitical factors across continents.

Universal human rights, greed, and criminal economic gain

Health and social service professionals have long known the correlates of poverty, race, and gender discrimination with the health status of people they serve. But successful integration of these factors in service planning for survivors demands deep awareness of the human rights issues underpinning the complex health, social, and legal issues faced by migrants and the victims of criminal trafficking of women and adolescents. The slavery-like exploitation of trafficked women and girls is "one of the world's fastest growing crimes and most significant human rights violations" (WHO, 2003, p. 1). This necessitates looking beyond the immediate psychological symptoms presented by survivors in primary care and other social service agencies to recognize the roots of the survivors' problems in greed, sexism, and the satisfaction of unbridled male sexual drive as the chief motivations for the atrocities wreaked against trafficked women and adolescents.

Global politics and economic policies in the post-colonial era have resulted in glaring in-equalities based on race, gender and ethnicity, and international tensions associated with mass migration of indigenous populations toward societies which historically have known economic and political privilege. These policies have also aided and abetted the work of trafficking perpetrators in obtaining money by deceit and criminal means from unwitting, innocent and usually poor women and girls. These survivors share many characteristics of those from other circumstances, (for example, domestic violence and sexual assault in dating relationships) such as shame, self-blame, and skepticism about would-be helpers. The next section summarizes the WHO (2003) guiding principles identified from the multi-country London School of Hygiene & Tropical Medicine study (Zimmerman *et al.*, 2003) for interviewing survivors of trafficking. These principles apply broadly to health and social service providers working with other survivors as well.

Interviewing survivors of trafficking: WHO recommendations

Research and clinical experience in the past few decades with survivors of domestic violence, sexual assault, and war trauma reveal characteristics also common among the survivors addressed in this and other chapters. Most prominent are fear, self-blame, and the desire to shed a "victim" identity despite their harrowing situation (see Hoff *et al.*, 2009, Chapters 11 and 13).

The cautions of would-be helpers or rescuers are also similar to what was learned from early work with battered women who had encountered this kind of question from lay persons and some professionals alike: "Why don't you leave?" – a question signifying major ignorance or misunderstanding of the women's situation, for example, there could be threats to find and kill her if she leaves; she might have nowhere to go and have only limited means to support herself and her children. As one abused woman noted about why she did not share her plight with fellow-nursing staff: "I used to come in [to my hospital job] with bruises and they [the nurses] would talk about it: 'How can a woman be so stupid and stay with a guy like that?' .... I couldn't have been bothered talking to any of them about my situation. But I couldn't help seeing how the doctors would put them down and they stood there and took it" (Hoff, 1990, p. 105; see also Chapter 11). One plausible explanation of this and similar revelations from abused women is that some health professionals (and students) are themselves survivors of abuse and violence from which they have not healed – put another way, they are *wounded healers*, who may be shutting down in self-protection when encountering horrendous traumas in their clients; another explanation may be burnout and vicarious traumatization, as discussed in Chapter 12.

For women and adolescents who have been trafficked, their cruelly constrained circumstances are exponentially more complex. Here, then, the WHO (2003) interviewing recommendations from the Zimmerman *et al.* (2003) study of trafficking are summarized with this twofold understanding: 1) such interviewing is the role of specialized and experienced professionals in mental health, social, and legal services designed *explicitly* for survivors of torture and trafficking (see the "Specialized services" below and the online resources in Part IV); 2) survivors of bondage and torture situations who present in general healthcare agencies for their medical problems may have *no intention* of disclosing the likely and extraordinary source of their current health issues, out of fear, shame, etc., as already noted. Health and social service providers in primary care and front-line crisis work must therefore be generally knowledgeable about the specialized services for such patients in order to make safe and trusted referrals for further care (Hoff, & Morgan, in press). In communities where such specialty services are not available, informed and experienced mental health professionals should nevertheless be consulted for appropriate service, as should the full WHO document for further information about how to proceed in the best interests of such client survivors.

For ethical and safe interviewing of women who have been trafficked, WHO researchers (WHO 2003, pp. 2–27) offer Ten Guiding Principles – whether a woman is still in the trafficking situation or has left it. These are briefly elaborated here as they apply as well to other survivors in high risk situations:

1 *Do no harm*: this means no interview if it will in any way make the woman's immediate or longer-term situation worse, and assuming that the potential for harm is extreme unless there is explicit evidence to the contrary. For example, the trafficker may have told her he would kill her or her children if she divulges her situation.
2 *Know your subject and carefully assess the risks* before undertaking an interview. Consult as necessary with agencies serving refugees, women's rights, and immigrants.
3 *Prepare referral information – do not make promises that cannot be fulfilled*: this includes accurate knowledge about legal, health, shelter, church groups, and security services offered in the woman's own language, and assistance with referral process. Be certain that any referral sources will be on the same page regarding these principles.
4 *Prepare interpreters and co-workers*, including assessing the risks and benefits of such services, for example, a trafficker or pimp might pose as a relative.
5 *Ensure anonymity and confidentiality* through the entire process in accordance with the woman's wishes about making details of her case public or in academic publications.
6 *Obtain informed consent*, and all that this implies regarding rights about refusal to answer questions and how the information will be used. Academic and other researchers are

reliable sources for obtaining informed consent meeting ethical standards, as required, for example, by the US National Institutes for Health (as noted in Chapter 2).

7   *Listen to and respect a woman's assessment of her situation and risks to safety.* As in other instances of abuse and violence, each woman's concerns and decisions about her plight may be different from how others might view them, and if she is not ready for outside intervention for whatever reasons or risks, her choices must be respected. It is very important to pay very careful attention to what the client says around readiness to disclose feelings and memories about the abuse that she has learned to contain. This involves balancing help from counselors in the healing process with the client's self-regulation strengths. As one battered woman in a high risk domestic situation stated: "I had to practice how to leave." Regarding long-term recovery, it is empowering for a traumatized person to take credit for the decision to leave not only the risky situation but also the identity as a "victim." Put another way, we should offer information and support, but refrain from telling a woman what to do, and contain any out-sized "rescue" fantasies (see Chapter 12). This principle may also evoke attention to the "Stockholm syndrome": when released from a hostage situation, some survivors expressed gratitude to the hostage-takers for NOT killing them.

8   *Do not re-traumatize a woman* by provoking an emotionally charged response that may push her to relive the ordeal she has been through. Respect cultural differences that may include spoken or unspoken rules about sharing traumatic or humiliating experiences. "Catharsis" as used in Western psychoanalytic theory is not universally applicable (see Madrigal, 2005, regarding risks for victims as well as providers in pressing people to "talk about it in order to heal" if cultural values proscribe such divulging, or in the case of combat veterans who feel comfortable sharing only with fellow veterans; see also Hoff *et al.*, 2009, Chapter 13). In the case of a tortured person's seeking asylum, counselors can use asylum evaluations to learn about traumatic past experiences, offer empathetic support, and refrain from pressing the client to retell his or her story.

9   *Be prepared for emergency intervention* if and when a woman asks for urgent or immediate help. This includes appropriate and reliable linkages to professional emergency medical, legal, and other crisis responders, plus follow-up after emergency intervention.

10 *Put information collected to good use.* This includes engaging with a woman in a neutral way about how others in her situation might benefit from sharing her plight, and the value of such information to health, social service, and legal professionals concerned with ending trafficking, torture and other violations of basic human rights.

Practice implications

Services for those women who are out of the trafficking situation and into the integration and re-integration process commonly fall into three stages: (1) crisis intervention and meeting practical needs; (2) meeting medical and psychological needs stemming from the physical, sexual, and psychological abuse, and setting personal and tangible goals based on professional assessment and active collaboration with the trafficked woman; (3) recognizing and planning with the woman for longer-term mental health issues and a future free of terror and abuse (Zimmerman *et al.* 2003, pp. 6–7 and see Chapter 3 in this book).

Health and mental health providers offering support and specialized services to survivors of torture and trafficking of women, while attending to their own physical and psychological health in this poignant field of work (see Chapter 12), may find solace in these words from noted sociologist C. Wright Mills (already cited in Chapter 2 as a theoretical underpinning of this book, and addressed further in Chapter 12): "It is the political task of the social scientist – as of any liberal educator – continually to translate personal troubles into public issues, and public issues into the terms of their human meaning for a variety of individuals" (1959, p. 187).

Translated at a practical level to front-line workers and every professional and student of health and social services, this wisdom of a renowned social scientist suggests the following for contemporary practitioners: while extremely busy and time-constrained, and perhaps physically and psychologically exhausted from dealing with the enormity of suffering, pain, and sorrow of our clients, we should try to reserve a few minutes each day to *reflect on this question*: why does violence against women continue apparently unabated? After decades of UN- and Member State-enacted platforms of action at international conferences on the rights of women, strategic plans to end violence against women, publication of atrocities revealed by WHO-sponsored research, numerous NGOs, and the studies cited in this book – why does such violence, including rape as "spoils of war" continue apace in the twenty-first century? A plausible answer to this question lies with all people of goodwill. Only concerned and outraged citizens of the world, and educated professionals confronted with the enormous price paid by victims of such carefully planned violence and exploitation of women and children, may be in a position to organize and make a difference to stop such human rights atrocities.

Case example: an immigrant abused by family and the mental health system

Leela is a 31-year-old woman who emigrated from an Asian country with her extended family twelve years ago, two years before her marriage. She was married for eight years and has a son, Ashok, age five. Ashok witnessed his father's violence and is now in the care of his maternal grandparents since Leela's psychiatric hospitalization experience three years ago following beating episodes by her husband over several years. Divorce is very much frowned on in Leela's culture, and in her very tight-knit family, even when there is violence. Leela hoped though, that if she got an education and some financial independence she might at least succeed in getting away from her violent husband since she was unable to divorce him. Thus Leela started taking evening classes toward a social work degree at a local university. On one occasion following a beating, Leela confided in a professor, also an immigrant from the same country, teaching a class in social welfare. "He told me, 'By all means don't go to a White social worker.' I was really stunned and said, 'I'm really surprised to hear a comment like that from you.' And he said to me, 'You don't understand how people look at us.' And he was trying to encourage me to keep it within the family. He also said that he was giving a good example [of keeping things within the immigrant community]: 'Just look at my situation, my wife started working and I go home and I'm all alone.'"

As the beatings escalated, Leela's isolation also deepened. Once after a beating she went to a hospital emergency department, but did not get the help she needed. So she left her husband and went back to her family home. "I thought I would go down the road of psychologists because they don't really have as much power ... like they'll help you if you have problems emotionally but they can't give you a prescription and can't have you admitted on their word, because psychiatrists have a lot of power." But after the psychologist fell asleep on her, Leela said: "To heck with it, I'll just buy some books, I'll read, what's good for me I'll take, what's bad for me I'll leave and that's it, because what else do you do?"

Describing her admission to a psychiatric ward, Leela said: "My family brought the police on me. I was cooking for them, cleaning for them and I was acting normal listening to all those religious things. At least they were educated so they are afraid to say so, but the more religious the family the more they think you're crazy, the more they think you are possessed by the devil and I don't know what else." Leela's family called her sister from Chicago to help them get Leela in the psychiatric hospital. During an apparently normal family evening, Leela's mother became ill and Leela tried to call the doctor. "My sister bangs the phone down because she's scared .... She's told all these doctors that '[Leela's] crazy and you have to put her in the hospital,' so she's ashamed, because here I am calling the doctor for my mother like anybody would."

Leela said that after several years of abuse from her husband and family, "I started getting messages from the TV, which is my mind working on me, first saying all the nice things about me and then saying, 'Yes, of course something happened,' and then they started saying 'You are no good .... Everything is so bad about you,' – that I was no good and I had better die. And I was scared. So I wrote to my sister 'Please help me. I am getting messages from the TV that I should kill myself.' But that is the proof that they needed. So the Justice of the Peace said: 'I think you should go to the hospital.'" Leela said that though the physical abuse from her husband "became tenfold bad, it was a lot more psychological, because every time he did it he would say 'She is imagining, she's hallucinating.' How can I hallucinate beatings?"

Asked how she explained the TV messages to herself, Leela said: "Somebody must be doing some investigation of me, how else would they know? But then later on, these two kind feminist ladies explained to me when you are under too much pressure your mind confuses you and I understand all that. After that initial thing, I had never seen things, I had never got messages from nowhere but of course my mind has been worked on now, it has been screwed up so I do get paranoid now and then ... paranoid in the way that I am scared .... Why is that person maybe asking me that such and such a thing happened? But then I straighten myself out .... How do I straighten myself out? I just ask them." Leela said that her "mind playing games" on her with the TV messages "happened only for a week or two, that's the only time it ever happened .... It can be cured because when it happens to children it's because they are living in an unbearable situation and they start imagining things, but they are not crazy. Yeah, it's the same thing that happened to me. There were some compassionate people who explained things to me and gave me some compassion, and I was okay. I was lucky enough that I had gone to the Women's Career Centre and the lady said one thing is once you are on medications your brain doesn't work, you can't talk, your body has no energy. Whatever the drug was I told the psychiatrist, and I even told my family and the police: 'You kill the soul and you are making the body live. This is what they do to all the psychiatric patients, they kill the soul. And I said, you will kill me inside if you give me drugs, because I tell you I don't want it .... See they know, and still they give you drugs. And this was the reason why they took me off that medication. If they hadn't taken me off that medication I wouldn't have talked to that lady .... She was willing to listen to my story. And caring and listening from a stranger is enough for you."

Key concepts and practice implications

In the case of Leela and her family, Leela's visible immigrant minority status renders her doubly vulnerable to the crises and psychological aftermath of violent abuse. Major issues and concepts illustrated by this situation include:

- Minority status leaves people vulnerable, but "visible immigrant" minority status taps into deep-seated racial bias. Unlike immigrants of the same racial group, it is not possible for visible immigrant people to "pass" as would-be members of mainstream culture. As a result, the social isolation experienced by most visible immigrant groups is exacerbated. And if they report abuse, they may be alienated within their own community.

- Current international data reveal attention to victimization and/or the threat of violence as a consideration for refugee status. Health professionals need awareness of these policy issues in relation to advocacy on behalf of abused immigrant minority persons.
- Responses to and interpretations of stress such as Leela's vary cross-culturally. Such cross-cultural variation cannot be used to obscure basic human rights of freedom from violence and abuse. The concept of cultural relativism vs. universally recognized principles of behavior, regardless of culture, is central to understanding situations like Leela's (see Chapter 2). In other words, when Leela's family members say "But he's your husband," (see below) implying she must tolerate his abuse, the health provider's response must include recognition of Leela's basic human right to freedom from violence regardless of cultural variation in respecting this right. Nor should a psychiatric history, including hallucinations, be used to mitigate or obscure this right.
- The primarily Western model of responding to both medical and psychosocial problems with drugs appears in Leela's case to be particularly objectionable, since most traditional societies have a long-standing and successful record of non-medical healing approaches to psychosocial problems. Thus, while numerous psychiatric survivors cite the abuse they have received through over-use of drugs, immigrant minority women were the most poignant in their objection to what, as Leela noted, was a means of "killing the soul."
- The psychiatric concept of paranoia must be carefully distinguished from the reality-based fears of many battered women that someone is "out to get them." Labeling theory clarifies the double jeopardy of any victimized person perceived as "crazy." Language barriers or differences might also result in the misapplication of psychiatric labels (see Hoff *et al.*, 2009, Chapter 3).
- While a psychiatric diagnosis can serve a purpose in treatment plans, it should not become a tool to discredit a person's disclosure of abuse. The diagnosis of "borderline personality disorder," can be particularly hazardous for survivors of abuse.
- Mental health legislation which authorizes involuntary psychiatric containment needs careful examination and monitoring for possible abuse or misapplication. The individual, family, and system abuse of Leela affects not only her mental health, but also that of her child Ashok.

Clearly, Leela had learned to handle the psychological aftermath of her abuse. Apparently she had also adjusted to independent community living following the "hallucinatory" or delusional episode with the TV. Asked about her current family situation she said: "Because I left my husband he was out of the picture. But it was my family who continued the abuse and now they are so ashamed. So now my mother keeps saying, 'But he was your husband, but he was your husband.' And now I say 'Yes he was but you people continued,' and they don't want to hear that. My family would see me beaten up by my husband and my older brother would say to me, 'Yeah, well you know kid, I know the way you are.' More or less, like you know, you deserve a beating once in a while. My brother and I needless to say do not communicate very often any more."

Values and diversity issues

The fact that Leela's son was in the care of his grandparents during her bouts of psychiatric hospitalization points to the strong value in Leela's culture that assumes the extended family's responsibility for children. This value is more common in non-Western societies.

The attitudinal stance revealing belief in cultural relativism is central to understanding women like Leela, her family, and related situations. When it comes to the abuse of women, many are still willing to use "culture" as an excuse to look the other way, rather than recognizing abuse as a universal human rights violation, regardless of the cultural group in which it occurs. Another value revealed in this situation is the influence of racism and its contribution to the social isolation felt by many immigrant and Native groups: "You don't understand how people look at us." While Leela saw her professor's advice not to talk to a White social worker as misguided, nevertheless caregivers must recognize the origin of his fear and advice in his probable experience of racist attitudes in mainstream culture.

Practice implications and interdisciplinary applications

Besides the clinical skills needed for any victimized person, this and related situations among visible minority clients reveal the need for:

- institutional staffing patterns that reflect the composition and values of the community served;
- enhanced skills in listening to people of another language group;
- language ability or accessibility to translator services;
- crisis assessment and intervention as a strategy to *prevent* the kind of cognitive disturbance appearing after years of unalleviated stress from spouse and familial abuse;
- advocacy to protect people like Leela from inappropriate application of mental health laws;
- community organization and networking skills to increase accessibility and appropriateness of service for diverse cultural groups;
- applying culturally-specific interventions such as the Medicine Wheel approach to dealing with violence as advocated by the Ojibwa and Sioux Nations (see Chapter 8).

The interdisciplinary/generalist role in this situation underscores the need for awareness by *all health and mental health providers* of the special needs of disadvantaged groups. Also, vigilance is needed to avoid cultural relativism and interpreting cross-cultural differences in a narrow psychopathological framework (see Chapter 2). *Specialists* here include mental health professionals prepared not only to assess and treat persons with psychopathological disturbances (i.e. clinical psychologists, clinical social workers, occupational therapists, psychiatric nursing specialists, psychiatrists) but who do so with knowledge of how the victimization experience can result in psychopathological disturbances, and with sensitivity to gender and cultural issues in psychotherapy. Other specialists are community groups with expertise in the problems and issues of visible minority and/or immigrant groups, and psychiatric survivors. *Students* would assist with and participate in the above generalist roles; graduate students also participate in specialist roles.

As with the very complex examples above, analysis, teaching, and practice about these situations address several categories: global facets of violence against women and children; cross-cultural, legal, and diversity issues; mental health policy and practice with survivors; family and community support resources.

Specialized services for immigrants and survivors of torture and trafficking

The actual and potential crises of immigrants and refugees have become more visible as ethnic conflict and international tensions have grown. People persecuted or sought out for their public protest against injustice seek refuge and political asylum in friendly countries with greater frequency. Cooperation between private and public agencies on behalf of these people is paramount to avoid unnecessary distress and crisis. In addition to legal, housing, language, and immediate survival issues, refugees experience the psychological pain of losing their home-land. No matter how they may have been treated, most people have a strong attachment to their country of birth. Whether this bond is broken voluntarily or by torture or threat to life, refugees need an opportunity to heal their wounds, mourn their losses, and find substitutes for what was left behind. They also should not have to endure prolonged detention in sub-standard facilities which the UN defines as a denial of basic human rights. Following are some examples of agencies dedicated to refugee services, healing, and protection of human rights.

Travelers Aid Family Services

This US agency began as the Travelers Aid Society and has been doing crisis intervention work with people in transit for years. It arose from nineteenth-century social movements formed to help immigrant single women and families find housing and jobs. Caseworkers of this agency see travelers at the peak of their distress. The traveler who calls the agency is often without money or resources and is fearful in a strange city. In extreme cases, the person may have been beaten, robbed, or raped in country of origin or the host country. The agency caseworker gets in touch with relatives; ensures emergency medical services, food, and emergency housing; provides travel money; and ensures the traveler a safe trip home. A close working relationship with 24-hour crisis services has bolstered the agency's preventative and advocacy goals on behalf of families at risk. The relative isolation of this agency often results in its staff handling suicidal or emotionally upset travelers by themselves, without the support of crisis specialists who should be available. Similar agencies are available across cultures.

International Institutes

International Institutes and special refugee groups are pivotal in helping people in crisis related to immigration. In the US, the International Institutes' unique contribution is crisis work with refugees and immigrants who do not know the local language. Inability to speak a country's language can be the source of acute distress related to housing, employment, health, welfare, and legal matters. Institute workers, most of whom speak several languages, assist refugees, asylum seekers, and other immigrants in these essential life areas. The International Institute of Boston serves over 7,000 immigrants and refugees annually. Its major goal is to promote self-sufficiency through legal services, resettlement and social services, and workforce development (including educational service, language training, employment assistance, and a lending and financial literacy service).

There is an International Institute or comparable agency in nearly all major metropolitan areas of the United States, Canada, and Western European countries, where most refugees and immigrants first settle. Health and social service personnel can refer immigrants who are unaware of this service on arrival. The language crisis is so acute for some immigrants that they may be mistakenly judged psychotic and taken to a mental hospital, or they may have to rely inappropriately on their own children for translation. Intervention by a multilingual person is a critical part of care in such cases. Unfortunately, this important social service agency may have low visibility in the community and may not always be linked adequately with 24-hour crisis services. Such linkages may become routine as health and crisis services become more comprehensive and cosmopolitan.

Medical and social services for torture survivors

In major cities in Canada, the United States, and Western European countries there are centers dedicated specifically to the needs of refugees and survivors of torture. Some of these (in Toronto, Minneapolis, Boston) are affiliated with university medical centers. For example, the Boston Center for Refugee Health and Human Rights (BCRHHR) functions within Boston Medical Center that is affiliated with Boston University's Schools of Medicine, Dental and Public Health, and Law. Its mission is to "provide comprehensive healthcare for refugees and survivors of torture, to educate and train agencies and professionals who serve these communities, to advocate for the promotion of health and human rights in the United States and worldwide, and to conduct clinical, epidemiological, and legal research for the better understanding and promotion of health and quality of life for survivors of torture and related trauma." The BCRHHR serves survivors of persecution and human rights violations looking for a new life from dozens of countries through the gateway of Boston. Key emphasis is on holistic care and healing from the damaging physical and psychological effects of torture. Here is a citation from their informational brochure: "As our patients feel better, learn English, attain asylum, go to work, are reunited with their families, are accepted to university, and extend kindness to others after being brutally tortured, we witness the victory of the human spirit over despair and brutality. This inspires our work." (See online resources).

References

Amnesty International (2000). Pass the Refugee Protection Act. *Amnesty International*, Summer, 21.

Aubry, J. (1994, March 5). Exiled to a forsaken place. *Ottawa Citizen*, p. 1, B1–6.

Gozdziak, E. M., & MacDonnell, M. (2007). Closing the gaps: The need to improve identification and services to child victims of trafficking. *Human Organization*, 66(2), 171–84.

Greene, J. M., Ennett, S. T., & Ringwalt, C. L. (1997). Substance use among runaway and homeless youth in three national samples. *American Journal of Public Health*, 87(2), 229–35.

Hausman, K. (2005). Moving to new homeland doesn't ease trauma. *Psychiatric News*, 40(17), 17.

Hoff, L. A. (1990). *Battered Women as Survivors*. London: Routledge.

Hoff, L. A. (1994). *Violence Issues: An Interdisciplinary Curriculum Guide for Health Professionals*. Ottawa: Health Programs and Services Branch.

Hoff, L. A., Hallisey, B. J., & Hoff, M. (2009). *People in Crisis: Clinical and Diversity Perspectives* (6th edn.). New York: Routledge.

Hoff, L. A., & Morgan, B. (in press). *Psychiatric and Mental Health Essentials in Primary Care*.

Jaranson, J. M., *et al.* (2004). Somali and Oromo refugees: Correlates of torture and trauma history. *American Journal of Public Health*, 94(4), 591–8.

Madrigal, K. B. (2005). Treatment beliefs of combat trauma survivors with posttraumatic stress disorder. *Practicing Anthropology*, 27(3), 37–40.

Maria, S. (2004). *Mulheres Sobreviventes de Violacao*. Lisboa: Livros Horizontes.

Marshall, G. N., *et al.* (2005). Mental health of Cambodian refugees 2 decades after resettlement in the United States. *Journal of the American Medical Association*, 294(5), 571–9.

Mills, C. W. (1959). *The Sociological Imagination*. London: Oxford University Press.

Robertson, C. L., *et al.* (2006). Somali and Oromo refugee women: Trauma and associated factors. *Journal of Advanced Nursing*, 56(6), 577–87.

Sparks, A. (1990). *The Mind of South Africa: The Story of the Rise and Fall of Apartheid*. London: Mandarin.

Vulliamy, E. (2005). Streets of despair. *Amnesty International*, Winter, 10–16.

WHO – World Health Organization (2003). *WHO Ethical and Safety Recommendations for Interviewing Trafficked Women*. Geneva: WHO.

Zimmerman, C. *et al.* (2003). *The Health Risks and Consequences of Trafficking in Women and Adolescents.* London: London School of Hygiene & Tropical Medicine.

10 Perpetrators of abuse and violence

Individuals and states

Magueye Seck and Lee Ann Hoff

- Views on battering and offenders
- The scope of the problem
- Emerge: a treatment and group education program for batterers

  — History
  — Philosophy
  — Ability and motivation for change
  — Program approach
  — Collaboration and contact with battered women's programs

- Male violence and alcohol abuse – an "excuse" or a context?
- Training for nonviolence and abusers' resistance
- Primary, secondary, and tertiary prevention from the perspective of perpetrators
- International and multicultural perspectives

  — Cross-cultural field approaches to male violence issues
  — Botswana: healthcare workers' views regarding violence
  — Cuba: Domestic violence policies regarding patriarchal ownership and control
  — Senegal and Ghana: Violence and health providers' role in refugee camps

- The role of social institutions in curbing violence

  — The O. J. Simpson case: an example of race, class and gender issues in domestic violence
  — South Africa: violence cannot be the solution

  > Whereas recognition of the inherent dignity and of the equal and inalienable rights of all members of the human family is the foundation of freedom, justice and peace in the world ...
  >
  > (Universal Declaration of Human Rights, Preamble)

Studies about the perpetrators of abuse and violence and their impact on women, children, refugees, and the assailants themselves, have recently taken center stage as a public issue of worldwide concern. Important questions regarding the perpetrators of abuse and violence are: What is it about a society that increases or decreases the likelihood of violence and abusive behaviors? How does social life shape, encourage, or discourages violence? Why is it critical to analyze health policies relating to perpetrators of violence and their victims? Why do some women respond to abuse with retaliatory violence?

This chapter examines the issues of perpetrators of abuse and violence from a multidisciplinary and international perspective. Using ethnographic examples of various types of violence, it addresses issues of interpersonal and institutional violence in a multicultural context, with a focus on increasing the knowledge of health professionals on issues of interpersonal and institution-based violence. The programs that are now being developed and implemented for dealing with perpetrators of violence are possible because of the evolution in thinking about how we view these offenders. The most successful programs combine services for individual offenders with community intervention and criminal justice efforts. Throughout this chapter we attempt to come to grips with these issues.

Views on battering and offenders

Early work in the violence literature depicted wife battering as the norm in marriage and batterers as incorrigible, with character disorders or a problem with alcohol that excused them from accountability. Gondolf's research (1987) with violent men reveals four types of batterers – sociopathic, antisocial, chronic, and sporadic. Gondolf suggests that sociopathic batterers need continual restraint to stem their violence, whereas those with antisocial behaviors need a variety of coordinated interventions. In a controversial experimental study, Sherman and Berk (1984) found that arrest had the greatest impact on reducing recidivism (repeat battering) as compared with mediation and crisis intervention. Edleson and Tolman (1992, p. 132), citing later studies, note that community intervention such as the Minneapolis Intervention Project *combined with* criminal justice efforts may offer more protection to women. Similar findings have been reported in Canada, despite its aggressive arrest laws (MacLeod, 1989).

This view is supported by Klein's (1994) study of 664 men who were issued civil restraining orders by the Quincy, Massachusetts District Court. Reliance on such orders alone did not prevent more abuse, especially among younger, unmarried abusers with prior criminal records who also abused alcohol. Klein, chief probation officer of the Quincy Court, asserted that these male batterers looked, acted and re-abused like criminals. As discussed in Chapter 8, this study revealed how little control women have in preventing re-abuse.

Klein's study supports earlier critiques of the criminal justice system that has failed to treat domestic violence as criminal behavior. Newspaper accounts also reveal that restraining orders have not prevented the murders of women. In fact, clinical work with abused women reveals that they are perhaps in greatest danger after filing for a restraining order, particularly in cases in which the woman's partner feels that he owns her and is now confronted with an external force threatening his need to control her. This underscores the need for caution in persuading a woman to seek court protection and for trusting the woman's own judgment of the man's potential for violence and the contextual factors that may inflame him (Hoff *et al.*, 2009, Chapter 11).

The scope of the problem

Only recently have sociology textbooks directly presented the issue of violence to students in the social sciences. For example, typically, incidents of physical abuse from violence, rape, and even attempted murder – involving severe, bitter violence – have been addressed as serious *individual personal* problems. To be defined as a *social* problem, violence must also arouse widespread societal concerns. That is, many people must see the violence as reducing their quality of life and want something to be done about it (Henslin, 2006, p. 128). Violence was one of the first social problems that sociologists studied. Emile Durkheim, the first University professor to be formally identified as a sociologist, examined the murder rates in Paris and the suicide rates in European countries between 1897 and 1904. For Durkheim, communities undergoing rapid social change, which consequently loosen social bonds, causes "anomie" – the feeling of being unconnected and uprooted, and prone to violence. Although it is important to understand the roots of violent behavior and the personality of perpetrators, we also need to critically examine the underlying issues regarding offenders and their treatment, particularly from a health and social service perspective. Healthcare providers, like their criminal justice counterparts, have been struggling to respond to the problems of violence in communities around the world.

Violent and emotionally abusive men come from all socioeconomic, racial, religious, and age groups. One of the most common characteristics among male offenders is that they tend to minimize and deny their violence. According to many experts in this field, it is very embarrassing for some men to discuss their violence, and they purposely avoid talking or even thinking about it (Sonkin, 1985, p. 39). Another characteristic is that they tend to blame their partners for their violence. If they abuse drugs or alcohol, they tend to forget their violence because they were under the influence of the substance. Some clinical work shows that abusive men tend to be dependent on their partner's support, so that the partner is seen as part of them. They often do not have other close relationships (Seck, 1995, p. 4).

Emerge: a treatment and group education program for batterers

Emerge was established in Boston by a group of six men at the request of women who were working in a battered women's program in the Boston area. Since then, at least 1,500 programs for abusive men exist in the United States alone, with growing numbers developing internationally. Because of controversy among some professionals about the principles guiding services for abusive men, we present the Emerge program here for its emphasis on *accountability* and prevention of violence, while recognizing offenders' *individual* problems such as alcohol abuse, but which should not serve as an excuse for abuse of their partners. (The following excerpts are reprinted with permission and minor editing from Adams, & Cayouette, 2002.)

History

Until Emerge's founding in 1977 as the nation's first batterer intervention program, notions of men taking responsibility for their violence remained untested. The initial emphasis of the battered women's movement had been on calling attention to domestic violence, redefining it as a crime against women, and promoting safety and justice for women (Schechter, 1982). But many victim advocates argued that men must join women in this effort, not only to communicate the message that violence against women was a human rights issue of equal importance to men, but also to play a unique role in educating and confronting men who abuse women. Emerge was established at the behest of women who had founded the first battered women's programs in Boston. Hotline staff at Transition House and Respond [shelters for battered women] were receiving an increasing number of calls from batterers; some requesting information about their partner's whereabouts and others requesting help for themselves. Since it was not their mission to work with men, staff from these programs publicized a request for men to establish a program for batterers. Nearly all the ten men who attended the first planning sessions of Emerge were friends or relatives of workers at Transition House and Respond. While most of the founders were social workers or counselors, the others included a teacher, a community organizer, a lawyer and a cab driver.

The founding members of Emerge committed their first 6–12 months to studying the issue of domestic violence as a first step in formulating an intervention program. A review of the literature revealed that while several books and articles had been published which specifically addressed men who batter, nearly all of these put forth theories which mitigated men's responsibility for violence. In "The wifebeater's wife: A study of family interaction", published in 1964, the authors concluded that the majority of the 37 battering men they interviewed were "provoked" or otherwise incited to become violent by "manipulative," "domineering," "irritating," or "sexually frigid" wives (Snell *et al.*, 1964). Three separate articles about batterers published in 1977 all advanced the notion that batterers were not fully responsible for their violence. Faulk (1977) found that the most prevalent type of batterer was a "dependent, passive type," who "characteristically gave a good deal of concern and time trying to please and pacify his wife, who tended to be querulous and demanding." Geller and Walsh (1977) concluded that battering will not stop "unless both partners are involved in counseling." Shainess (1977) asserted that men "lash out from frustration" and typically exhibit "poor ability to tolerate frustration."

By 1979 however, several published articles presented a different view of batterers; one held that men's violence toward women was not provoked or irrational behavior, but was behavior which served as an instrument of *control* (Warrior, 1976; Martin, 1976). In studying actual cases of domestic violence, Dobash and Dobash (1979) concluded that the use of violence against wives is "an attempt to bring about a desired state of affairs .... When a husband attacks his wife he is either chastising her for challenging his authority or for failing to live up to his expectations or attempting to discourage future unacceptable behavior."

While these latter writings were helpful, the most critical sources of information for the founders of Emerge were battered women themselves. Staff from the three existing battered women's programs in Boston encouraged battered women to share their experiences with Emerge – and dozens did so. From this testimony arose an understanding of battering as a *pattern of coercive behavior* that included physical, sexual, psychological, verbal, and economic abuse. Just as compelling as the actual abuse was the "re-victimization" that these women had experienced at the hands of police, courts, medical centers, and social service agencies. It became apparent that by minimizing domestic violence and by discouraging or blaming women who sought help, mainstream institutions often *colluded with batterers to avoid accountability*.

Philosophy

The Emerge philosophy about battering behavior can be summarized as follows:

- Battering is not merely physical violence but a range of coercive behaviors that often consists of physical, sexual, psychological, verbal, and economic abuse. These behaviors serve to undermine the victim's self-esteem and independence.
- Battering is purposeful behavior. Rather than being impulsive, spontaneous, or irrational, battering is intentional behavior that serves to gain and maintain control in relationships and other social interactions. The individual batterer need not be fully conscious that he uses violence to gain control; in fact he may believe that he is not in control and that others are controlling him. Whatever his stated intentions, violence is always an attempt to force the other person to do, or not do, something (Adams, 1989). Except in cases of self-defense or insanity, violence is always a choice made by the person committing the violence.
- Battering is learned behavior. According to social learning theory, behavior is learned in two ways; through modeling and positive reinforcement (Bandura, 1977). Men's behavior, attitudes, and expectations concerning women are most often originally influenced by how

their fathers (or other male caretakers) treated their mothers. These behaviors and attitudes are additionally shaped by male peer pressure as well as by societal messages concerning gender roles and the legitimacy of violence as a means of resolving differences (Adams, 1988). Violence can also be 'positively reinforced' when it enables a person to establish control and dominance in his intimate relationships. While violence also leads to negative outcomes, such as the loss of closeness, some men come to prioritize control over closeness.

• Domestic violence occurs within a social context of male dominance over women in social, familial, institutional and economic spheres. In male/female interpersonal relations, male dominance is shaped by traditional sex roles in which men come to expect subservience and deference from women.

Sexism does not exist by itself, however, but intermeshes with other forms of oppression such as racism, classism, ageism and heterosexism. All of these forms of oppression serve to reinforce hierarchical divisions and to devalue categories of people. Another integral aspect to the social context of domestic violence is the social acceptance of violence as a means to achieve ends. The widespread use of violence in international relations, workplaces, popular media, and in families (e.g. use of physical discipline), make violence and coercion seem normal, natural, and in the case of popular media portrayals, even glamorous.

Ability and motivation for change

We believe that violent men can change, that they all have the ability, and that some have the desire to change their behavior and attitudes toward those they abuse. We believe that these men know how to be non-abusive in most situations, yet choose to be abusive toward their partners and children in situations that benefit themselves in the short term. For the majority of offenders, most of their abuse is focused on their intimate partner and/or children rather than a generalized violent response to everyone in their life.

We believe that batterer intervention programs work best for participants whose violence is primarily intimate partner violence. Many batterers conduct some, if not most, of their non-familial relationships in a respectful manner, which indicates that they already know how to practice respectful treatment of others when they *decide* to. We believe that batterers decide that it is socially acceptable to use abuse and control with their partner and/or children in order to get what they want in the immediate situation. They believe that the short-term gain is more important than the long-term losses they might experience because of the abuse. Batterer intervention programs should therefore challenge batterers' belief systems and offer alternatives to their destructive beliefs. Non-abusive responses are based on the beliefs that abuse of a partner and child are not acceptable, that respect is not predicated on the responses of others, and that the long-term costs of abuse are high to both the abuser and the abused.

While we recognize that most of our clients are externally motivated to seek our services, particularly in the beginning stages, we believe that ultimately each client must develop internal motivation to make any *lasting* changes. We recognize that people are motivated by different factors. Some of these include anxiety, excitement, pleasure and the anticipation of positive experiences, and the memory of a positive or negative experience. Some people believe that pain and negative memories or anticipation are more effective motivators of behavior, and some studies of operant conditioning in laboratory animals seem to bear this out (McMahon, & McMahon, 1982). Many motivational speakers believe that people will do much more to avoid pain than to gain pleasure, if both factors are equally balanced (Robbins, 1991). In contrast, some authors believe that internal motivation comes from methods that are based more on treating people with respect, rather than conditioning them to respond based on fear or pleasure (McGregor, 1960; Perlmuter, & Monty, 1977). In his book, *Punished by Rewards* (1993), Alfie Kohn suggests a new approach to thinking about internally motivated change, since the cultural dialogue has been dominated by the carrot/stick dichotomy.

Kohn suggests that "authentic motivation" occurs in a context of "the *collaboration* that defines the context of work, the *content* of the tasks, and the extent to which people have some *choice* about what they do and how they do it (Kohn, 1993). Emerge's philosophy fits within Kohn's motivational framework since we believe that the alternative to collaborative group work is authoritarian leadership that teaches more abuse. We further believe that the educational content of the groups must resonate with the group members, and be representative of their life challenges, whether or not they choose to act and make positive changes. Until abusive men are presented with the reality that *they* choose their behavior, they will invariably abdicate their responsibility, blame others, and think of themselves as victims.

Batterers who continue to be non-abusive (or in some cases, less abusive) after they leave a program will do so on an ongoing basis because of internal motivation. In other words, they have gone beyond changing because they *have* to, to changing because they *want* to. Those who stop being abusive *only* because they are responding to external controls are in danger of re-abusing. They often do not work on changing the negative thinking or "self-talk" that perpetuates their belief system that they have the right to be abusive. They are merely tolerating behavior that makes them want to abuse until such time that they can once again get away with it. This time will inevitably occur, so to prevent this, we believe that perpetrators of violence must work on changing their belief system which tells them that they are entitled to abuse someone, given the right set of circumstances.

We agree with Kohn's argument that "carrot" approaches to change, even so-called positive approaches, ultimately demean the individual because they assume that a reward actually appeals to the same selfish desire to have others make decisions about how one should act. Kohn sees reward and punishment as opposite sides of the same coin, which ultimately assumes the worst of people and appeals only to their own sense of self-interest, rather than also to their ability to respect others.

We recognize that we cannot change abusers but can only provide information and documentation in a manner that does not jeopardize the safety of victims. By teaching about the effects of abuse, stressing personal responsibility, and helping to identify the elements and benefits of respectful behavior, we can help batterers to *choose* nonviolence, but it will always remain their choice.

A unique aspect of the Emerge model is that it provides opportunities for each group member to practice accountability by discussing his own abusive and controlling behaviors and by receiving feedback from others. Emerge clients are expected to recognize and to critically examine their own patterns of abuse and control. This contrasts with other approaches that only require clients to identify various kinds of abusive behavior in general. When abusive men are merely required to recognize and analyze abusive behavior in *others*, or in the abstract, it does not necessarily lead to recognizing or confronting their *own* abusive behavior. In fact, some simply become better at judging other people's behavior, while continuing to justify or rationalize their own.

In our view, the effectiveness of any approach that promotes personal responsibility and accountability depends on men giving detailed reports of their ongoing interactions with partners and children. It also depends upon their receiving meaningful and constructive feedback about this behavior from fellow group members. Both of these things have to be actively promoted in groups, since abusive men often do not give helpful self-reports or feedback. Without active prompting and/or coaching from group leaders, abusive men tend to give superficial or highly skewed reports of their interactions with their partners. Superficial reports such as "Things were fine; we had no problems this past week" or "We had a few conflicts but nothing serious"; do not give enough information to allow for meaningful feedback from others. Skewed reports such as "She was on my case all week" or "She yelled at me for no reason" are designed to put oneself in the best possible light and one's partner in the worst possible light.

Program approach

Clients are asked to attend Emerge for a minimum of 40 group sessions. The program is divided into two phases: an 8-session First Stage, followed by a Second Stage which clients are expected to attend for at least 32 additional sessions. Group sessions are weekly and of two hours duration.

Approximately 75 percent of Emerge's clients are court-referred and it is a condition of their probation that they attend the minimum 40 sessions and satisfy all other conditions for completion of the program. The remaining 25 percent of Emerge clients are referred by the Massachusetts Department of Social Services and other agencies, or are self-referred. Voluntary clients are also asked to attend a minimum of 40 sessions. Those voluntary clients who state that they don't wish to attend 40 sessions are asked to attend the 8-session First Stage in order to sample the program and make a more informed decision about whether they would benefit from additional time in the program. All clients are told that they must attend at least 40 sessions to be eligible to complete the program, however.

Groups at Emerge are co-facilitated by a male and a female group leader. One advantage of this approach is that abusive men are more likely to exhibit their negative attitudes toward women in the presence of a female group leader. Particularly in the beginning stages of the program, they are more apt to interrupt, challenge or ignore their female group leaders. Previously, when Emerge groups were co-facilitated by men only, it was more difficult to identify their abusive or disrespectful behavior toward women since they less frequently exhibited these behaviors or attitudes toward male leaders and often came across as friendly and eager to learn. Abusive men's more negative responses to female group leaders are helpful since we can call attention to them as they are happening in group. These group behaviors can then be likened to the men's negative actions and attitudes toward their partners. Another advantage of male/female co-facilitation is that it offers a model for male/female cooperation and sharing of leadership. We believe this modeling to be of equal importance to the content of our educational curriculum in terms of what we are teaching our clients. Ideally, this modeling enables clients to observe how men can listen to, share power, solve problems, negotiate time, and communicate with women. Emerge therefore devotes considerable attention, in staff meetings and supervision sessions, to helping group leaders consider how well they are modeling male/female co-leadership (Cayouette, 1996).

Group leaders at Emerge are not required to have professional degrees, since we believe that this condition would limit the pool of otherwise qualified and effective group leaders. All group leaders are required to meet the Massachusetts Certification Standards of having received 24 hours of initial training on batterer interventions, as well as an additional 12 hours of group observation and debriefings. Group leaders must have been free of violence in their personal lives for a minimum of three years (Massachusetts, 1995). Those who have been violent must also have completed a certified batterer intervention program.

To assess abusiveness in the personal lives of job applicants, Emerge requires their consent for checking their criminal record, and asks them to do a self-inventory of abusive and controlling behaviors in their intimate relationships. We do not expect prospective group leaders to have been free of all controlling behaviors but to be aware of these behaviors, take responsibility for them, and be committed to a process of self-examination concerning this. For a personal reference, Emerge also requires group leaders to include their partner, or most recent partner.

Collaboration and contact with battered women's programs

Emerge participates in numerous collaborations and special projects with local battered women's programs. These include preventive education projects aimed at young people, joint trainings of criminal justice, social service and healthcare workers, special initiatives aimed at organizing religious leaders and congregations, and community outreach and education efforts (see the online resources in Part IV for a brief summary of some of these collaborations).

In 1985, the Massachusetts courts started referrals of batterers to Emerge for treatment and education. Also in 1985, about 80 percent of the batterers who came to Emerge for treatment were voluntary clients. Since 1985, Emerge has contracted with local battered women's programs to observe its groups and to provide written feedback, particularly in terms of our potential impact on victims. The state of Massachusetts now requires all certified batterer intervention programs to contract with their local battered women's programs for this kind of group observation and feedback.

By 1987, most states began to enact pro-arrest and prosecution policies regarding perpetrators of domestic violence. Emerge began to expand rapidly during these years as the courts were inundated with domestic abuse cases, and consequently toughening of the laws began to occur. New laws expanded police powers of arrest for domestic violence and created liability for police who failed to protect victims. In 1993, Governor William Weld declared a state of emergency for women in Massachusetts in response to the murders of 28 women and 6 children at the hands of their husbands or boyfriends. Most killers have previously battered their victims.

At the beginning, Emerge provided services to an average of 21 clients per week, compared to 350 clients in 1993. Only 1 percent of the clients who came to Emerge were court-mandated in 1983. By 1993, more than 60 percent of the clients who came to Emerge were court-mandated (Seck, 1995, p. 14). Clients must agree that Emerge would contact their partners (battered women) every eight weeks for a more accurate evaluation and assessment of the batterer's behaviors. These partner contacts are done by battered women's advocates and counselors for Emerge. Also, Emerge does collateral contacts and refers batterers to other services such as alcohol, drugs, gambling rehabilitation, etc. When children are involved in the case, the Department of Social Services will provide child care services, and in many cases collaborate with Emerge and the battered women shelters for the safety of children. Emerge sends a weekly attendance report to the courts, and notifies the courts of any non-compliance by the batterer (see the online resources in Part IV for the rules and details of Emerge intake and assessment procedures).

Male violence and alcohol abuse – an "excuse" or a context?

Worldwide, before the institution of programs such as Emerge, among the general public as well as health professionals there was a common, simplistic, and reductionist "cause and effect" association between alcohol abuse and intimate partner violence. The view (shared even by some victims) was addressed in early sociological work suggesting that alcohol should be interpreted more as an "excuse" to avoid responsibility for violence, rather than as a "cause" of it, as in "I was drunk and didn't know what I was doing" (Gelles, 1974; Hoff, 1990, p. 132).

In an effort to understand the perpetrators of abuse and violence, a study conducted at Emerge compared the differences in behaviors between the batterers who had dual problems (of substance abuse and battering) and those who did not abuse substances (Seck, 1995). The study examined differences within and between the groups. Several issues which are crucial to treatment of violent behaviors were addressed: first, the frequencies of abusive behavior; then, the length of program attendance and the rate of absenteeism during treatment; next, the rate of program completion with regard to compliance with program rules, and group participation.

In addition, the Emerge program supporting this study included important questions such as the real effect of alcohol and drug abuse in the treatment of perpetrators. For example: Do men who abuse alcohol have higher frequencies of abusive behavior while in treatment than men who do not? Do alcohol abusers who batter have poorer attendance and more repeated lateness than batterers who do not abuse alcohol? Are men who abuse alcohol less likely to complete the batterer program? The results indicated that 44 percent of the batterers at Emerge had drinking problems. Alcohol abusers had higher frequencies of abusive behavior. Surprisingly, the non-alcoholic abusers had higher attendance rates than substance abusers only in the first 8 weeks of treatment. Non-alcohol abusers were also more likely to be terminated for absence, although overall they had the longest period of attendance in the program. Last, the findings indicate that although the overall successful completion rate, based on Emerge standards, is low for both groups, the non-alcohol abusers had a higher rate of completion than problem drinkers (Seck, 1995).

Work with men in the Emerge program revealed the importance of coordination between the policies of batterers' programs on the one hand, and substance abuse programs on the other. Such coordination would encourage offenders to take responsibility not only for their overt physical violence, but for all their abusive behaviors, including the abuse of alcohol. However, there are often more complications when victims rationalize the drinking of their perpetrators by saying "He is violent only when he is drunk."

Records of Emerge clients also revealed how some misused the program's attendance policy. An offender may well complete all the required meetings, but continue substance abuse and display abusive attitudes and behaviors against women. This letter sent to the Boston District Court by Emerge documents why one batterer dropped out of the program:

> Mr. John Doe has been participating at the Emerge Program for a year now. He has attended 45 meetings and has been absent from 7. Although he has therefore completed the minimum 44 meetings that Emerge recommends we continue to have concerns about his progress here.
>
> Our concerns focus on Mr Doe's apparent explosiveness at his home. He continues to report frequent occurrences of verbal abuse toward his partner and long periods of refusing to talk to her. This use of silent treatment can often be more frightening to an abused woman than the verbal abuse, because the abuser appears to be building up pressure inside him. We also worry because of his history of alcohol abuse and failure to address it in a substance abuse treatment program .... He also continues to minimize the effects of the fact that he was caught having an extended affair with another woman, and refuses to understand why his partner now no longer trusts him. Additionally, we are concerned that he has been extremely neglectful of the two children he has from two previous relationships, visiting them by his own admission as little as once every three or so months, although they live locally. This to us is hardly evidence of a man who is taking a path towards responsible behavior.
>
> Mr Doe has been a constructive group member when he is present, and has been willing in words to take responsibility for his behavior. I wish these words would translate into more positive change in his abusive behavior on the home front.

All across the United States, new guidelines relating to police and court responses on domestic abuse began to enforce the idea of protecting the victims and increasing accountability for perpetrators. Police are now required to advise victims of their rights, offer them assistance and referral, and arrest the alleged perpetrator if there was probable cause to believe that domestic violence had occurred. Subsequently, many states began implementing a policy called "victimless prosecution" policies in which prosecution of the offender does not depend upon the testimony of the victim. This would significantly reduce the probability of retaliation to victims after they testify against their abusers.

Training for nonviolence and abusers' resistance

Emerge became the leader in training police officers, prosecutors, doctors, nurses, and other professionals (Adams, 2003). Among the experts who led this incredible shift in policies to curb violence against women was Dr David Adams, co-founder of Emerge, who also conducted an in-depth study of imprisoned men who agreed to tell their stories of why they killed their intimate partners (Adams, 2007). His study revealed five types of killers, with considerable overlap among these types: jealous; substance-abusing; materially motivated; suicidal; and career criminal. More than half of the thirty-one murderers interviewed for this study belonged to more than one of these types (p. 35).

Training for nonviolence is one of the most challenging aspects of this work. It is true that counselors in treatment programs for batterers, and counselors in battered women programs generally, understand the principles of nonviolence since it is primarily what they do – preventing violence through communication and education. Dr Adams (2003) describes how Emerge teaches men to identify their "negative self-talk," or internal dialogue, that typically precedes physical or verbal violence (Pence, 2002). Examples of negative self-talk include, jealous thoughts, habitual negative beliefs about one's partner (e.g. "She never gives me credit" or "She is so stupid"), jumping to conclusions (e.g. "There she goes again"), or blaming thoughts (e.g. "She makes me so angry" or "She should do things the way I want her to"). Clients are taught to interrupt these habitual thoughts and to replace them with positive self-talk or more constructive ways of thinking (Hamberger, 2002). Overall, offender programs cite these major goals (Adams, 2003, pp. 6–9):

- Overcoming denial
- Taking responsibility for abuse
- Refraining from abuse
- Learning alternatives to abuse
- Supporting gender equality

 See the online resources in Part IV for various applications of these cognitive behavioral strategies used in programs for offenders.

Primary, secondary, and tertiary prevention from the perspective of perpetrators

Broadly, treatment and re-education programs for offenders illustrate the public health concepts of primary, secondary, and tertiary prevention principles cited in Chapter 3, with a focus on victim/survivors. Applied to perpetrators, prevention strategies might include the following:

Primary prevention

- Teach and model parenting roles that do not perpetuate rigid gender roles of male aggression and female subordination.
- Address bullying in schools which, if ignored, can serve as a foundation for later interpersonal violence.
- Educate both male and female teens on how to recognize *early* the signs of control and abuse in their dating relationships.
- Conduct public education programs on self-protection and non-violent conflict resolution in colleges, work sites, churches, civic and neighborhood groups.

Secondary prevention

The aim here is to address immediate threats and alleviate trauma and pain already present. Emerge, for example, has for many years helped violent men deal with and learn from the "pain" of losing their spouse as a result of violence and being threatened with jail time. For others it means not "looking the other way" about violence. This includes consulting police and specialized violence and abuse hotline services when suspecting a family member or neighbor is either a victim or perpetrator, and learning how to respond without putting oneself in danger by action that might exacerbate a potentially life-threatening situation. If programs for offenders do not exist, it means advocacy to develop one through joint efforts with the police, courts, healthcare agencies, victim/survivors programs, churches, and neighborhood groups through education, partner contact, and collaboration with the probation courts as discussed throughout this chapter.

Tertiary prevention

Since abuse has already occurred and offenders have sincerely engaged in programs aimed at learning non-violent responses to family conflict, the focus here is to assist offenders in a determination not to repeat themselves in a relationship they have managed to salvage by stopping their abusive behavior and/or in a new relationship in which they commit themselves to non-violence – perhaps thanks to a program like Emerge, the courts, and the public which no longer tolerates the tradition of excusing intimate partner violence.

International and multicultural perspectives

Counselors from Emerge have taken their experiences and practice skills from the United States to areas around the world, in Europe, Asia, Africa, and the Caribbean. In an e-mail newsletter, Emerge provides information on ending domestic violence to a national and international audience. (See the Emerge website (http://www.emergedv.com) and Part IV for further information around international collaboration, including Harmony House in Hong Kong which is working to adapt the Emerge model to Chinese culture.) Extensive experience (and some minefields!) in cross-cultural research documents the caution and sensitivity required for successful adaptation of practice models from one culture to another – even when firmly grounded in the principle of universal human rights.

Cross-cultural field approaches to male violence prevention

The valuable insights gained from these qualitative field studies (Seck, 2000, 2002) highlight both the theoretical and practical aspects of the problems of violence as they relate to perpetrators.[1] Field sites included Botswana, South Africa, Senegal, Guinea, Egypt, Ghana, Haiti, Cuba, China, France, Canada, and the United States, which led to greater understanding of both male intimate partner and State-sponsored violence in all their complexities.

A fruitful avenue in this endeavor, especially for avoiding cultural offense or dismissal, was expanding on the concept of *social support* through workshops and seminars in various communities with questions such as: "Where do women and children go when they are victimized by violence in this community?"; "Are there shelters or clinics for battered women and children?"; and "What services for abusive men are available in this community?" Answers to such questions, among others, revealed scenarios illustrated in the following ethnographic examples which reveal commonalities and differences in addressing violence in cross-cultural context.

Botswana: healthcare workers' views regarding violence

A group of four high ranking Botswana healthcare workers learned that the philosophy of programs such as Emerge for abusive men are pro-feminist and emphasize gender equality. Issues of patriarchy, power, authority, coercion, and sexism in communities were stressed in a seminar. Here was a typical reaction: "Do you really believe that you can change the African men with these theories?" one asked, with this follow-up question: "How do you define the African man?" Answer: "Well, getting the men into treatment for behavioral change is something that is hard to imagine in this society – even if they are guilty of violence." Question: "What is the definition of being guilty in this country? If you can find a man guilty in the court of law for abusing his partner, that is a good start which means that there is room for behavioral change if the community demands it." When asked "Is rape a criminal act?" one participant responded: "If proven, yes, but it is very difficult!" The next question was "Why is it difficult?" followed by "There are many women infected with AIDS in this country as a result of rape. And behind the act of raping a virgin some men believe this is a way to find treatment for their ills ... how do you explain this?" Such interchanges strongly suggest that social and medical service providers must take the lead role in redefining and stopping perpetrators, and assume a leading role in redefining rape as a criminal act.

Since there is no universally accepted definition of rape, the African Commission on Human and Peoples' Rights is arguably the most important regional body for responding to gender-based violence in these circumstances. To date however, many observers, and health professionals, and community activists believe it has been ineffective in this respect. A potentially successful avenue for teaching about honorable, non-violent behavior of men and gender equality in Botswana is Alexander McCall Smith's contemporary fictional portrayal of mechanic Mr J. L. B. Matekoni in the internationally acclaimed series, *The No. 1 Ladies' Detective Agency*.

Cuba: domestic violence policies regarding patriarchal ownership and control

During an academic and cultural tour in Cuba with a colleague and a group of American students, a female student came with her father who physically and emotionally abused her almost everyday. On the third day in Cuba, the level of violence increased around 10 p.m., and the girl suddenly ran away from her apartment to the next apartment where the academic faculty were staying. She was crying and scared from the father's attack.

At this point, two male faculty members met to find an intervention strategy. The father was still in his room. It was not a good idea to try to settle everything that night. The two professors convinced the student to stay with the other girls for the night. The next day, after long conversation, the two professors decided to confront the father's behavior. As expected, he took control immediately, saying "Hey, now, what I am going to hear from the two professors?" One of the professors (author Seck) with many years of experience working with abusive men, told the man "You are the father but you are not the authority here. Since we are all new in Cuba and we have not yet informed anyone on this campus regarding the incident, we want you to cool it for now! We will inform you today about the Cuban policies on domestic abuse." His reply was "What do you mean Cuban policy – this is me and my daughter!" This ended our very short dialogue, with a lot of tension! Jealousy was this man's reason for abusing his daughter.

Early the next day, during breakfast, we decided to learn about domestic violence policies from other Cuban staff and faculty by asking several basic hypothetical questions: "How do you deal with domestic violence in Cuba?" "How do you deal with violence on campus?" and "Who are the authorities in charge of domestic violence?" The scenario as presented was identical to what was at hand. It was fascinating to find out how similar almost all the responses were: "Domestic violence is not tolerated in Cuba"; "You would not want the Cuban authorities involved"; "The punishment for perpetrators are extremely severe"; "It's an automatic arrest if there are injuries involved"; "If you are a visitor it's even harsher."

The information was clear, and illustrates a key concept in this book: *Knowledge is non-violent power*. Together, we two professors conveyed the exact information to the father. There was no question asked. He lost all his controlling tendencies after he received the facts, and the realities became clear. He was then informed: "There will be no second chance with another assault. The next incident will be reported, and we can predict with certainty, what the outcome may be." Also made clear to the man was that there were no social supports here other than the State. There were no battered women programs, and no treatment programs for batterers or abusive men. The Cuban government does it all. There was not a single abusive incident afterward. Interestingly, the man apologized to the professors after they returned to Boston. This incident illustrates the powerful use of *facts* – when employed strategically – to prevent violence. But it also suggests the need of further interaction with the abused student for how she might protect herself in the event of her father's retaliation against her, once leaving Cuba. As it turned out, the student returned safely to her college dormitory, and the professors strongly advised her to seek follow-up support from student counseling services.

Senegal and Ghana: violence and health providers' role in refugee camps

Colonialism laid the foundation for the rape and depletion of African resources that continues past the independence movement. Since the end of the Cold War, many African scholars now realize that Africa is no longer a strategic asset in a global struggle between superpowers. Likewise, it is widely known that there is a close link between illegal resource extraction, arms trafficking, human trafficking, human rights violations, humanitarian disaster, and environmental destruction. Now, the immense problems of emigration are added to the load. (See Chapter 8 for similar exploitation among indigenous people on other continents and its intersection with interpersonal violence today.)

Senegal

Within Senegalese society, as in most countries of the world, violence against women is as difficult to solve as it is to measure. Almost always, the violence occurs within the privacy of the home – into which friends, relations, neighbors, and authorities are reluctant to intrude. The victims themselves voice fewer complaints, and have less recourse to the law than other victims of violence. Many of the victims come to accept beatings as an inevitable accompaniment of a woman's inferior status in home and society. Conditioned from birth to esteem themselves only in terms of their ability to serve and satisfy others, many women respond to violence by looking first to their own failings, blaming themselves, justifying their attackers, and hiding the marks of their shame, the tears and the bruises, from the outside world (UNICEF, 1995).

Field observations suggest that Senegalese violence is more often related to the social and economic conditions of youth than to women. In Senegal, people view action on gender issues and male violence against women as less urgent than finding jobs for both boys and girls. Rather than advocating for battered women's shelter, they argue for a visa to leave the country instead. In this quest, known as *Bursa ou Bursak*, many thousands are jailed for illegal emigration, abused, or die in refugee camps or on the high seas in an attempt to reach Europe in a contemporary scene that harks back to the slave trade centuries ago and the tragic intersection of race and class as factors affecting inequality and violence. (See Part IV for the aims and outcomes of a 2007 international colloquium on this and related issues held in Senegal at the Université Gaston Berger.)

Ghana

Traditional Western definitions of violence would not adequately explain the failure or lack of policies when it comes to responding to violation of the most basic human needs as revealed in the Ghanaian refugee camp of Buduburam. Although it is useful to ask these important policy questions, it is equally important to put the questions into perspective. How are they related to State violence and to human rights? How are they related to war? What role does culture play in policy making about violence and human rights?

In Ghana, like most places around the world, one of the most common forms of violence against women is that perpetrated by a husband or other intimate male partner. As in most other places, intimate partner violence takes a variety of forms, including physical, emotional, psychological, economic and sexual. The level of violence against women inside the refugee camps is considerably more elevated than in other areas. It appears that mainstream values are carried to the camps where there are fewer or no institutional controls or accountability for violent behavior. The role of medical and rescue workers is challenging enough in stable societies, but in refugee and war environments it can be nearly impossible with limited funding and the near or total collapse of standard healthcare and other institutions – another reason for embracing peace and non-violent strategies to resolve interpersonal and political conflict situations.

Interviews in these case studies relied on information provided by the camp authorities who were concerned with women's safety, but admitted that no consistent data were being collected. Since the Ghanaian government in general has inadequate ways of tracing victimization of women even in urban or rural areas, it is not surprising that no such tracking would be conducted inside refugee camps. The authorities in the camps did, however, notice a huge difference in the mistreatment of women inside the camps in comparison to what they experienced anywhere else. The reasons or justification they gave were numerous: Stress, war related anxiety, overcrowding, and economic despair, among many other sociological variables. There were no places within the camps for women to go to if they were victims of either physical or sexual abuse, particularly if the perpetrator was also a partner or husband. What role did the organization of the camp have in this situation? What impact does this have on women's health and safety?

Across Sub-Saharan Africa, professionals from various disciplines have explored the prevalence of violence in most of its forms. The big question remains: how do we explore the opportunities and challenges related to developing an active response to domestic violence within reproductive and other health services? To ensure that women are not further victimized or blamed during the process of consultation and disclosure, aid workers and health staff must first confront their own biases, misconceptions, and fears about violence against women – factors that may further reduce effective action in constrained circumstances. In their Sub-Saharan Africa study, researchers Charlotte Watts and Susannah Mayhew (2004) found that violence and reproductive health often are treated as separate rather than related entities, despite the framing of both issues as essential components of women's human rights and the growing evidence connecting them.

To identify women at high risk, health providers must incorporate into their practice evidence-based questions about unexplained injury or maternal bleeding, preterm labor, etc. – critical indicators in any situation (McFarlane *et al.*, 1992). International relief workers like "Doctors Without Borders" know about Western-based research regarding the "health/mental health" impact of violence. But the stark reality in refugee camps is that life-saving medical interventions (e.g. in response to cholera) take priority over psychological trauma from intimate partner violence. However, even in busy US hospital emergency rooms battered women know and understand they are not the only ones there if a nurse has to leave them to attend to an acute heart attack patient, a brief statement such as "Please stay, I'll be back soon" or some such is reassuring. Thus, in a refugee camp where the combination of medical and social/psychological needs can be overwhelming, one can at least make an empathetic comment such as "I'm so sorry this has happened to you," and offer to inquire whether possible mental health relief workers might be available on site or during post-refugee status.

While social services for abused refugees may be out of reach in refugee camp situations, women everywhere would welcome having healthcare providers, social workers, or community organizers who understand domestic violence and *listen, provide information, and advocate* for them. As for the fundamental question about what to do with the perpetrators, the Emerge model offers some hopeful guidelines if introduced, adapted, and sensitively applied cross-culturally. The program at Emerge (now extended internationally) and the work of David Adams (2007) demonstrates a promising way forward, including training throughout community and government agencies – for health and social services, mental health, the courts, and police.

Knowledgeable and skilled trainers and social activists enhance the prospects of successful outcomes when casting their work in a universal human rights framework. They also are keenly sensitive to cultural differences and how various societies define and deal with criminal, social, and medical matters, and how cultural relativism may be used as an explanation for either violence or victim status, as in "My culture made me do it" (Torry, 2002). The Cangleska offender program (see Chapter 8) illustrates the blending of mainstream and indigenous models while assuring Native Sioux control of training, etc. without using "culture" as an excuse to overlook violence from a universal human rights perspective. (See Chapter 2 for discussion of how a psychopathology framework has served to attach a psychiatric diagnosis to battered women, and to excuse the perpetrator (Stark *et al.*, 1979)).

In our analysis, the role of the community in general, and the role of professionals in particular, are intertwined. Solving the problems of the perpetrators through behavioral changes within a complex system is not easy. Such an endeavor needs to be coordinated with solid planning, and integrated through clear rules, regulation, and policies. This constitutes another major challenge. In programs like Emerge one is convinced that community involvement in the process of organizing training is a must.

The role of social institutions in curbing violence

Both Herbert Spencer and Talcott Parsons defined *social institution* as a sort of "super-custom," a set of mores, folkways, and patterns of behavior that deals with major social interests: law, church, hospital, police, and family. A social institution consists of all the structural components of a society through which the main concerns and activities are met. Another critical concept is *social control*, a term widely used in sociology, referring to the social processes by which the behavior of individuals or groups is regulated. Who really controls the hospitals when health professionals signal that genocide is taking place somewhere? Are there authorities within the health and social service professions who assess a situation and determine that there is a genocide occurring? Based on the information that health professionals have on the field, should others decide for them any course of action? Or should such reporting be left to the diplomats and other bureaucrats, and the military? Can healthcare professionals take a more decisive role in such instances? Why and how? This was the case in Rwanda. The perpetrators were overwhelmingly men who tried to hide behind the institutions, while the international community played the deaf ear. Consequently, over one million people were murdered, and countless were raped.

As introduced in Chapter 2, in 2007, the United Nations General Assembly (UNGA) urged Member States to ensure that all human rights and fundamental freedoms are respected and protected – actions that comprise primary prevention. The UNGA also urges States to review, revise, amend or abolish all laws, policies, practices and customs that discriminate against women. The UN resolution also sought to ensure that States take positive measures to address structural causes of violence against women. Here, such "structural" causes include built-in laws and policies that allow outright discrimination against women, or otherwise serve to oppress disadvantaged groups; for example, failing to prosecute violent domestic partners, or other crimes against women. Furthermore, States must integrate a gender perspective into national plans of action on the elimination of violence against women. Next, States must recognize that gender inequalities and all forms of violence against women and girls increase their vulnerability to HIV/AIDS. Then, States must protect women and girls in situations of armed conflict, and in post-conflict settings for refugees and internally displaced persons. Finally, States must allocate adequate resources to promote gender equality and to prevent and redress all forms and manifestations of violence against women (Delport, 2007).

The O. J. Simpson case: an example of race, class and gender issues in domestic violence

On June 12, 1994, Nicole Brown Simpson, age 35, and Ronald Goldman, age 25, were stabbed to death. Their bodies were found in the front courtyard of Nicole's condominium in Brentwood, California. The intense media coverage of the case revolved about the question: why? Both victims in this case of a double homicide were unmarried Caucasian residents of the community. The victims knew each other but were not believed to have been romantically involved. O. J. Simpson was the prime suspect. Nicole had been married to Simpson, and was the mother of his two children. Simpson was a batterer known to many, including the police and hospital. Unfortunately, this did not become relevant because of race and class factors, according to many observers. In the criminal case, Simpson was found not guilty of the murder of his ex-wife

Nicole. But in the civil case, which has a lower burden of proof, he was found liable for both deaths.

In spite of Simpson being known to the hospital, the medical community remained silent all along. The Simpson case was a classic murder case where sexism (with shades of an "honor" killing), racism, classism, and police incompetency all colluded, and eventually captivated the attention of the American public and the international community – it was not just about a perpetrator of violence and their victims, but rather an endless number of devious behaviors which took the violence that was involved out of context. Although several experts on domestic abuse were called to testify, not much was useful because the focus was no longer on domestic abuse as we knew it then; it was much bigger, including growing tension between the Black and White communities, and infighting in the Los Angeles Police Department.

Today, many would ask what lessons have we learned from this case, as a society? From every aspect, or perspective, one can look at the State, the courts, the police, the hospital, and see a gap within the system. Unfortunately, the perpetrator almost always sees the gap and takes advantage of it. Thus the O. J. case was a very unfortunate one which many observers believe did not do justice to how society should respond to violence. These and other questions remain:

- How can the system respond in a synchronized way to intervene in domestic violence?
- Who is in charge? To answer these questions, certainly one would have to move beyond the concept of personal responsibility to include institutional responsibility.
- Did racial composition of the two juries (criminal and civil) play a role, and how does this reflect the centuries-old racial tension in the US: i.e. a Black-dominated jury exonerates (revenge for past racial injustice?) or a White-dominated jury condemns – maybe not on "objective" evidence and merits of the case?
- Given O. J.'s battering history, how does it comport with other "ownership-of-wife" (or in this case "ex-wife") murder cases regardless of race, and with historic White stereotypes of the "violent Black male"? (see Chapter 11 which shows that the majority of assailants in school-based violence are affluent White males and Chapter 8's discussion of the Cangleska program for Native American offenders).

South Africa: violence cannot be the solution

They questioned me extensively on the issue of violence, and while I was not yet willing to renounce violence, I affirmed in the strongest possible terms that violence could never be the ultimate solution to the situation in South Africa.

(Nelson Mandela)

Few countries have experienced as much violence and abuse as South Africa under apartheid, and post-apartheid. We cannot talk about modern South Africa and violence in any form without starting with *Rolihlahla*. The colloquial meaning of this Xhosa word is "troublemaker." *Rolihlahla* is the real name of Nelson Mandela. For four decades, he challenged the international community to explain the apartheid system, and to help resolve the government's violent policies against Blacks in South Africa. He became a "troublemaker" for asking serious political questions that slowly but surely helped in the deconstruction of the violent apartheid system. Nelson Mandela was and is a fierce advocate for social justice and a fearless social and political activist who fought for decades to maintain the mental health of Blacks in South Africa.

In the long run, it was incredible that both the government and the African National

Congress did listen to Mandela's idea for talks and negotiations. The paradox in South Africa today is that Mandela symbolizes both violence and nonviolence. Violent and abusive behavior constitutes a considerable toll on the physical and mental health of South Africans. Although child abuse and spouse abuse continue to threaten the health of thousands of South African families, the consequences of past apartheid violence are still a major preoccupation at every level in South African society. Poverty, AIDS, and homicide are the leading causes of death. Survey and ethnographic research on violence against South African women and children across the life cycle attests not only to traditional values that place all women at risk of violence, but also how apartheid exacerbated rates of rape, intimate partner and other violence in South Africa (Dangor *et al.*, 1998). Participant-observation visits in Johannesburg, Cape Town, and Robin Island affirmed this scenario about South Africa (Seck, 2002). The level of insecurity, or street violence, anger, frustration, crimes of all sorts, and animosity overwhelm the city of Johannesburg. What happened?

During apartheid, by law, Blacks were not allowed to stay in the city after 5 p.m. Thus, historically, violence has been the responsibility of the field of law enforcement. In the post-apartheid era, there is no curfew but Blacks are without skills, education, or opportunity. The visibility of alcohol abuse, drug abuse, mental illness, and crimes spread from the townships into the cities. Drivers in the city of Johannesburg were afraid to stop on red lights for fear of being attacked in many areas of the city. Many of the victims were women drivers. Paramedics and police will not go to many areas of the city after dark. The South African example is the classical example where individual violence draws a parallel with State violence. Similar to the situation in the United States, historically, violence had been the responsibility of the field of law enforcement, social services, and mental health; and now it has become a national public health priority (the Healthy People 2010 program). The psychosocial consequences of decades of State-sponsored violence in South Africa extend far beyond the physical injuries. Unfortunately, the availability and quality of data on morbidity and disability associated with State violence are poor. (See Part IV for the anti-violence work of NISAA – the Institute for Women's Development – in Southern African nations.)

In conclusion, our examination of issues regarding perpetrators of abuse and violence, using international, multidisciplinary, and multicultural perspectives, as well as ethnographic examples, serves our deep commitment to social justice. Apparently, violence cannot be the solution to social problems, thus our understanding of both interpersonal and institutionally sponsored violence should direct prevention guidelines for counselors, social services managers, government organizations and health professionals in their responsibilities. For educators and their students in health and social services to respond adequately to violence, multidisciplinary approaches become absolutely necessary. The major breakthrough in the 1995 Women's Conference and Forum in Beijing helped to move the issues beyond punishment of perpetrators and victim's assistance. Accordingly, the ultimate goal is to eliminate prejudice, all forms of violence and exploitation, and practices based on stereotypes or ideas of superiority and inferiority.

References

Adams, D. (1989) Treatment models of men who batter: A profeminist analysis. In K. Yllo, & M. Bograd (eds.), *Feminist Perspectives on Wife Abuse*, pp. 176–99. Beverly Hills, CA: Sage.

Adams, D. (2003). Treatment programs for batterers. *Clinics in Family Practice*, 5(1), 159–76.

Adams, D. (2007). *Why Do They Kill? Men Who Murder Their Intimate Partners*. Nashville: Vanderbilt University Press.

Adams, D., & Cayouette, S. (2002). Emerge: A group education model for abusers. In E. Aldarondo, &

F. Mederos (eds.), *Programs for Men Who Batter: Intervention and Prevention Strategies in a Diverse Society*, pp. 4-1–4-23. New York: Civic Research Inc.

Bandura, A. (1977) *Social Learning Theory*. Englewood Cliffs, NY: Prentice-Hall.

Cayouette, S. (1996). Safety issues for female group leaders. Unpublished. Available from the Emerge website (http://www.emergedv.com).

Dangor, Z., Hoff, L. A., & Scott, R. (1998). Woman abuse in South Africa: An exploratory study. *Violence against Women: An International and Interdisciplinary Journal*, 4(2), 125–52.

Delport, E. (ed.) (2007). *Gender-Based Violence in Africa: Perspectives from the Continent*. Pretoria: Centre for Human Rights.

Dobash, R. E., & Dobash, R. (1979) *Violence against Wives: A Case against the Patriarchy*. New York: The Free Press, Macmillan.

Edleson, J. L., & Tolman, R. M. (1992). *Intervention for Men who Batter: An Ecological Approach*. Thousand Oaks, CA: Sage.

Emerge (2000). *Batterer Intervention Program Manual for First and Second Stage Groups*. Available from the Emerge website (http://www.emergedv.com).

Faulk, M. (1977) Men who assault their wives. In M. Roy (ed.), *Battered Women: A Psycho-Sociological Study of Domestic Violence*. New York: Van Nostrand Reinhold.

Geller, J., & Walsh, J. (1977). A treatment model for the abused spouse. *Victimology: An International Journal*, 2(3–4), 630.

Gelles, R. J. (1974). *The Violent Home*. Beverly Hills: Sage.

Gondolf, E. (1987). *Research on Men Who Batter*. Bradenton, FL: Human Services Institute.

Hamberger, K. (2002). The men's group program: A community-based, cognitive-behavioral, pro-feminist intervention program. In E. Aldarondo, & F. Mederos (eds.), *Programs for Men Who Batter: Intervention and Prevention Strategies in a Diverse Society*, pp. 7–1-7-46. Kingston, NJ: Civic Research Institute.

Henslin, J. (2006). *Social Problems*. Upper Sadlle River, NJ: Pearson, Prentice Hall.

Hoff, L. A. (1990). *Battered Women as Survivors*. London: Routledge.

Hoff, L. A., Hallisey, B. J., & Hoff, M. (2009). *People in Crisis: Clinical and Diversity Perspectives* (6th edn.). New York and London: Routledge.

Jencks, C. (1993). *Rethinking Social Policy: Race, Poverty, and the Underclass*. New York: Harper Perennial.

Klein, A (1994). Re-abuse in a population of court-restrained male batterers after two years. Development of a predictive model. Unpublished doctoral dissertation. Northeastern University, Boston.

Kohn, A. (1993). *Punished by Rewards: The Trouble with Gold Stars, Incentive Plans, A's, Praise and Other Bribes*. Boston: Houghton Mifflin.

McFarlane, J., Parker, B., Soeken, K., & Bullock, L. (1992). Assessing for abuse during pregnancy: Severity and frequency of injuries and associated entry into prenatal care. *Journal of the American Medical Association*, 267(23), 3176–8.

McGregor, D. (1960). *The Human Side of Enterprise*. New York: McGraw-Hill.

MacLeod, L. (1989). *Wife Battering and the Web of Hope: Progress, Dilemmas, and Visions of Prevention*. Ottawa: Health and Welfare Canada. National Clearinghouse on Family Violence.

McMahon, F. & McMahon, J. (1982) *Psychology: The Hybrid Science*. Homewood, IL: The Dorsey Press.

Martin, D. (1976). *Battered Wives*. San Francisco: Glide Publications.

Massachusetts Department of Public Health (1995). *Standards and Guidelines for the Certification of Batterer Intervention Programs*. Massachusetts Department of Public Health. Batterer Intervention Programs.

Pence, E. (2002). The Duluth domestic abuse intervention project. In E. Aldarondo, & F. Mederos (eds.), *Programs for Men Who Batter: Intervention and Prevention Strategies in a Diverse Society*, pp. 6–1-6–46. Kingston, NJ: Civic Research Institute.

Perlmuter, L., & Monty, R. (1977) The importance of perceived control: Fact or fantasy? *American Scientist*, November–December, 759–65.

Robbins, T. (1991). *Awaken the Giant Within: How to Take Immediate Control of Your Mental, Emotional, Physical and Financial Destiny.* New York: Fireside.

Schechter, S. (1982). *Women and Male Violence: The Visions and Struggles of the Battered Women's Movement.* Boston: South End Press.

Seck, M. (1995). *Substance Abuse Among Male Batterers.* Ann Arbor, MI: University Microfilms International.

Seck, M. (2000, 2002). Field study notes: Violence and migration. Africa. Unpublished.

Shainess, N. (1977) Psychological aspects of wifebeating. In M. Roy (ed.), *Battered Women: a Psycho-Sociological Study of Domestic Violence*, pp. 114–15. New York: Van Nostrand Reinhold.

Sherman, L. W., & Berk, R. A. (1984). The specific deterrent effects of arrest for domestic assault. *American Sociological Review*, 49, 261–72.

Snell, J., Rosenwald R., & Robey, A. (1964). The wifebeater's wife: A study of family interaction. *Archives of General Psychiatry II*, August, 109.

Sonkin, D., & Martin, L. (1985). *The Male Batterer: A Treatment Approach.* New York: Springer.

Stark, E., Flitcraft, A., & Frazier, W. (1979). Medicine and patriarchal violence: The social construction of a "private" event. *International Journal of Health Services*, 9, 461–93.

Torry, W. I. (2000). Culture and individual responsibility: Touchstones of the culture defense. *Human Organization*, 59(1), 58–71.

UNICEF. (1995). New York: UNICEF.

Warrior, B. (1976). *Wifebeating.* Somerville, MA: New England Free Press.

Watts, C., & Mayhew, S. (2004). Reproductive health services and intimate partner violence: Shaping a pragmatic response in Sub-Saharan Africa: International family planning perspectives. *Encyclopedia Britannica, Book of the Year, 30*, p. 372. Chicago: Encyclopedia Britannica, Inc.

Williams, O. (2000). An enhanced treatment perspective with African American men who batter. *Wisconsin Coalition against Domestic Violence*, 19(2), 5–9.

Note

1 The bicultural identity – Senegalese and American – of researcher Magueye Seck was an apparent advantage in addressing male violence cross-culturally.

Part III

Professional, continuing education, and practice applications

As a whole, this book integrates clinical and public health perspectives, with the foundation laid in Part I, while Part II addresses the spectrum of interpersonal and State-sponsored violence – focusing on clinical aspects of individual health, the socioeconomic costs of violence, and the service implications for victim/survivors and their families. Part III shifts toward the arena of workplace and learning environments and professional issues, including the stressful impact on health and social service providers themselves exacted by this demanding work. Such stress is exacerbated when professionals and front-line providers do not feel adequately prepared and supported for meeting the complex service needs of victim/survivors – with burnout and compassion fatigue some of the predictable results. This Part assumes that clinical skills and public health endeavors on behalf of victim/survivors and perpetrators may falter without simultaneous attention to self-care and support of caretakers themselves.

Chapter 11 focuses on violence in schools and the workplace where (in addition to students and employees as victim/survivors in "normal" not "clinical" settings), understanding violence and its prevention includes an Assessment Tool for early identification of dangerous persons and the risk of assault and/or homicide applicable to clients, abusers, their families, and service providers. Chapter 12 then addresses professional issues encountered in providing service to victims and providers, including the possibility of vicarious traumatization. Chapter 13 describes the health and criminal justice interface, and illustrates this with examples of interdisciplinary comprehensive service. Online Resources supplement the material in these three chapters.

11   Violence, bullying, and abuse in schools and the workplace

- Violence and abuse: from home and mainstream culture to learning and work environments
- Accountability for violence: intersection of mental health and criminal justice
- Case example: September 11, 2001 – understanding and pathologizing violence
- Threats to safety in learning environments

  - Bullying as abuse and precursor to violent backlash
  - Primary prevention of violence in schools and colleges

- Violence and abuse in the workplace

  - Types and extent of workplace violence

- Case example: abuse and disrespect of immigrant workers – cleaning and restaurant industries
- Nursing: a high risk profession
- Promoting healthy and safe employment in healthcare – the PHASE study
- The context and consequences of violence against nurses
- Recognizing signs of danger and potential for assault and homicide

  - Violence prevention strategies
  - Assessment of individuals for danger
  - Case examples: assessment and service planning (Australia)

- Crisis care and support of injured or threatened workers

  - Critical Incident Stress Debriefing (CISD): values and cautions

- Personal and institutional strategies for violence prevention

Several common assumptions about violence and abuse in learning and work environments bear attention by the everyday student and worker, as well as by parents, teachers, job supervisors, and the public at large. Children coming from either a protective or abusive home assume that school is a primary place for learning and freedom from abuse – not for bullying or violent assaults by fellow students. A teenager hoping to escape the fury or revenge from a community-based gang member envisions school as a refuge from possible attack. A female worker abused at home hopes she will be safe at least temporarily while doing her job – only to cringe in fear when her abusive partner pursues her at work for further abuse or even murder. In one case a nursing professor's trusted secretary was the only one privy to the professor's "secret" of abuse by her husband, a physician – it was too shameful to share with her nursing colleagues. Thus, when the professor did not show up for work one day, the secretary went to the professor's house and encountered a "murder-in-process" – the husband stabbing his wife to death. This chapter addresses violence and abuse issues and their relevance to educational and workplace settings.

Violence and abuse: from home and mainstream culture to learning and work environments

Many of the same principles and practice strategies discussed in other chapters apply to learning and work environments as well, with a particular emphasis on early warning signs of danger. For example, in publicized accounts of school, college, or workplace incidents of violence – some involving the murder of several or dozens of students and workers – a common response is to attribute the tragedy to the purported "mental illness" of the identified assailants – "He had to have been crazy to do something like that." This response is akin to ones discussed earlier in this book about intimate partner violence, e.g. "She must be crazy to stay with a man like that," or excusing the assailant on similar grounds of psychopathology. Indeed, analysis following these tragic events usually reveals a history of troubled individuals. But does this mean they "just happened" and were not preventable? History suggests the sad reality that we cannot prevent all violence despite our best efforts. But schools and ordinary work places are not and should not become fortresses, when prevention efforts based on available evidence should be emphasized over "pulling up the drawbridge" after the fact.

As already addressed in Parts I and II, violence and abuse are not "private" acts emanating from impaired cognitive functioning (a sine qua non of serious psychopathology) but for the most part are *social*, consciously-planned actions aimed at *power and control* of their victims, or a final "no-lose-game" of finally gaining attention around troubling issues (see Hoff *et al.*, Chapter 9). This does not negate the fact that some perpetrators are indeed cognitively impaired (and therefore may be excused from accountability for their violent behavior), but research documents that this is the exception, not the norm, in most instances of violence and abuse. Discussion of these issues follows, with international illustrations.

Accountability for violence: intersection of mental health and criminal justice

Historically, violence has been the concern primarily of the police and specialized psychiatric and crisis personnel. Indeed, most research on assessing risk of violence has focused on psychiatrically disturbed persons presumed as the main perpetrators of violence (Monahan, & Steadman, 1994). The idea of a "mental illness/violence" link is deeply embedded in US popular culture and international media coverage of horrifying violence such as school shootings and the September 11, 2001 terrorist attacks.

Forensic psychiatry is a specialized field intersecting between criminal justice and psychiatry which focuses on the mental status of a person apprehended or on trial for an alleged crime. If evidence suggests "insanity" the person is entitled to leniency under the law – in other words, is not "morally" accountable for injurious or murderous behavior. *Insanity* is a legal, not a mental health, concept. It implies impairment of cognitive functioning to the extent that it renders a person incapable of rational and morally accountable decision making and conduct in accordance with established social norms. Many insanity pleas, however, leave much room for doubt.

Forensic psychiatry is not an exact science, and relies heavily on the *Diagnostic and Statistical Manual of Mental Illness* (APA, 2000), an ever-expanding and currently 943-page compendium of psychiatric diagnoses that is influenced by political and cultural factors, and is critiqued by social scientists on its questionable scientific grounds (Cooksey, & Brown, 1998) and indeed within the psychiatry profession itself (McHugh, & Clark, 2006). While there is a deplorable lack of adequate and humane treatment for the mentally ill (Earley, 2006; Ustun, 1999), one cannot have it both ways; that is, on the one hand, exercise the freedom to reject treatment and hospitalization for behavioral disorders and, on the other hand, plead temporary insanity when failing to control violent impulses and committing a crime. In instances of assaulting staff members in psychiatric or emergency settings, the accountability issue is compounded by the commonplace assumption that such injuries are just "part of the job" (O'Sullivan *et al.*, 2008).

Case example: September 11, 2001 – understanding and pathologizing violence

It is one thing to recognize the interface between violence and a particular individual's personal turmoil and psychic pain. On the other hand, a university professor offers this dramatic example of the deep-seated tendency to interpret political and culturally tinged violence as evidence of psychopathology.

In a graduate class on politics and culture in health affairs on September 12, 2001, the teacher facilitated student discussion of the attack, their fears, and attempts to make meaning of the event, much as many American people asked, "Why do they hate us so much?" (A few years later, survivors of the London and Madrid transit bombings asked similar questions.) The grief and psychological pain was almost palpable. One student, trying to grapple with the enormity and rarity of such an event on American soil, said "I can only think that at the moment of impact [on the World Trade Center] they had 'lost their minds ... they were insane.'"

Fellow students and the teacher were stunned at this analysis. The gently led discussion concluded as follows:

1 It is something of an affront to all persons with diagnosable mental illness to suggest that the pilots whose own lives ended along with the victims were psychotic. That is, psychosis by definition includes serious impairment of normal cognitive and emotional functioning which also affects behavior. The attackers met none of these criteria. Rather, they systematically planned and prepared for the attack over time, including obtaining legitimate US visas and taking lessons in US licensed schools for flying jet aircraft. The night before, they stayed outside of Boston – presumably to avert detection – their planned site for flight take-off from Logan International Airport. Such deliberately planned and carefully executed actions are not typical of psychotic persons.
2 Violence in most instances is a conscious action directed toward exerting power and control, which is contrary to some popular conceptions. This case and those in London and Madrid are examples of "Holy War" or what some describe as a "clash of civilizations" rooted in many earlier "Holy Wars" such as the medieval Crusades.
3 These global, mostly religious-based clashes are extensively addressed elsewhere and are beyond the scope of this book except to note research (Friedman, 2006) that the presumed "sea of psychotic violence" is clearly unfounded (Pies, 2008).

Unfortunately, the question "Why do they hate us so much?" is afforded much less attention than more wars in response, resulting in many thousands more deaths and the untold suffering of millions. Such deaths and widespread suffering could be avoided if diplomacy were valued more, and if the everyday person and leaders attended to this lesson from research on intimate partner and other violence: *Violence as a response to violence begets more violence* (Hoff *et al.*, 2009, Chapter 12).

Threats to safety in learning environments

It is wrenching for parents, students, their teachers and whole communities to learn from national and international media of yet another shooting of students by one of their own class-mates. The sad mourning rituals have become familiar by now, and raise serious questions for the communities and nations in which these tragedies occur.

Bullying as abuse and precursor to violent backlash

Aggressive, anti-social, and violent behavior among children and adolescents is gaining inter-national attention. Overall crime rates in the United States and Western Europe have declined sharply for several years, while dramatic shootings by school children have captured inter-national attention. Bullying and mobbing – usually child-on-child aggression – continue to create terror in schools and have even been associated with suicide. Paralleling adult patterns, the majority of bullying and anti-social behavior is perpetrated by males against both males and females, while females also increasingly behave similarly (Ellickson *et al.*, 1997; Hoover, & Juul, 1993, p. 28; Walker, 1993, p. 21).

Youth violence has moved parents, social scientists, journalists, legislators, and others to debate and deep soul-searching about the cultural climate and other factors that have spawned these tragedies. Research on bullying in Europe traces such behavior to a combination of inter-acting factors: in the home (for example, inconsistent discipline, alcohol); in the school (more anti-social behavior in the worst schools); and issues confronting the individual victims and perpetrators (for example, low self-esteem stemming from parental indifference or abuse).

Broadly, bullying has been defined as abusive behavior by children and adolescents against their peers. The bully may be motivated by bias based on race, ethnicity, religion, sexual ori-entation, etc., while the person bullied may already feel disadvantaged by any of these same factors marking him or her as "different" and an easy "target" for ridicule, teasing, intimidation, exclusion, or spreading rumors – in essence, a negative "rite of passage" at a vulnerable age that includes a deep need to "belong" (Hoff *et al.*, 2009, Chapter 6). Recently, the term bullying has been used for abusive behavior among adults as well. There it is congruent with Type 3 violence: Worker-on-Worker behaviors that include verbal put-downs and threats of physical violence – sometimes referred to as *lateral* or *horizontal* violence (see "Types and extent of workplace violence" below and Chapter 12 for the culture of nursing).

Addressing the seriousness of school-based bullying and its prevention, the Massachusetts Department of Public Health has produced *Direct From the Field: A Guide to Bullying Prevention* (Parker-Roerden *et al.*, 2007), designed particularly as an aid to teachers and school administra-tors. It builds on a 2002 report, *The Safe School Initiative*, compiled by the US Secret Service National Threat Assessment Center in collaboration with the US Department of Education. A major challenge in addressing this threat to children's safety is breaking the silence and undoing the long-standing myth that bullying "is just part of growing up," with the bullied child or adolescent left to nurse in private the psychological wounds of this kind of abuse that occurs primarily out of adults' sight – on buses, in locker rooms, at sporting events, or walking home. And if this were not enough to defy preventive solutions, the well-known code of se-crecy among teenagers – even if not bullied – is exacerbated by fear of retaliation if they report the abuse.

This code of silence, intersecting with teachers and administrators who are unprepared to intervene effectively, serves to embolden the bullies and compounds the task of bullying prevention. The challenges to effective prevention and intervention around bullying have much in common with other forms of violence and abuse – intimate partner violence, sexual assault, trafficking, and abuse of older persons. *Direct From the Field* is also akin to the Cangleska program for offenders (see Chapter 8) for its inclusion of strategies to engage teachers, counselors, families and students themselves – those bullied and witnesses afraid to intervene – in collaborative efforts to address this serious and widespread form of abuse. For example, it lists for students "20 Things You Can Do When Someone is Being Bullied" (e.g. tell a trusted adult, include young people who are usually excluded, invite a targeted student for lunch). A worksheet entitled "My Bullying Buster Pledge" provides a structured aid for defining what one pledges to do and how to do it.

Many young people act out aggressively because they feel disempowered and alienated in a society that does not meet their needs. But as frightening as bullying, youth aggression and violence can be, it is crucial to remember this major theme from research and clinical data: *Violence begets violence* (Carlsson-Paige, & Levin, 2008). As with prevention of other forms of violence, knowledge is power, and comprises a first step in addressing this form of abuse (see Garbarino, & deLara, 2002; Hoover, & Oliver, 1996; and Part IV).

Primary prevention of violence in schools and colleges

On April 16, 2007, a 23-year-old student at Virginia Tech University in the US killed two students in a dormitory, then killed 30 more (mostly students) two hours later in a classroom building. His suicide brought the death toll to 33, making the shooting rampage the worst of its kind in US history. The following summary reveals what was already known and what primary prevention measures might have been taken to prevent these deaths and similar massacres in other learning environments where guns are more regulated than in the US (excerpted and edited from Hoff *et al.*, 2009, Chapter 12):

- Over some period of time, the student shooter provided e-mail and other clues to his distress. Although fellow-students reached out to him, adults and classmates apparently did not know how to take further steps in response to his clues of loneliness and distress. Significantly, it was the student's creative writing teacher who sensed most accurately this student's distress. Yet, systematic information and front-line action plans for crisis response are not routinely made available for faculty who are not crisis or mental health professionals.
- The student had been psychologically evaluated, revealing "mental health" problems. After one episode of psychiatric treatment, he was discharged with mental health professionals' estimate of no suicidal or homicidal danger, and no formal follow-up care.
- Despite the student's psychiatric history, he was easily able to purchase guns over the Internet with no background checks or constraints on these purchases – an issue of particular relevance to the controversial "gun culture" in the United States.
- Nation-wide, colleges and universities have instituted tighter police security measures and immediate notification to student bodies of potential danger. Yet, college communities are vulnerable to results of national policies regarding easy availability of guns, and a culture of "reaction" after the fact vs. comprehensive prevention and counseling programs that often take second place in identification and follow-up of students in distress or crisis.
- In a comparable situation of a failing student threatening (through the Internet) murder of

the faculty member in response to his grade, the frightened teacher was ignored through various chains of reporting. Since this student in fact was failing all his courses, the apparent assumption was this: he will soon be "out of here" and then he will be someone else's problem. But since colleges are not impregnable fortresses – nor should they be in a "free" society – there seems little awareness that this failure to offer counseling and career advice for such students might result in a student returning to campus in murderous revenge.

• Suicidology and crisis experts have long known that threats of suicide following murder (plus for some, a history of being physically abused and/or bullied) *increases* the risk of dangerousness to others. Yet this knowledge and need for systematic incorporation of life-threatening risk assessment into routine health and mental health protocols has yet to reach many primary care providers and others such as school counselors.[1]

Violence and abuse in the workplace

Violence as an occupational health hazard has gained international public attention (Christmas, 2007; Jackson, 1998; Levin *et al.*, 1992; Lipscomb, & Love, 1992; Merchant, & Lundell, 2001). Police officers, health, mental health, crisis, and other workers make up a special category of victims. Among women who died as a result of workplace trauma, 41 percent were homicide victims (Jenkins *et al.*, 1992). With greater skills in applying danger assessment knowledge in the workplace, many instances of workers' injuries from violence might be avoided.

Types and extent of workplace violence

Broadly, the term "workplace violence" is used to describe actions ranging from offensive or threatening language to emotional abuse to physical assault and homicide directed toward persons at work (NIOSH, 2006).

In April 2000, to assist in the design of appropriate strategies to prevent workplace violence, the University of Iowa Injury Prevention Research Center's Workplace Violence Intervention Research Workshop proposed the following 4-type classification based on a perpetrator's relationship to the workplace:

• Criminal Intent (Type 1): the perpetrator has no legitimate relationship to the business or its employees, and is usually committing a crime in conjunction with the violence.
• Customer/Client (Type 2): the perpetrator has a legitimate relationship with the business and becomes violent while being served by the business.
• Worker-on-Worker (Type 3): the perpetrator is an employee or past employee of the business who attacks or threatens another employee(s) or past employee(s) in the workplace.
• Personal Relationship (Type 4): the perpetrator usually does not have a relationship with the business but has a personal relationship with the intended victim (UIIPRC, 2001).

Although most physical and verbal assaults in healthcare settings are perpetrated by patients (Type 2), nurses and other healthcare workers also cite verbal abuse and sexual harassment by physicians, co-workers, and supervisors (Type 3). An example of Type 4 violence is that of an abusive husband in the childbirth department who threatens a nurse after she attempts to set limits on his abusive behavior toward his wife who is in labor. Additionally, nurses' histories of childhood abuse and intimate partner violence (Type 4) have been shown to increase their vulnerability to workplace violence (Anderson, 2002).

Other contributing factors to workplace violence include low staffing levels, lack of effective staff training in recognizing and coping with potentially dangerous patients, lack of violence prevention programs, inadequate security, the tendency for some to view hospitals, clinics, and pharmacies as sources of drugs and money and thus targets for robbery, and, in the US, the presence of guns and other weapons among hospital patients and visitors. In addition, historically, hospitals were places of safe refuge, but with easy access to guns, and domestic conflict spilling over to the workplace, unrestricted movement of the public within hospitals makes it difficult to determine who has a legitimate reason to be in the hospital and who does not (Clements *et al.*, 2005). This reality underscores the urgency of preventive measures and early detection of potential danger and abuse.

Case example: abuse and disrespect of immigrant workers – cleaning and restaurant industries

The following are vignettes from interviews with immigrant women from Central and South America who work as housecleaners and waiters in a large eastern city of the United States.

> With my boss from the cleaning company, I was 5 months pregnant and arrived at the appointed time at the client's house in a leafy suburban neighborhood of wealthy home owners. Only on arrival did we learn that the home's water supply was temporarily shut off, resulting in a toilet filled to the brim with human waste. Despite this fact, the client insisted that the house be cleaned "now," minus any available water. He was verbally abusive and in the presence of children ages 2, 4 and 6, while pointing his finger in accusation, repeatedly yelled at me to "clean the house."

> Upon arrival to work, the client kept following me around through the whole time. When she noticed I was pregnant (about 4 months), she called the agency director stating she wanted someone non-pregnant, apparently completely insensitive to the reality that poor women who are pregnant need to work. I finally left the cleaning company for a better paying job, but received no pay for the work already done. I did not pursue the matter, because I was afraid of being deported as I only had a visitor's visa.

> After cleaning a woman's house, two weeks later she called my boss to report that a set of earrings were missing, and that if she couldn't find them there would be no further work for me and she would call the police. I had been cleaning this woman's house for a long time. A week later she called to say she found the earrings. There was no apology for accusing me, and I continued to work for her because I needed the job.

> The cleaning boss took me to the third floor and told me to clean "on my hands and knees." I know that mopping floors is now a standard for cleaning companies, and she did this only because I'm an immigrant and afraid of being deported .... It made me feel like a dog on all fours. One client also insisted I clean toilets without rubber gloves because she thought that ungloved hands were better for really getting at the dirt.

> I was offered a job as a waitress, and the first day of training, he (the owner) was a gentleman, the second day he offered compliments and alcohol, and the third day, asked me for a date (I'm happily married and have two children). When I returned for payment, he made seductive advances, asked me to "close the books" for the night and while doing that he fixed a dinner for me at 1 a.m., and asked everyone else to leave so he could be alone with me.

He told me if I wanted the job, I'd have to sleep with him. I refused ... he expressed surprise and as I got ready to leave he said "You can think about it." I went to the immigrant service center and filed a complaint, and won!

These women and the leader of a support group for immigrant women in the house cleaning industry also described this double exploitation and abuse: 1) being forced by some company "bosses" or their clients to use toxic and harmful cleaning substances – a practice in clear violation of safety standards of NIOSH – the US National Institute of Occupational Safety and Health; and 2) if working for one of these "bosses," here is the typical scenario: a team of three (the boss, the driver, and the cleaner) go to an appointment. The "boss" introduces the cleaner, and moves on to the next job with another cleaner. A typical day for each cleaner is 12 hours of labor. The "boss" collects an average of US$500 for such a 12-hour day: out of this total, the boss retains $300, the driver gets about $100, and the cleaner gets less than $100 for 12 hours of work, just barely above the minimum wage (2008 wage figures).

In contrast, if each housecleaner is her own "boss," in whatever payment option she negotiates with an individual client, she keeps the total amount of pay per job. For example, $60 for a 3-hour job, times a total of three jobs over 9 hours, and total income of $180 per day (a stark difference from $100 or less for a 12-hour day!)

As immigration debates continue across the globe, it often appears too easy for affluent users of cheap immigrant labor (in jobs that many would disdain doing themselves) to forget their own immigrant origins. These vignettes are also a reminder of the basic rights of all human beings for an opportunity to support themselves and their families; to be treated with respect while they do so; and to be free of toxic substances, financial exploitation, and psychological and sexual abuse by their employers.

Nursing: a high risk profession

In hospitals, violence occurs most frequently in psychiatric wards, emergency departments, waiting rooms, and geriatric units. Despite widespread perceptions noted above regarding crime and psychiatric illness, mental patients are probably no more violent than they were in the past, and their rates of violence are comparable to those of the general public (Friedman, 2006). Yet, nurses and others may be getting hurt more often by patients who should never have been admitted to a mental health facility in the first place.

A number of studies in recent years have pointed to the prevalence of workplace violence experienced by healthcare workers. Among those injured, professional nurses (RNs) and nursing assistants in hospitals and long-term care facilities are prime targets in their role as direct care providers:

- The Bureau of Labor Statistics (US) reported that in 2000, 48 percent of all non-fatal injuries from violent acts against workers occurred in the healthcare sector with nurses, nurses aides and orderlies suffering the highest proportion of injuries (McPhaul, & Lipscomb, 2004).
- Among health personnel, nursing staff are most at risk of workplace violence with the student nurse, staff and charge nurses and ambulance staff leading the way (ICN, 2001).
- Erickson and Williams-Evans (2000) reported that 82 percent of nurses surveyed had been assaulted during their careers (ICN, 2001).
- In a study across clinical settings by Anderson (2002), 71 percent of nurses reported emotional types of workplace violence, 42 percent reported sexual types, and 39 percent reported physical types.
- In 2000, the Alberta Nurse Survey of 8,780 Canadian staff nurses from 210 hospitals

revealed that over their past five shifts worked, 46 percent of nurses experienced one or more types of violence and that between 17 and 21 percent experienced a physical assault (Duncan *et al.*, 2000);

- The Minnesota Nurses' Study reported annual adjusted rates of 13.2 percent for physical assault and of 38.8 percent for non-physical violence among all participants (Gerberich *et al.*, 2004).

Yet, these studies do not tell the whole story, due to variations in study designs and reporting systems, and that many nurses are reluctant to report violent incidents. The Alberta Nurse Survey found that 70 percent of nurses do not report violent incidents. Some studies estimate that more than 80 percent of all assaults on registered nurses go unreported (ANA, 2002). Reasons for this underreporting may include: (a) a lack of institutional reporting policies; (b) the perception that assaults are part of the job; (c) employee beliefs that they may be blamed for the incident, or that the assaults might be viewed as a result of poor job performance or worker negligence.

Adverse consequences of workplace violence against nurses span short- and long-term physical and psychological symptoms. Even in the absence of physical injury, results of the epidemiological Minnesota Nurses' Study revealed that nurses' moderate to severe reactions to assault lasted for six months to one year, while the case study findings cited job changes, chronic pain, and depression as long as four years after the assault (Gerberich *et al.*, 2004). Like the stories of victim/survivors of intimate partner abuse, nurses say it is easier to heal from physical wounds than from the psychic trauma of angry and assaultive words (Herman, 1992).

Promoting healthy and safe employment in healthcare – the PHASE study

Responding to national and international attention to workplace violence issues, researchers from the University of Massachusetts Lowell conducted a five-year federally funded study of health disparities among healthcare workers titled PHASE: Promoting Healthy and Safe Employment in Healthcare (Slatin, 2006). This interdisciplinary multi-methods study included epidemiological survey data and extensive qualitative methods such as case studies and focus group inquiry. Two hospitals and two long-term care facilities collaborated in the study. An additional collaborative partnership with the Massachusetts Nurses Association (MNA) provided the opportunity to learn about the working conditions nurses face in a range of healthcare settings.

Key questions addressed how healthcare system restructuring has affected workers' health and safety across a range of healthcare workers representing race, class, gender, and age differences. In the MNA segment of the study, nearly 50 nurses (including elected leaders, local unit leaders, occupational health advocates and staff nurses, employed mostly in hospital environments), participated in a series of seven focus groups on the following topics: General health and safety; violence and abuse; diversity and discrimination issues; post-injury return to work experiences; and healthcare system restructuring. The following are the highlights of findings from analysis of focus group data with particular relevance to workplace violence and implications for prevention (Hoff, & Slatin, 2006).

The categories of assault and abuse included physical but non-life threatening, life-threatening, and verbal and emotional abuse. Violence occurs across practice settings, with patients as primary perpetrators and direct care staff the primary targets. Nurses attribute increasing assaults and abuse to lack of preventive programs and management support, inadequate staffing and security measures, admission of patients with histories of violence, the "free flow of people and [generally] increased aggressiveness of patients and families," short staffing and long waits for service leading to patient frustration. Abuse included verbal attacks by physicians and the emotional toll of "constant negative evaluations" by management, labeling them as "malingerers" if injury was not physically apparent, and humiliating them in front of patients and other staff.

Nurses distinguished the trauma from abuse in relation to the cognitive status of the perpetrator: if the patient is impaired, it is easier to excuse the assault. Yet, there is a tendency to interpret assaults in healthcare settings as "part of the job," unlike, for example, recognizing assault in a supermarket as a "criminal act." For example, when complaining about a sexually assaultive patient, a supervisor said, "We can't do anything. He has a right to be here until a court order is obtained." Similarly, in a dramatic and *life-threatening hostage situation*, management was apparently oblivious of the emotional toll on the nurse trying to bring a very violent patient under control and save her own and others' lives when cowering for safety in a room. The patient had threatened to kill the hostages by releasing the contents of a fire extinguisher he had ripped off a wall. The nurse manager pressed the traumatized nurse to continue in her care-giving role with "Hurry up, let's go" and no opportunity was offered for post-incident debriefing or support after such a traumatic experience. Also noted was a rank indifference in management's response to assault of workers, with more attention paid, for example, if the assaulted victim was a physician.

Nurses cited management indifference, blatant victim-blaming, or even hostile rebuke of a reporting nurse; for example, management sent a nurse-educator to "teach somebody what, obviously, she did wrong," implying "You really did it yourself", or "You don't know what you're doing," or "It's in your head, you're overreacting" or "You must have psychiatric problems." Another nurse said that the nurse manager would "rip up the incident reports" and verbally attack nurses for "trying to cause trouble", saying "Why are you making out these incident reports just because someone got punched in the face? What's the big deal?" Nurses therefore get to the point of saying "Why bother?" [reporting]. In an instance of verbal abuse with no physical injury by a surgeon, management indifference was exemplified by the remarks "He's like that," or "He talks to everybody that way .... It's like a no-win situation."

Overall, nurses said that "lack of support almost is worse than the illness or what happened to you." When the burden of responsibility for documenting injury is on the injured party instead of the agency, nurses felt re-abused by the system. They also cited the money that could be saved by solving the occupational health problems vs. legally intimidating the injured worker. In a similar vein, they cited "throwing away experienced nurses." Rather than dealing with what nurses experienced as the inadequate Workers' Compensation system, a nurse said, it's easier to "just take Motrin [ibuprofen] and go on working." On the other hand, one nurse acknowledged that "We put ourselves in harm's way" [in contrast to others who assert themselves], while another said "Adaptation is a terrible thing, you do it because it's expected of you. And eventually you don't even realize how bad it is for you."

The context and consequences of workplace violence against nurses

Most people are surprised to learn that nurses rank with police officers and fire fighters in rates of injury on the job. Public perception squares with the fact that policing involves interaction with persons who have already broken laws or are deemed dangerous to others, while the risks of fighting fires are self-evident.

But the reasons for risks faced by nurses are more complex and intertwined with sociocultural factors similar to those addressed in other chapters. Attention to these risks is underscored on several counts: (1) worldwide, nursing personnel are predominantly female; (2) within the healthcare industry itself, nurses and nursing assistants comprise a significant majority in sheer numbers compared with myriad categories of other workers; (3) in addition to injuries suffered by other victim/survivors of assault, workplace violence results in negative organizational effects such as low worker morale, increased job stress, increased worker turnover, reduced trust of management and co-workers, a hostile work environment, significant costs associated with lost workdays and wages, and a serious undermining of the healing mission of the healthcare organization (AACN, 2004; NIOSH, 2002).

From the hospital's perspective, consequences of workplace violence against nurses can lead to deterioration in the quality of care to patients, increased errors, worsened patient outcomes, lower patient satisfaction, and negative effects on recruitment (Arnetz, & Arnetz, 2001). Results from a 2001 survey of registered nurses by the American Nurses Association (ANA) revealed that health and safety concerns played a major role in nurses' decisions about leaving the profession (Nachreiner *et al.*, 2005). In the US, a government estimate is that by the year 2020 there will be a nursing shortage of nearly one million. This has global health and ethical recruitment implications in that trained nurses from poor countries come to the US in hope of a better job, only to deplete poor countries' educated work force and join the ranks of abused American nurses. Violence against nurses, the associated crisis of recruitment, and analysis of this issue in sociocultural context is continued in Chapter 12.

Recognizing signs of danger and potential for assault and homicide

Too often the signs of impending assault or homicide are either not recognized or are ignored until it is too late, as documented in widely publicized massacres at schools and worksites. Professionals and the lay public need reminders that murder does not occur in a cultural or social vacuum; it does not "just happen." Rather, it is planned, although impulse may play a part. Thus, for example, occasions for job terminations are a reality in the work environment. But wise administrators know from organizational theory that the *humane treatment of workers* when delivering news of discipline or layoff is a violence-prevention measure needing attention, if for no other reason than self-interest. When this principle of respect for workers is ignored, some fired workers who are treated like criminals – whatever the reason for job termination – come back to terrorize their former workplace with all-too available guns or explosives.

Fortunately, the days of assaulted health workers' having to absorb their injury and emotional trauma as "part of the job" appear to be coming to an end (O'Sullivan *et al.*, 2008). This and other research has uncovered the relationship of workplace injury to gender, race, and class factors, as well as to the work environment itself – for example, inadequate staffing and lack of structured supervisor support. Governmental and labor union action portend the prospect of redressing the neglect of many victimized workers who have been largely on their own in the process of recovering from the trauma of such mostly preventable violence (Jenkins *et al.*, 1992; Levin *et al.*, 1992; Lipscomb, & Love, 1992; Miller, 1999; Rosen, 2001; Runyan, 2001).

In the US there are no federal regulations or mandates for employers to offer training in workplace violence. The federal government by way of the *Occupational Safety and Health Administration (OSHA)* has issued *voluntary* guidelines for healthcare and social services employers. At the state level, only California and Washington have enacted regulations aimed at reducing patient-employee (Type 2) violence in healthcare settings (McPhaul, & Lipscomb, 2004). Worker training is often recommended as part of a comprehensive approach to workplace violence, yet few interventions have been evaluated for their effectiveness (Nachreiner, *et al.*, 2005).

Also, there are very few scientific studies on how to *prevent* violence toward healthcare workers. The ANA, the International Council of Nurses (ICN) and the American Academy of Nursing (AAN), as well as healthcare labor unions, are calling for increased intervention effectiveness research and more widespread protective regulations. The American Association of Colleges of Nursing (AACN) issued a Position Paper in 1999 emphasizing the inclusion of violence-related content as "essential" in nursing curricula, while the American Psychiatric Nurses Association (APNA) issued a Position Paper on Workplace Violence in 2008. These are all promising signs of potential action on this urgent issue.

Violence prevention strategies

Several strategies could reduce the hazard of workplace violence: (1) routine application of danger assessment techniques; (2) implementation of the principles and strategies for creating a therapeutic milieu; and (3) use of social network techniques and community-based services to defuse highly anxious and hostile behavior by non-chemical means (Cowin *et al.*, 2003; Dyches *et al.*, 2002). Staff in these highly charged situations also need to reserve time and energy for considering the impact of managed care policies on treatment of the seriously and persistently mentally ill. Some of the results of these policies include the current focus on pharmacological and very brief hospital care and reduced staffing by skilled professionals; in response, staff may then resort to more authoritarian approaches to disruptive behavior, which in turn escalates tension and violence potential among patients.

Traditionally, nurses and psychiatric professionals have been taught that if they get hurt by mentally disturbed people, it is probably because they missed cues to rising anxiety levels or they antagonized or otherwise dealt inappropriately with the disturbed person. For example, when mental health professionals use chemical or physical restraint before trying time-tested inter-personal approaches, retaliative attacks on the staff can result. Only a small percentage of mental patients are dangerous, and psychiatric facilities usually have precise protocols for preventing and responding to those who are. Police procedures are also precise and comprehensive. A basic principle in both disciplines is to avoid force and physical restraint except for protecting oneself and others. This interpretation is strongly supported by Bard's (1972) precedent-setting research and subsequent training for New York City police officers. The number of NYC police injuries and deaths on the job were significantly reduced as a result of the application of crisis intervention techniques and tightening readily accessible linkages with mental health professionals, especially in family disturbance (domestic violence) calls. These techniques have been expanded to deal with terrorists through hostage negotiation strategies (Hoff *et al.*, 2009, Chapter 12).

Based on Monahan's (1981) pioneering research, risk assessment criteria include:

1 *Statistics* – for example, men between the ages of 18 and 34 commit a much higher percentage of violent crimes than older men or women of any age. Statistical indicators, however, should be viewed with the same caution as in suicide risk assessment (see Hoff, *et al.*, 2009, Chapter 9).
2 *Personality factors*, including motivation, aggression, inhibition, and habit. For example, once a habit of response to upsets by verbal threats and physical force is established, it lays a foundation for further, potentially lethal violence.
3 *Situational factors*, such as availability of a weapon or behavior of the potential victim.
4 *The interaction* between these variables.

In another pioneering work on violent men, Toch (1969) claims that the *interaction* factor is a crucial one influencing violence. The interactional process begins with classifying a potential victim as an object or a potential threat to the man's ego and need to control, as in a hostage situation or in rape crisis, if the rapist has a deadly weapon. A most basic principle then in defusing a potentially dangerous crisis is *time and keeping communication open*. Precipitous action, taunts and counter-threats may only heighten the danger.

Clearly, assessing danger – at home, at school, at work – is no simple matter, but lives can be saved by taking seriously the fact that only potentially dangerous people make threats of assault or homicide. A careful read of newspaper accounts of murders reveals almost invariably the assailant's verbal and other cues that were either ignored or misinterpreted as not being serious. The major *verbal clues* that alert us to possible danger from others include: speaking loudly or yelling, swearing, a threatening tone of voice. Major *non-verbal or behavioral clues* include: heavy breathing, pacing or agitation, arms held tight across chest, a fixed stare, aggressive or threatening posture, thrown objects. In addition, it is important to be sensitive to when one's own "flight or fight" response has been triggered, for example, involuntary shaking of hands, hyperventilation and breaking out in a sweat.

Awareness of these clues, therefore, and how to respond to them is paramount for co-workers, teachers, various professionals, and among one's own family and friends to identify disturbed or potentially violent people. This includes always inquiring about the *meaning* of verbal threats that too many times are dismissed by family, friends, and associates, as in "Oh, he just talks like that when he's angry," thus foregoing an opportunity to find out more and engage outside help before it is too late.

When the indicators of dangerousness discussed here, and the assessment tool illustrated in Table 11.1, were introduced decades ago and routinely applied in crisis and counseling clinics in western New York state, staff were astounded at how many clients were entertaining violent fantasies. But crisis workers in that public mental health system also noted the clients' openness to receiving help in dealing with their anger and violent impulses. The key elements of that danger assessment approach are recommended for application across the spectrum of dangerous and even life-threatening situations: (1) in learning environments among bullying classmates or ambitious college students enraged by a failing grade they may perceive as a death knell for their future careers; (2) in the workplace where threats of violence and abuse occur from a number of sources (see the 4 types of workplace violence), and (3) in domestic dispute situations with women fearful of their abusive partners, and in programs for men who have battered and emotionally abused them.

For the second and third situations in the above list, here are some potential responses for someone aware of verbal and behavioral clues signaling possible danger:

Nurse: I'm sorry, Mr Jones, you can't see your wife just now. How about I meet you in the waiting room when we finish the procedure?

Patient's husband, in angry threatening tone: What do you mean, "wait"? I'm her HUSBAND and I want to see her NOW!

This response might signal an abusive husband who is still trying to control his wife – even in the hospital where she is in labor and giving birth to their child. Or if an abused woman has enacted a restraining order against her husband, he violates it, and says "If I can't have you, no one can," she recognizes this as his claim to "ownership" of her and as a serious and imminent threat to her life. She "keeps communication open," and looks for opportunities to escape or call for help. For example, a battered woman taken hostage was allowed to go to the "ladies room" in a restaurant enroute to where he was taking her "away from her new boyfriend"; on the way she whispered her plight to a waitress who called the police, and she was rescued.

These examples illustrate a crucial part of safety and crisis intervention planning: Awareness of clues to violent and life-threatening behavior, include the following principles. While violent people can learn other ways, past abusive and violent behavior is still a *powerful indicator of future behavior*. As the triage questions in Exhibit 4.1 (Chapter 4) indicate, routine screening for assault and homicide potential is gender neutral; therefore, the abused woman's own potential for assaulting or killing her assailant following abuse must also be ascertained. And since significant numbers of female health professionals are also survivors of domestic violence that spills over to the work environment, all should be alert for evidence-based assessment of potential for all 4 types of violence in the workplace.

Table 11.1 Assault and Homicidal Danger Assessment Tool

Key to danger	Immediate dangerousness to others	Typical indicators
1	No predictable risk of assault or homicide	Has no assaultive or homicidal ideation, urges, or history of same; basically satisfactory support system; social drinker only
2	Low risk of assault or homicide	Has occasional assault or homicidal ideation (including paranoid ideas) with some urges to kill; no history of impulsive acts or homicidal attempts; occasional drinking bouts and angry verbal outbursts; basically satisfactory support system
3	Moderate risk of assault or homicide	Has frequent homicidal ideation and urges to kill but no specific plan; history of impulsive acting out and verbal outbursts while drinking, on other drugs, or otherwise; stormy relationship with significant others with periodic high tension arguments
4	High risk of homicide	Has homicidal plan; obtainable means; history of substance abuse; frequent acting out against others, but no homicide attempts; stormy relationships and much verbal fighting with significant others, with occasional assaults
5	Very high risk of homicide	Has current high lethal plan; available means; history of homicide attempts or impulsive acting out, plus feels a strong urge to control and "get even" with a significant other; history of serious substance abuse; also with possible high lethal suicide risk

Assessment of individuals for danger

Translated into everyday practice, the following criteria are helpful as guidelines to assess dangerousness and the risk of assault or homicide (Hoff *et al.*, 2009, Chapter 12):

- history of homicidal threats;
- history of assault;
- current homicidal threats and plan, including on the Internet;
- possession or easy availability of lethal weapons;
- use or abuse of alcohol or other drugs;
- conflict in significant social or clinical relationships – for example, infidelity, threat of divorce, labor-management disputes, authoritarian approaches to the mentally ill.

Threats of suicide following homicide.

Case examples: assessment and service planning (Australia)

The following examples refer to violent incidents involving members of the local White and Aboriginal community and how community mental health and other staff dealt with them. They are taken from the clinical experience of Joy Adams-Jackson.

The brief analysis is framed from the perspective of a crisis or mental health professional available as a consultant to staff healthcare workers threatened by Type 4 violence in the workplace. It suggests a preliminary level of risk according to the criteria and danger assessment in which domestic violence and other abuse spills over to the healthcare setting, and hospital workers are the secondary targets of controlling behavior and threats by the abuser.

Example 1

A female community mental health nurse was called by nursing staff to the local hospital ward and asked to settle a 24-year-old female substance abuser who was becoming increasingly aggressive and threatening to leave hospital contrary to medical advice. On arriving at the ward the patient's so-called boyfriend (pimp) aggressively confronted the nurse and told her in no uncertain terms where she could shove her medical advice. He offered to "punch her lights out" if she refused to let his girlfriend discharge herself into his care.

Assessment and service planning Using Table 11.1, based on available data, the preliminary assessment of risk level is between 3 and 4: moderate to high, with indication that a more reliable assessment of assault/homicide risk requires obtaining further information from the hospital patient as well as the aggressive boyfriend. The hospital nurse had learned from the patient that the mental health nurse knew this couple from her community-based work. Follow-up care of this client draws on principles discussed in Chapters 4 and 10, as well as collaboration with practitioners with expertise in substance abuse treatment.

Example 2

A nurse working in the hospital emergency room called the mental health crisis team to make a quick and urgent assessment of a 33-year-old male. The man was brought into the hospital by local police following a very public and violent altercation with his partner. The victim had called the police, who in turn arranged for her transfer by ambulance to the hospital for treatment of her injuries. The man had fractured his partner's ribs and broken her nose. Police also took the perpetrator to the hospital for a mental health assessment because they feared that his extremely unpredictable and violent outburst was due to an underlying mental illness. In the emergency room the man continued his aggressive and threatening behaviors. He was particularly angry at staff for denying him any access to his partner who was receiving treatment by emergency staff. Upon arrival of the mental health crisis team, they in turn were threatened and abused by the man. Their evaluation revealed no evidence of a mental disorder and therefore they returned the man to police custody.

Assessment and service planning: follow-up work on behalf of this violent man indicates the necessity of collaboration between police and mental health professional consultation, as discussed in the forensic psychiatry section above. This includes further assessment of his danger potential, with attention to the criteria described above, and outreach to his injured partner. (See Chapter 13 for illustrations of medical and criminal justice collaboration.)

Crisis care and support of injured or threatened workers

As noted from outcomes of the PHASE study, the failure of immediate support and attention to an injured or threatened worker can be as traumatic as the assault itself. Given the international momentum on preventing and ending workplace violence, the days of interpreting or dismissing work-related violence as "part of the job" should be over. It is not acceptable to expect emotionally traumatized workers to simply move on and nurse their psychological wounds in private.

As a result, most healthcare and other work settings have "employee assistance programs" that offer crisis intervention, immediate support, and referral for physical and psychological follow-up care. These programs vary widely in the extent and quality of service and satisfaction by injured workers. But however programs are structured for threatened or injured workers, the basic principles and strategies of crisis care apply, as in the case of *anyone* in acute distress or crisis. This means building in opportunities for listening to and supporting the worker in a collaborative plan for immediate medical and psychological service, and any follow-up counseling needed for post-traumatic stress in instances such as serious threat to life.

Original work with disaster survivors led to identification of three typical phases of the crisis experience: Impact, Recoil, and Post-trauma (Tyhurst, 1951). During the *Impact* phase, the focus is on rescue and immediate protection from further danger; during the *Recoil* phase, medical care and basic human needs are the focus; the *Post-trauma* focus is on counseling around psychological after effects of the disaster. These helping strategies correspond broadly to the intervention and counseling strategies of contemporary crisis theory addressing the *emotional*, *biophysical*, *cognitive*, and *behavioral* responses to traumatic life events. Research with survivors of domestic violence (Hoff, 1990) led to an elaboration of early crisis theory. This included the unique consequences of critical events originating from one's disadvantaged position in social structures, and deeply entrenched values that supported not only the acceptability of violence against wives and rape as "the spoils of war" but also "pathologized" or excused perpetrators on flimsy grounds. Intervention and care of survivors in such instances must explicitly acknowledge these sociocultural origins and plan services accordingly. The Crisis Paradigm (see Chapter 13) illustrates the crisis response and helping process aimed at preventing negative crisis outcomes such as depression or violence against others at work, in schools, or home (Hoff *et al.*, 2009).

Critical Incident Stress Debriefing (CISD): values and cautions

Mental health professionals trained in grief work, crisis intervention, and assessment of psycho-pathology will be careful not to pathologize what is essentially a *normal* response to an event that is beyond the range of events experienced by most people (see Neria, 2007; Zunin, & Zunin, 1991). Caution is also in order around formalized debriefing, known as Critical Incident Stress Debriefing (CISD), after disaster or with workers injured on the job, especially for survivors who might interpret structured debriefing as a sign they are going crazy.

Regehr's (2001) review of research evidence on this debated topic suggests that the highly ritualized CISD process incorporates into a very formal structure the basic elements of crisis intervention long-known from the work of crisis theory pioneers like Tyhurst (1951) and Caplan (1964), and others. As noted in Chapter 9 regarding work with torture or trafficking survivors, mental health professionals and victimology experts know about the potential damage of eli-citing expression of deep psychological trauma prematurely or without appropriate follow-up and support during the aftermath of divulging certain feelings such as shame and rage. Regehr's review suggests evidence of secondary trauma or "vicarious traumatization" among some CISD participants from hearing other participants' graphic descriptions. In a related cautionary note, Jacobs *et al.* (2004) discuss the personality characteristics of some emergency personnel conduct-ing CISD sessions: high need for control, a need for immediate gratification, and a strong need to be needed (see Chapter 12 for the Victim-Rescuer-Persecutor Triangle).

Adapting CISD in its subset, Critical Incident Stress Management (CISM), Mitchell (2003) summarizes established crisis care strategies and implies with "management" a theme from medical practice. That is, "managing" diabetes or heart disease, for example – as is well known in medical circles – will almost inevitably fail if evidence-based treatment sidelines the patient's own role in "managing" his or her illness. "Management" suggests control and taking charge, but means little without the active collaboration of those "managed" – as corporate and other leaders have experienced.

Applied to the aftermath of workplace violence, survivors need respite from danger, im-mediate support, time to heal, and linkage to appropriate counseling, workers' compensation, and legal services. Considering that feelings of disempowerment are a common response to violence, the highly structured CISD process may not be what injured workers and witnesses might choose as the most helpful route for regaining a sense of control and personal mastery – particularly if it is a formal administration *requirement*.

Personal and institutional strategies for violence prevention

Clearly, since the consequences of violence are so injurious to individuals, families, and whole societies, prevention should ideally be front and center in comprehensive approaches to the problem. But how do we get beyond emergency measures? How do we conserve energy to avoid burnout and disillusionment from the demanding work of caring for victim/survivors? Many strategies have already been addressed regarding the needs of individual victim/survivors and perpetrators. The following are primary prevention strategies specific to learning and work environments (Hoff *et al.*, 2009; see Chapter 12 for self-care and vicarious traumatization).

Personal and sociopsychological strategies

While one person cannot singlehandedly address the massive problem of violence, everyone committed to making a difference on this issue can incorporate primary prevention into everyday life. For example, using non-violent language in ordinary social interaction and refraining from physical discipline of children; avoiding sex-role stereotyping in child-rearing and other interactions with children; providing employees and fellow workers with violence prevention information and emergency protocols, including how to recognize and respond humanely to an upset or disgruntled worker with anti-social tendencies.

Sociopolitical strategies

These include, for example, educating the public through schools, community organizations, and churches; contacting legislators and organizing for changes in the laws regarding violence accountability that may be outdated; using advocacy and systematic organizing to seek equality and protection for disadvantaged groups (immigrants, and gay, lesbian, bisexual, or transgender youth) at particular risk of violence; addressing the media and its influence on violence. These strategies are most successful when combined with personal and sociopsychological approaches on the premise that people need grounding in information and self-confidence in order to stand firm against obstacles in the political arena.

The vast knowledge already available about this poignant topic can be widely disseminated to the public; it can be harnessed to change the values and attitudes that have served as fertile soil for nurturing violent and anti-social behavior; and it can affect broad policy and functioning of social institutions through the political process necessary to bring about needed change.

References

AACN – American Association of Colleges of Nursing (2004). *Policy Statement on Workplace Violence Prevention.* Washington, DC: AACN.

ANA – American Nurses Association (2002). *Preventing Workplace Violence.* Washington, DC: ANA.

Anderson, C. (2002). Workplace violence: Are some nurses more vulnerable? *Issues in Mental Health Nursing,* 23(4), 351–66.

Anderson, C. R. N. (2002). Past victim, future victim? *Nursing Management,* 33(3), 26–32.

APA – American Psychiatry Association (2000). *Diagnostic and Statistical Manual of Mental Illness* (4th edn.). Arlington, VA: American Psychiatric Publishing, Inc.

Arnetz, J. E., & Arnetz, B. B. (2001). Violence towards health care staff and possible effects on the quality of patient care. *Social Science and Medicine,* 52, 417–27.

Bard. M. (1972). *Police, Family Crisis Intervention, and Conflict Management: An Action Research Analysis.* Washington, DC: US Department of Justice.

Bureau of Justice Statistics (2001). *Special Report: Violence in the Workplace, 1993–99.* Washington, DC: US Department of Justice.

Caplan, G. R. (1964). *Principles in Preventive Psychiatry.* New York: Basic Books.

Carlsson-Paige, N., & Levin, D. (2008). *Taking Back Childhood: Helping your Kids Thrive in a Fast-Paced, Media-Saturated, Violence-Filled World.* New York: Hudson Street Press.

Christmas, K. (2007). Workplace abuse: Finding solutions. *Nursing Economics,* 25(6), 365–7.

Clements, P. T., *et al.* (2005). Workplace violence and corporate policy for health care settings. *Nursing Economics* 23(3), 119–24.

Cowin, L., *et al.* (2003). De-escalating aggression and violence in the mental health setting. *International Journal of Mental Health Nursing,* 12, pp. 64–73.

Duncan, S., Estabrooks, C. A., & Reimer, M. (2000). Violence against nurses. *Alta RN,* 56(2), 13–14.

Dyches, H., *et al.* (2002). The impact of mobile crisis services on the use of community-based mental health services. *Research on Social Work Practice,* 12(6), pp. 731–51.

Earley, P. (2006). *Crazy: A Father's Search Through America's Mental Health Madness.* New York: Berkley Books.

Ellickson, P., Saner, H., & McGuigan, K. A. Profiles of violent youth: Substance use and other concurrent problems. *American Journal of Public Health*, 87(6), 985–1.

Emergency Nurses Association (2006), *Position Statement on Violence in the Emergency Care Setting*. Available online at: http://www.ena.org/about/position/pdfs/violenceintheedpositionstatement2006. pdf (accessed July 7, 2006).

Erickson, L., & Williams-Evans, S. (2000). Attitudes of emergency nurses regarding patient assaults. *Journal of Emergency Nursing*, 26(3), 210–15.

Freire, P. (1989). *Pedagogy of the Oppressed*. New York: Continuum.

Friedman, R. A. (2006). Violence and mental illness – How strong is the link? *New England Journal of Medicine*, 355(20), 2064–6.

Garbarino, J., & deLara, E. (2002). *And Words Can Hurt Forever: How to Protect Adolescents from Bullying, Harassment, and Emotional Violence*. New York: Free Press.

Gerberich, S. G., *et al.* (2004). An epidemiological study of the magnitude and consequences of work related violence: the Minnesota Nurses' Study. *Occupational and Environmental Medicine*, 61, 495–503.

Herman, J. (1992). *Trauma and Recovery*. New York: Basic Books.

Hoff, L. A. (1990). *Battered Women as Survivors*. London: Routledge.

Hoff, L. A. (1994). Comments on race, gender, and class bias in nursing. *Medical Anthropology Quarterly*, 8(1), 96–9.

Hoff, L. A., Hallisey, B. J., & Hoff, M. (2009). *People in Crisis: Clinical and Diversity Perspectives* (6th edn.). New York & London: Routledge.

Hoff, L. A. & Slatin, C. (2006). *Workplace Health and Safety: Report of PHASE/MNA Focus Groups*. University of Massachusetts Lovell.

Hoover, J., & Juul, K. (1993). Bullying in Europe and the United States. *Journal of Emotional and Behavioral Problems*, 2, 25–9.

Hoover, J., & Oliver, R. (1996). *The Bullying Prevention Handbook: A Guide for Principals, Teachers, and Counselors*. Bloomington, IN: National Education Service.

ICN – International Council of Nurses. 2001. *Anti-Violence Tool Kit*. Geneva, Switzerland: ICN.

Jackson, J. (1998). Violence in the workplace. In J. Horsfall (ed.), *Violence and Nursing*, pp. 49–58. Australia: Royal College of Nursing.

Jenkins, E. L, Layne, L. A., & Kisner, S. M. (1992). Homicide in the workplace: The U.S. experience, 1980–1988. *American Association of Occupational Health Nurses Journal*, 40, 215–18.

Levin, P. F., Hewitt, J. B., & Misner, S. T. (1998). Insights of nurses about assault in hospital-based emergency departments. *Image: Journal of Nursing Scholarship*, 30(3), 249–54.

Lipscomb J., & Love C. (1992) Violence toward health care workers. *American Association of Occupational Health Nurses Journal*, 40(5), 219–28.

McPhaul, K., & Lipscomb, J. (2004). Workplace violence in health care: Recognized but not regulated. *Online Journal of Issues in Nursing*, 9(3), Manuscript 6. Available online at: http://www.nursingworld. org/ojin/topic25/tpc25_6.htm

Merchant, J., & Lundell, J. (2001). Workplace violence intervention research workshop, April 5 -7, 2000. Washington, DC: *American Journal of Preventive Medicine*, 20(2), 135–40.

Miller, L. (1999). Workplace violence: Prevention, response, and recovery. *Psychotherapy*, 36(2), 160–9.

Monahan, J. (1981). *Predicting Violent Behavior: An Assessment of Clinical Techniques*. Thousand Oaks, CA: Sage.

Monahan, J., & Steadman, H. J. (eds.) (1994). *Violence and Mental Disorder: Developments in Risk Assessment*. Chicago and London: University of Chicago Press.

Nachreiner, N. M., *et al.* (2005). Impact of training on work-related assault. *Research in Nursing & Health*, 28(1), 67–78.

Neria, Y., *et al.* (2007). Prevalence and psychological correlates of complicated grief among bereaved adults 2.5 – 3.5 years after September 11th attacks. *Journal of Traumatic Stress*, 20(3), 251–62.

NIOSH – National Institute for Occupational Safety and Health (2002). *Violence: Occupational Hazards in Hospitals*. NIOSH Publication No. 2002–101.

O'Sullivan, M., *et al.* (2008). It's part of the job: Healthcare restructuring and the health and safety of nursing aides. In L. McKee, E. Ferlie, & P. Hyde (eds.), *Organizing and Reorganizing: Power and Change in Health care Organizations*, pp. 99–111. Houndmills, Basingstoke, Hampshire, UK: Palgrave MacMillan.

Parker-Roerden, L., Rudewick, D., & Gorton, D. (2007). *Direct From the Field: A Guide to Bullying Prevention*. Boston: Commonwealth of Massachusetts.

Pies, R. (2008, February 25). Mentally ill unfairly portrayed as violent. *Boston Globe*. Op. ed.

Regehr, C. (2001) Crisis debriefing groups for emergency responders: Reviewing the evidence. *Brief Treatment and Crisis Intervention* 1, 87–100.

Rosen, J. (2001). A labor perspective of workplace violence prevention: Identifying research needs. *American Journal of Preventive Medicine*, 20(2), 161–8.

Runyan, C. W. (2001). Moving forward with research on the prevention of violence against workers. *American Journal of Preventive Medicine*, 20(2), 169–72.

Slatin, C. (2006). Social Context of Occupational Health Disparities for Healthcare Workers: Findings of the PHASE in Healthcare Research Project. Paper given at the 134th Annual Meeting & Exposition of the American Public Health Association, Boston, MA, November 4–8.

Toch, H. (1969) *Violent Men*. Chicago: Aldine Publishing Co.

Tyhurst, J. S. (1951). Individual reactions to community disaster. *American Journal of Psychiatry*, 107, 764–9.

UIIPRC – University of Iowa Injury Prevention Research Center (2001). *Workplace Violence – A Report to the Nation*. Iowa City, IA: University of Iowa. Available online at: http://www.public-health.uiowa.edu/news/pubs/special/workplace-violence/ (accessed July 24, 2006).

Ustun, T. B. (1999). The global burden of mental disorders. *American Journal of Public Health*, 89(9), 1315–21.

Walker, H.M. (1993). Anti-social behaviour in school. *Journal of Emotional and Behavioral Problems*, 2(1), pp. 20–4.

Zunin, L. M., & Zunin, H. S. (1991). *The Art Of Condolence: What to Write, What to Say, What to do at a Time of Loss*. New York: HarperCollins.

Note

1 Researchers and university student affairs personnel are invited to contact the author regarding collaboration in further use of a pilot-tested survey tool on "Student Stress and Crisis" providing a database for planning crisis prevention, intervention, and mental health services for college students. (See online resources.)

12   Implementation issues

Personal/professional victimization

- Personal abuse history, provider stress, and relationship to caretaking
- The "wounded healer" in diverse roles: practitioner, teacher, student
- Abuse of practitioners: gender, class, and race relations
- The culture of nursing and lateral violence
- Health providers' abuse of patients
- Vicarious traumatization and boundary issues

    — The Victim-Rescuer-Persecutor triangle

- Case examples of vicarious trauma and compassion fatigue

    — A family therapist
    — A professor of nursing
    — A humanitarian aid worker
    — An immigrant student from a poor country

- Self-care and support programs for providers
- Social change and professional strategies complementing self-care and support

It is one thing to embrace and master the essential knowledge, attitudes, and skills needed for violence prevention and the humane professional care of victim/survivors but there are related issues for consideration as well, without which personal and professional efforts may well not succeed. These include:

- The general stress and conflicted feelings that may be aroused from working with victim/survivors and perpetrators of violence.
- The potential for burnout and vicarious traumatization from violence-related work, especially without support from colleagues.
- Physical abuse by patients, especially of female providers like physical therapists, nurses, and physicians whose work involves much hands-on contact.
- Tension, conflict, and sometimes abuse along gender, race, and class lines between and within professional groups – a situation historically most pronounced between medicine and nursing, but by no means limited to these professions.
- Abusive behavior by providers in personal and/or professional relationships.
- Faculty/student/counselor roles and personal victimization histories among health providers – faculty as well as students, and practitioners who are role models for students and volunteer workers.

This chapter addresses these issues and the preventive measures – both personal and institutional – that can alleviate the considerable stress on health and social service providers dedicated to violence prevention and dealing with the consequences of violence experienced by so many victim/survivors and their families.

Personal abuse history, provider stress, and relationship to caretaking

During focus groups and interviews conducted across disciplines for this book, as well as in survey data and in the emerging literature on the topic, two themes repeatedly emerged: (1) the caregiver's personal abuse history and provider stress; and (2) abuse of individual practitioners, and provider abuse of patients.

When interpersonal violence emerged from the historic "private" realm and was declared a public health issue, early research revealed that the incidence of physical and/or sexual abuse among the general female population was very high (Russell, 1990). And since women constitute either majorities or large numbers of those doing direct care within the health and social service professions, it is highly probable that abuse histories exist among practitioners, students, and faculty of these professions as well. But since the male/female power disparity and the cloak of silence that has preserved women's abuse "secrets" until recently are reflected in the health professions, it is also probable that many traumas from such abuse may not have been worked through by faculty, clinical preceptors, or counseling services for students. In addition, a person who is currently in an abusive situation may find that barriers surface in one's work with other victim/survivors. One nursing student discusses the situation of a classmate:

> One of my girlfriends just dropped out of the course. She was sexually abused by her two older brothers when she was younger and it was a really big problem for her. She dropped out after the first year [because] she hadn't resolved it. When she moved away from the small city she was in and came here, she started to see a counselor and it was all being re-lived and it was just not a good time for her at all but the counselor was helping her a lot. She said she came into nursing because she thought it would help with her problems, but it just didn't work out that way until she got some help.

Similar dynamics may be present among male providers who were physically or sexually abused as children and have not healed from the experience (Hunter, 1990; McManiman, 2000).

Since this is a clinical book, not a therapy manual, the intent here is to make explicit a factor which for some, if perviously hidden, can interfere in successful practice and in the teaching/learning process. From a prevention perspective, this entails a focus on the issue *before* assuming professional practice roles in the challenging health and social service arena that inevitably will include care of victim/survivors. For example, when a student – at least midway in clinical courses – bursts into tears and leaves class during a film on child abuse, it may signal an issue about the curriculum/personal trauma interface. Students make it very clear that they expect an early introduction to potentially disturbing topics like abuse and their possible connections to students' personal histories. They do not expect counseling or therapy from faculty around troubling abuse histories but they *do* expect easily accessible services with a contemporary approach to the problem, and non-intrusive understanding from instructors as they deal with the issue. One student said the problem is that information is "disseminated all over the place. It would be nice if there was some sort of printed pamphlet where it could be at your fingertips, to have handy if you need it." Such a resource should include policies on sexual harassment.

Of course, faculty can neither predict nor prevent student upsets during discussion of emotionally laden topics. But their probability can be reduced by explicitly informing new students that later clinical learning experiences may trigger unanticipated personal responses. Such an introduction early in the curriculum may motivate a student to seek counseling for belatedly uncovered problems which have not been resolved as had been assumed. When such anticipatory guidance fails, however, crisis intervention by faculty for distressed students is appropriate, while ongoing counseling is not (see the online resources on role and boundary issues in Part IV).

Aids to such anticipatory guidance include incorporation of explicit attention to personal history as one of several criteria underpinning assessment protocols in clinical work where victimization is a key concern. Thus, if one has *not* dealt with a personal history of victimization or abuse, success in creating a climate for victimization assessment and empathetic work with other victim/survivors may be compromised. A provider whose own abuse issues are still raw or unresolved over years may "close down" as a veil of self-protection. When this happens, it should not be simply ascribed to a callous or indifferent attitude. Rather, it is more likely that listening to another survivor's story of abuse may re-open long-repressed psychological wounds, or that the person lacks the knowledge and skills needed for this challenging work.

The "wounded healer" in diverse roles: practitioner, teacher, student

Even more challenging than dealing with students' possible history of abuse is facing the prospect that fellow faculty and professional colleagues may be living in high risk situations daily but may feel even more reluctant to disclose their plight than students might. This scenario is compounded by several factors:

- There is a lingering myth that violent behaviors occur only among the poor, people of color, and other disadvantaged populations – most certainly not among health professions faculty and practitioners. While violence statistics do correlate strongly with social disadvantage, poverty does not *cause* violence, and most poor people are not violent.
- Society expects people privileged on class grounds to conform more closely to behavioral norms and use "private" means to resolve their conflicts and problems – a norm which reinforces the "privacy" myth about domestic violence and which may serve as an additional deterrent to people of means seeking help.
- Health professionals have an intense socialization process and ethic to place their clients' needs before their own. While most certainly preserving this service ethic, self-care should not be neglected.
- Boundaries are sometimes blurred between professional and therapeutic relationships. While it is widely accepted that professionals cannot act as therapists to family members, friends, students and associates, this usual boundary gives way in crisis and other situations in which *every citizen* has a human duty to act and help link the person to other resources.

Regardless of a possible personal history of abuse, the treatment, care, and support of abuse survivors takes a toll on health providers similar to that experienced by police officers who witness and must follow up on some of the worst manifestations of our common humanity. And like disaster victims, health professionals observing the brutal results of violence are themselves shocked. Their "sense of coherence" (Antonovsky, 1980), i.e. making sense and meaning out of horrific life events, is shaken (Hoff, 1990). In a vein with holocaust or Hiroshima survivors, they may experience "survivor guilt" (Lifton, 1967), even while their clients' violation starkly reminds them of their own vulnerability (Hoff *et al.*, 2009, Chapter 13).

As health providers confront their own feelings, they may discover identification with either the victim or assailant, depending on past experience and other factors. Physicians and nurses in trauma and emergency centers, and social workers in child and adult protective services, are most frequently exposed to the shocking reality of violence, though no health workers are immune. And so if a "wounded healer" avoids some victims, it may be less from indifference or neglect than from the need for self-protection and support. Another prospect to be faced is that some members of student, clinician, or faculty groups may themselves be abusing their partners, children, or frail elderly parents. These grim realities must be built into educational and personnel services for students and professionals, and should include fostering a climate for appropriate disclosure and accountability, and planned avenues for peer support, time-out, and self-care activities as essential prerequisites for effective service on behalf of victims.

Abuse of practitioners: gender, class, and race relations

Discussion here complements Chapter 11 on violence in work environments, with an emphasis on gender issues and the culture of nursing, and an elaboration of Types 2 and 3 violence. As in the case of women generally, women in the health professions can easily be deluded about female equality because of external freedoms such as driving a car, obtaining a credit card, and entry to traditionally male professions such as medicine, law, and engineering (Faludi, 1991).

Unfortunately, gender stereotypes and workplace inequalities from the larger society are often reproduced in the healthcare system. For example, in the high status profession of medicine, women physicians suffer sexual harassment (Phillips, & Schneider, 1993) and pay inequities, while areas of specialization (e.g. family medicine, psychiatry, pediatrics) tend to support traditions about "women's work." In the lower status profession of nursing, the minority of male nurses advance to higher paying administrative jobs more rapidly. One White male nurse – sensitized to gender issues – noted that he has to consciously struggle not to take advantage of privileges that come his way daily only because of his gender and race. Gender inequalities in nursing, for example, could not be sustained without collusion – and sometimes reverse sexism – by the female majority (Roberts, 1983). Some schools of nursing – apparently without benefit of a gender, race, and class analysis – are treating male students as a "minority" needing affirmative action protection (Barbee, 1993; Hoff, 1994).

In a similar vein, the abuse of individual practitioners usually falls out along gender, race and class lines. In general health and residential care settings, physical therapists, occupational therapists and female nursing staff have long been the object of unwanted sexual advances by male patients and staff (Kettl *et al.*, 1993; McComas, 1993). Physicians continue to be the major source of verbal abuse of nurses (Cox, 1991a, 1991b; Hoff, & Slatin, 2006). But in psychiatric and long-term care settings, where the incidence of physical attacks by patients against staff is generally higher, the most vulnerable are female nursing assistants – often women of color, and definitely the lowest paid group among the hierarchy of direct care staff; professional nurses are the next most frequently injured, and traditionally higher status staff least often injured. There is comparable disparity in the administrative attention paid to prevention, protection, and compensation for such abuse of nurses at various levels of practice (Lanza, 1992). In Massachusetts, for example, before recent legislation, physical assault of a physician by a patient was classified as a felony, while the same level of abuse against a nurse was "only" a misdemeanor (Quintal, 2002).

Some have noted with chagrin that formal nursing organizations were late in their support of the contemporary women's movement (Adams, 2008; Vance *et al.*, 1985). Less often, however, do writers note that nursing has been all but ignored by those feminists eager to open the doors of high status professions like medicine and law to women (Gordon, 1991). Nor is it often noted that women in medicine often suffer the same harassment and abuse as female nurses. While frequently discounted in the larger system, nurses have continued society's necessary work of caring for the sick – sometimes with risks to their own health and safety – though their work is often poorly compensated and "hidden" from policy makers and feminists alike (Rachlis, & Kushner, 1994). Meanwhile, most female health workers (regardless of discipline) face the additional stressors of doing the lion's share of society's unpaid work – child care, cleaning, cooking, and planning the family's leisure activities – even as they assume major leadership roles in health system services for victims of abuse. Progress in this field as a whole demands social change around the fact that violence is a *societal* problem, not just a woman's issue.

A broader-based analysis recognizes the inherent connection between the devaluation of women generally, and women's work in particular – whether performed by physicians, physical therapists, nurses, secretaries, nursing assistants, or others (Keddy, 1993; Waring, 1990). It would also make explicit that all women health professionals – as well as lesser paid women in the healthcare hierarchy – have more in common with one another than is apparent. Finally, a feminist and multicultural critique of the entire healthcare system would underscore the important principle that women, children, men, survivors of abuse and other clients, and society as a whole are not well served by inequalities based on gender, ethnicity, or other characteristics that make one "different."

Consider, for example, this analysis by a battered woman (employed as a nursing assistant) who was asked how nurses could be more helpful to abuse victims:

> I used to come in [to my hospital job] with bruises and they [the nurses] would talk about it: "How can a woman be so stupid and stay with a guy like that?" The nurses were so unsympathetic. I couldn't have been bothered talking to any of them about my situation. But I couldn't help seeing how the doctors would put them down and they stood there and took it. Women are too competitive with each other .... They [the nurses] would complain about how they were treated by doctors and the hospital, but in their relationships you'd have thought they were perfect the way they acted and talked.
>
> (Hoff, 1990, pp. 105–6)

This example is not cited to blame nurses, but to illustrate the continuum between the plight of women *generally*, vis-à-vis their unequal status in society's major institutions worldwide, and the majority of female nurses, i.e. nurses' work (and medical work such as pediatrics) traditionally has been regarded as an extension of women's work in the home for which they purportedly are more "naturally" disposed than are men. The example is also remarkable for the clarity of this battered woman's analysis. Without prompting or formal study of the issue, this abuse survivor intuitively was able to make the connection between her own plight and that of nurses with whom she worked. She laid bare the reasons why *any* professionals who feel abused may not be able to serve victims as they might: one is inhibited from caring for another victim when one's own abuse or oppression has not been confronted and satisfactorily resolved.

Thus, health providers might have mastered the ideals of the violence field vis-à-vis *knowledge*, *attitudes*, and *skills*. However, as is the case regarding prerequisites for crisis practice as a whole, one may be *personally* expert but *structural* barriers like these may effectively neutralize one's ability to practice. How can health professionals advocate for others if they have not first advocated for themselves? (Roberts, 2000). How can they empathetically enter an abused person's world and intervene in the disempowerment of victimization while feeling trapped themselves in rigid structures? A nursing student described her continuing concern over the directives she received regarding a teenage rape victim who gave birth:

> When I was on maternity [clinical placement] there was a 14 year old who had been raped and had the baby. She was in a private room and we would go in and take care of her but we couldn't talk about the baby ... like the family did not want the baby discussed. We could only discuss with this girl what changes were going on in her body and I had a big problem with it .... Like we were there just to practice some technical skills? The baby was being put up for adoption so she never saw the baby. And I thought "That's something that should be discussed, maybe not by me because I wasn't experienced enough, but you just don't pretend that nothing ever happened. Like when we walked into the room it seemed like she was so relieved because we were younger and we looked like her age. I think she was pretty scared, you know, 14 years old and having a baby. Like, wow!"

The attending nurse in this situation simply accepted the family's directive not to talk about the rape and pregnancy with the girl. She did what she was told, this time by the family. Most likely this was because the nurse lacked knowledge, skills, and comfort with the assertiveness needed to deal with this family – a family coping through denial and imposing social isolation on their daughter traumatized by rape and pregnancy.

These examples point to three commonalities between women in the health professions and abused women of all ages in other walks of life. First, the *origin* of battered women's plight and the struggles of female health workers lies in the worldwide social and economic inequality of women; the concomitant devaluation of women and their work (keeping abused women with violent men, and women – especially poor women of color – in inequitable service roles). A social worker, tired of oppressive hospital hierarchies, cited the following passage from a novel by a Zimbabwean author that illustrates what women have in common across continents. In the novel, a woman, Tambu, observes and reflects upon the beating of her female cousin:

> But what I didn't like was the way all the conflicts came back to this question of female-ness. Femaleness as opposed and inferior to maleness .... You can't go on all the time being whatever's necessary. You've got to have some conviction, and I'm convinced I don't want to be anyone's underdog. It's not right for anyone to be that. But once you get used to it, well, it just seems natural and you just carry on. And that's the end of you. You're trapped. They control everything you do.
>
> (Dangarembga, 1988, pp. 116–17)

Second, contemporary society has responded to both battered women and others by *blaming them* for their plight, e.g. "Women are their own worst enemies." Clearly, individual action by battered women and disadvantaged groups in the healthcare system to improve their lot is important. It is also wise to avoid a victimization framework as rationale (or excuse) for every unmet life challenge. Nevertheless, it is noteworthy that these *women are rarely if ever the authors/ creators of the unequal and oppressive structures* affecting their lives and work.

Third, rather than recognizing and responding to the reality that their oppression originates from sociocultural sources, historically battered women and others "get used to it," as Tambu says, and have typically responded to their plight by *blaming themselves* rather than looking "upstream" to the roots of their problem (Hoff, 1991; McKinlay, 1979).

So long as male and female faculty, practitioners, and students subscribe to the outdated myths about feminism, they will compromise the opportunity to forge necessary links with the community activists and caretakers who pioneered the development of appropriate models of victim/survivor care, and who have been the mainstay of victim service delivery (MacLeod, 1989; Schechter, 1982). And so long as traditional sexism and reverse sexism exists on the subject of men in nursing or women in medicine, the work of caring for abused people will suffer (Adams, 2008; Salvage, 1985). The ambivalent relationship between feminism and the health professions has shortchanged both arenas (Segal, 2000). Women and men, women's studies scholars and feminist activists have much to gain from collaboration around necessary work in one of the major domains of social life: treatment and care of the sick, wounded, and dying.

Traditionally, when the formal and informal boundaries of this work were less sharply drawn, women dominated in both realms; attendance at childbirth was the nearly exclusive task of women. But the systematic extinction of women healers and midwives followed by the social construction of formal medicine as the domain of men and lower status work that of women left in its wake the current hierarchical healthcare system, including the struggle of contemporary midwives for the right to practice (Ehrenreich, & English, 1973). Such disparities in a system "ordered to care" (Reverby, 1987) virtually defy coming to terms with the empowerment/disempowerment dynamics central to the collaborative treatment and care of victim/survivors.

The culture of nursing and lateral violence

From the historical perspective then, the plight of abused nurses can be compared to that of "battered women" and an era in which abuse and violence toward them was ascribed to their own purported psychopathology, and "victim blaming" was rampant. First, their injuries are comparable: broken bones, wounds, long-term chronic pain, muscle tension and soreness, sleep disturbance, flashbacks and other symptoms of post-traumatic stress disorder, fear of recurrent assault, anxiety, irritability, depression. In addition, nurses may feel sympathy for the patient perpetrator stemming from the professional caring ethic – in this case misplaced, but serving as rationale for excusing a patient perpetrator – and bury their bruises and psychological pain as "part of the job" (O'Sullivan *et al.*, 2008), not unlike the early assumption of the "marriage license as a hitting license." Or in the case of "smoldering anger" or professional "burnout," abused nurses may become callous and withdraw from patients; experience disruption of family and personal relationships; experience changes in their job performance and morale; and express themselves in bullying and abuse of fellow workers – what some have identified as "lateral violence" (Gerberich *et al.*, 2004; Levit *et al.*, 1998). (See Chapter 8 on oppressed group behavior.)

Emerging from qualitative analysis of the PHASE study focus groups with nurses (introduced in Chapter 11) was this overarching theme: in the healthcare restructuring process, healthcare agencies are redefined as *businesses*, patients are redefined as "widgets" in a factory-like line of production, and *service* delivered to these "widgets" is redefined as a *commodity*.

But as portrayed by the nurses in this study, patients are individual whole persons who need *nursing care*, not just piecemeal actions delivered in haste and recorded on the computer for reimbursement to support the hospital's "bottom line." Together, these redefinitions central to restructuring reveal that profit margins supersede concerns about and investment in basic training programs and policy implementation to protect the health and safety of healthcare workers. As already noted, vulnerability to injury and abuse is greatest among direct care workers and low paid ethnic minority employees whose English language deficits may limit their understanding of warning labels about hazardous materials, and/or who lack training in how to assess danger and respond to abusive patients.

The reality of healthcare restructuring is often the giant that is invisible to workers on the ground and faced with the grind and stress of daily duty. Nurses engrossed in everyday demands, rescue strategies, and survival (of themselves and patients) cannot readily see the "upstream" picture of healthcare restructuring and its pivotal role in their stress levels, safety, and threats to professional standards of nursing performance. Despite on-duty responsibilities and end-of-shift or double-shift exhaustion, nurses need time and support in order to connect their pain and "adaptation" to management demands about factors beyond their professional duty. Most notably, this includes nursing education curricula that may neglect or shortchange students' preparation in policy issues, social change strategies, and recognition that "wounded healers" are not in a strong position to enact their healing mission.

This presents an issue especially relevant to nurse educators and leaders in their capacity as catalysts for analysis and strategic action on behalf of rank-and-file nurses' safety and freedom from abuse, and the profession as a whole. That is, healthcare restructuring most likely could not have proceeded to the extent it has without the *adaptation*, *cooptation*, and *collaboration* of nurse managers as well as rank-and-file staff nurses. After all, the exploitation and disempowerment of nurses by powerful institutions like hospitals has been going on for more than a century. Yet, numerically, nurses comprise the largest single group of healthcare workers and, relatively speaking, they are paid more than social workers and beginning university professors, for example. Further, nurses are absolutely necessary for keeping healthcare institutions alive in their basic patient care mission – even when profit margins are the driving force.

These facts suggest, therefore, that aside from the powerful force of healthcare restructuring, nurses – educators, leaders, and those in front-line practice – need to critically examine curricula about violence and abuse issues, and reflect on how and why so many nurses have collaborated in the healthcare restructuring process – especially the elements so damaging to workers' health and safety and the quality of patient care. And – while not excusing institutional managers' exploitive profit-driven policies – nurse educators need to reflect on why after nearly 50 years of debate, nurses cannot agree among themselves, for example, on levels of entry to basic and advanced nursing practice, while "Rome burns" in the sacrifice of injured and/or burned-out nurses and the looming crisis of inadequate numbers of nurses to meet needs (Hoff, & Slatin, 2006; Smith, 2008).

Historical and contextual analysis suggests that the "culture of nursing" is a major factor in explaining the ongoing plight of the nursing profession. That is, the many decades' worth of values, beliefs, and behavioral norms influencing nurses' practice, health team interaction, self-care, and vulnerability to abuse provide a context for nurses' collaboration in implementing the policies and demands of powerful institutions. Put another way, the "culture of nursing" serves as an unwitting handmaiden of sorts to the political and economic process of healthcare restructuring. As in the case of "battered women," the issue is rooted in sociocultural and gender factors; when things go wrong, people in power "blame the victim;" and when victim/survivors absorb that verdict and blame themselves (rather than looking upstream to the sociocultural sources and holding abusers accountable) then depression, burnout, etc. are the predictable results (Hoff, 1991).

The plight of nurses and "lateral violence" (Worker-on-Worker, Type 3, see Chapter 11) can also be understood in the framework of "oppressed group behavior" as discussed in Chapter 8 concerning abusive behaviors among historically oppressed indigenous persons. A socio-structural and critical analysis of gender and class is necessary to understand the worldwide subordinate position of nurses in the larger healthcare arena where they and the relatively powerless nursing assistants they supervise are at particular risk of abuse. Professional nurses' potential power in sheer numbers and educational level (large numbers have graduate degrees) is often underutilized on behalf of safety in the workplace – not only their own, but that of the vast numbers of nursing assistants who are absolutely necessary for provision of nursing service (Freire, P., 1989; Hoff, 1994, 2009).

Health providers' abuse of patients

Despite the age-old ethic among medical and other providers to "do no harm" in the course of treatment and care, the sad reality is that some health professionals do take advantage of their power position vis-à-vis patients who have trusted them. Most notably this has occurred in psychotherapy and obstetrician/gynecologist (OB/GYN) practice contexts. The predominant pattern here has been male practitioners against female patients – similar to trafficking patterns that fall out along gender, class, and race lines: the traffickers are usually men, the trafficked are typically poor women (often of ethnic minority status), and the users of the sex services are usually affluent White males (see Chapter 9).

Power dynamics are dramatically revealed in the sexual exploitation of patients by health professionals and other providers such as clergy (Burgess & Hartman, 1986). The provider's abuse of his or her greater power in these relationships constitutes a profound violation of trust which survivors may spend a lifetime trying to regain. In some instances the client's present-ing problem is *prior* sexual abuse which compounds the trauma resulting from a provider's exploitation. One of the most unfortunate features of the victim-blaming legacy is a view of sexual abuse victims as "damaged goods" – a perspective which facilitates an abusive provider's sense of "entitlement" (Herman, 1981). Besides the damage to patients, as more survivors dis-close their exploitation and professional regulatory bodies tighten their disciplinary standards, professional careers are plundered, calling for increased vigilance among all professionals to prevent and report such abuse. Significantly in terms of gender and class, in the case of a male physician who was prosecuted for the crime of sexually abusing a post-surgical female patient, the attending nurse's testimony in the case was discounted in court and the testimony of an outside male forensic "expert" favored instead.

These stark realities must be faced and dealt with if health professionals are to actualize their enormous potential for interdisciplinary work on behalf of victimized clients. If all providers are sensitive to power dynamics and themselves feel empowered, they are in highly strategic positions to help break the cycle of abuse – among individuals, families, within professional relationships, and in society as a whole. It has been said that those who do not know history are doomed to repeat it (Ashley, 1976; Hoff, 1991; Roberts, 1983). The historical moment, as exemplified by the very production of this book, portends a turning point, an unprecedented opportunity for health professionals of both genders and various other identities to work to-gether and make an enormous difference on behalf of abused women, children, and others in Canada, the United States, and around the world.

Vicarious traumatization and boundary issues

When sincerely addressing violence issues and attending the trauma of victim/survivors, some individuals may become overwhelmed by the pervasiveness of violence and withdraw out of a sense of helplessness, burnout, or what is sometimes referred to as *vicarious traumatization* – also known as *secondary trauma* or *compassion fatigue*. In essence, this experience describes the process of internalizing the psychic pain that victimized clients share with empathetic providers.

Understanding this process and offering support requires examining not only one's personal history, as already discussed, but also the dynamics in one's "need to be needed," and a con-cept from transactional analysis: the Victim-Rescuer-Persecutor triangle. An apt lesson from Freudian theory applies here: among human needs, two of the most prominent revolve around love and work – someone to love and return love, and something worthwhile to do. In love relationships, excessive neediness or a lack of healthy independence on the part of either partner can spell trouble, including, for example, staying in an abusive relationship. As members of the human community, reaching out to others in distress is a universal impulse supported by civic and religious institutions and professional organizations. Among health and human service professionals, the desire to be of help to others is prominent and serves as a motivating factor to continue in very challenging work such as victim/survivor care and violence prevention – sometimes with minimal material returns.

The Victim-Rescue-Persecutor triangle

Depending on individual history and other circumstances, in one's basic need to pursue meaningful work an outsized "need to be needed" might be a pivotal motivating factor that can hamper the professional worker/client relationship. During the early years of community-based crisis and suicide prevention programs, agency organizers and administrators relied very heavily on trained volunteers to staff telephone hotlines. Significant numbers of these volunteers had at one time been suicidal themselves, were supported through the crisis, and sincerely desired to help others in similar suicidal crisis. But wise trainers and supervisors were careful to screen out applicants who were still too close to their own crises.

Similar scenarios emerged in developing services for victim/survivors of rape and intimate partner violence. As already discussed, if one's wounds as a victim/survivor are still raw, two interrelated factors may impede therapeutic success: 1) an over-identification with the victimized person (vs. an empathetic response); 2) a desire to "rescue" the suffering person. The result can be entrapment in the Victim-Rescuer-Persecutor (V-R-P) triangle (Hoff *et al.*, 2009, Chapter 4).

In such a triangle (Haley, 1969), one person allows or pressures another to define a relationship in a certain way. For example, if person A acts like a helpless victim and provokes person B to take care of him or her, person A is *actually in control* while being manifestly dependent. Translated to the helping relationship, if a counselor views a distressed person primarily as a *victim* (as in the case of a drowning person), the important process of re-empowerment is seriously compromised. Thus, while survivors of violence and abuse clearly need help, and should hear someone explicitly acknowledge that their victimization is "not right ... it's not your fault," regaining control is paramount in the healing process.

The V-R-P triangle which can hinder such healing occurs frequently in human relationships of all kinds, and is difficult to disrupt. This is because people viewed as victims are not rescued easily, so counselors who try it (perhaps from an excessive "need to be needed") are usually frustrated when their efforts fail. Their disappointment may move them to "persecute" their "victim" for failure to respond. At this point, the victim turns persecutor and punishes the counselor for a well-intentioned but inappropriate effort to help. Key concepts and practice implications of the triangle, adapted by the author from transactional analysis (Haley, 1969; James, & Jongeward, 1971; McKinlay, 1990) include:

Rescuer role:

*   Cannot be enacted without a complementary "victim."
*   May suggest provider's excessive "need to be needed."
*   Impedes growth and empowerment of client.

Victim role:

*   Threatens basic need for self-mastery and self-determination.

- Even if the overt message is demand for rescue, more help covertly leads to resentment and role switch to "persecutor."

Practice implications:

- Emphasize self-awareness and focus on empathy vs. sympathy.
- Conduct data-based assessment of client's actual needs.
- Provide neither more nor less than needed.
- Promote interdependence (vs. excessive dependence or independence).
- Be clear about necessary limits and rationale for same.
- Avoid power and control tactics.

Understanding vicarious trauma and attendant psychological dynamics in the helping relationship is central to maintaining appropriate boundaries in work with victim/survivors. But there are interconnections between boundary issues, secondary trauma, and the *therapeutic side-effects* of the research and writing process. In qualitative research with battered women and their families and in 5-year follow-up interviews (Hoff 1990), the study participants made it very clear that they did not expect to be rescued by health or other providers. On the other hand, they readily acknowledged how "helpful" it was to their healing to have an opportunity to share their life stories in-depth – especially if their experience and how they "survived" could help other women, thus affirming our common need to help others without entrapment in the V-R-P triangle. (See online resources.)

Case examples of vicarious trauma and compassion fatigue

Vicarious trauma spans the range of workers from academe to volunteers eager to do their best for victim/survivors and other disadvantaged fellow human beings. The following examples reveal the personal toll this work can exact and how sensitive supporters, colleagues and psychotherapists assisted in navigating the psychological shoals of this demanding but essential work.

A family therapist

Elena, a 55-year-old highly experienced and dedicated clinician with a graduate degree, thought she had done well in taking care of herself over years of working with seriously abused clients, including those who dealt with their trauma by indulgence in alcohol to dull the psychic pain. One of her clients, Anna, who had finally escaped an abusive marital relationship spent a short two weeks in a battered women's shelter, and was asked to leave after she brought alcohol and drugs to the shelter. She then called Elena's office for an emergency session for help with her issues related to years of living in an abusive marriage, including need for assistance with child care and household bills. The session ended with a plan addressing her complex needs, and emergency numbers to call if necessary. On her return to work the next day, Elena had a garbled message on her phone from Anna, including profanity and cursing Elena for "lying to her" and just not doing enough to help her. Although initially shocked by the foul language and with no previously experienced conflicts in the therapeutic relationship with Anna, Elena took the abusive message in stride, as it seemed obvious that Anna had been drinking and was perhaps "out of control" as a result. Through support from her supervisor, Elena dealt with Anna's outburst and continued with the therapeutic plan for Anna. The surprise for Elena, though, was the following: at home relaxing after work, and remembering the abusive phone message,

Elena began to weep uncontrollably as she experienced flashbacks to 30 years earlier when she was raped, and 15 years earlier when she had escaped an abusive marriage in which she was threatened with her life and suffered deeply wounding verbal abuse. During the weeping session, Elena also kept asking herself why she continued to work with abused clients.

As a professionally trained therapist, Elena recognized that her unusual weeping bout had less to do with Anna's problems than with the impact of her personal history as a survivor with wounds she had assumed were healed, but in fact were not. Complicating her own recovery as a rape survivor were these facts: Elena was a virgin at the time and engaged to be married. She was stalled on a highway during a storm and accepted a ride from a man who stopped to help. Instead of taking her to a service station, he ordered her to give him directions to her apartment. When she knew that rape was imminent, she told him she was having her period, hoping it would stop him. It did not, and he raped her orally instead. Elena had been incredibly traumatized, crying and vomiting for hours, but she did not define what happened to her as rape, since at that time the legal definition of rape did not include oral penetration. While Elena sought and received comfort (not blame) from her pastor soon after the rape, after reflection on the abusive telephone message from Anna and her flashback experience she engaged a psychotherapist for further help.

A professor of nursing

Martha, age 60, a long-time nurse dedicated to belief in the nobility and vital place of the nursing profession in world health, decided she had had enough of the bullying and in-fighting by her colleagues and what she and others perceived as the unfair treatment of her by the department chair. It seemed to Martha that no matter what she did it was never enough, and because of her "untenured" status she rarely received assignments commensurate with her clinical background and expertise. Martha was also keenly aware of the fact that her colleagues basically agreed with her around controversial assignment and other issues, but all were afraid to speak out and organize structural changes lest they meet the same fate as Martha. After repeated attempts to mobilize her colleagues, Martha, who was unwilling to relinquish her allegiance to the basic mission of nursing, concluded that the psychological price she paid for her university position was too high; she decided to leave her position and took a "peaceful" and very rewarding job as a hospice nurse. As a dramatic symbol of change, she planned a party, gathered all her nursing books, and burned them in a ritual bonfire in her front yard to the cheers of her supportive colleagues.

Not unlike others who have survived abuse or violence, this professor did not define herself as a helpless victim of her abusive colleagues, but made decisions that led to a more peaceful environment in which to use her knowledge and skills. In the framework of social change theory and readiness to enact such change, this is a sad but dramatic commentary on the personal toll of oppressed group behavior. It also speaks to the often untapped potential of the nursing profession to make a difference not only in stopping lateral abuse among their own ranks, but also on behalf of other abused workers and the masses of victim/survivors whose lives are touched by nurses (Adams, 2008; Roberts, 2000).

A humanitarian aid worker [from the experience of Glenda Dubienski]

Sarah, a compassionate third-year nursing student, is on a church-sponsored missionary trip to a Caribbean island nation. She connects easily with the local youth and young adults. Her keen listening skills, obvious empathy and desire to help draws out their deepest, darkest secrets. Daily helping sessions that include tales of incest, physical abuse, abandonment by parents, and substance dependency begin to take their toll on her. Symptoms of compassion fatigue are apparent: Sarah's normal cheery disposition is replaced with sullenness; her appetite is suppressed; sleep is not restful; and, she begins to isolate from the team. Recognizing these behavioral changes, it is the responsibility of the pastoral leader on the team to approach and help such an individual. In doing so, Sarah divulges, "I feel so small." The ensuing discussion opens the door for Sarah to share with the rest of her team (during a nightly debrief) how inept she feels and how overwhelmed she is by the vast needs of the island people. Her teammates respond by sharing in her sentiments, normalizing her experience and by no means minimizing it. They echo the comments of the "pastor" leading the mission in that they see the positive impact she is having on those with whom she sits and listens to. In the process, they affirm her and commend her for her ability to show such compassion. Sarah is encouraged to carry on and commits to talking about her thoughts and feelings with her teammates. Within three days of feeling "in crisis," Sarah begins to see for herself the fruit of her labors; the power of loving people well.

Working long hours in unfamiliar, unsanitary conditions, side by side with locals to help restore what has been lost through natural disaster, or to build what seems to those of us in affluent circumstances to be a basic need (like a hospital or school), there is an uncommon bond that occurs between the humanitarian aid worker and the local villager. Humility sets the stage for an opportunity to share intimately, fostering a relationship that is truly unexpected. The local villager is humbled by the fact that a total stranger would travel great distances to help, and the aid worker is humbled by the fact that this villager will share everything he/she has, which is usually less than enough. There is a profound recognition that "we" can't "do" life alone. Unhampered by the distractions of "stuff" so available in wealthy nations, the aid worker is drawn to the people of this strange land.

An immigrant student from a poor country [from the experience of Glenda Dubienski]

Isabella is an international student on full scholarship and President of her Student Union in a Canadian University. She openly expressed her passion about social justice issues. Within the first two days of the church-sponsored mission's trip, Isabella began exhibiting the following symptoms: difficulty concentrating, preoccupation, extreme tiredness, disinterest in food, and uncharacteristic apathy. Similar to Sarah's mission's experience, Isabella believed she was ill-equipped to provide assistance to the locals and felt paralyzed by the enormity of the task. Further discussion revealed that the root of this early response to mission field exposure was an unresolved issue related to the perspective that she had abandoned her Central American family to pursue a better life in Canada. "These people are just like the people at home," she claimed. The guilt she was feeling by lending assistance to strangers and selfishly ignoring the needs of her own people appeared insurmountable. Helping Isabella realize the unconscious correlation between these people and "her" people allowed her to open up to her teammates, and receive help in processing how this experience translates into her relationships with her family in Central America. At the same time, this experience and processing it with teammates afforded her clarity on her vocation by fueling her fire for social justice.

Similar to clinical and social service work with victim/survivors, international humanitarian aid work is intensive. With so much to do in such a short time frame (a short-term mission's usual run is 10 days to 3 months), there are heavy physical, emotional, and spiritual demands on every participant. Exhaustion is commonplace on the mission field and one often simply feels overwhelmed by the stories of injustice and atrocities, leading to questions about suffering and its purpose. Within that context for persons leading teams sponsored by churches or non-governmental organizations (NGOs) such as Amnesty International or Oxfam over many years, vicarious trauma or compassion fatigue is expected to surface on every trip. At the same time, volunteers and their leaders must resist the "victim rescue" impulse while supporting individuals in distress and keeping their eye "upstream" on broader society-wide and global changes that can foster prevention of so much individual suffering (McKinlay, 1979).

Self-care and support programs for providers

Few of us have the vision, charisma, and strength of people like Mahatma Ghandi, Nelson Mandela, or Mother Teresa for mobilizing the masses on behalf of the abused, oppressed, and dispossessed. Given the enormity and seeming ever-presence of interpersonal and State-sponsored violence across the globe, it is understandable that a sense of helplessness and cynicism about one's personal effort to "make a difference" can take hold, support withdrawal to a safe personal orbit, and thus inhibit fruitful action one might take.

The vision and wisdom of Professor David Gil of Brandeis University is instructive here. Professor Gil, a social worker and policy expert was instrumental in his pioneering testimony in the US Congress on the gender, race, and class correlates of child abuse and neglect that contributed to federal legislation on child protection. In a lecture to front-line social workers propounding on this theme, a case worker besieged daily by the tragedies of child abuse asked (paraphrased): "Well, Professor Gil, what do you want us to do ... quit our jobs and go out and start a revolution?" To which Professor Gil responded "No, but I hope you can take time to consider the roots of the everyday suffering of children and the sociocultural context of child abuse and neglect" – the classic "both-and" – not "either-or" – approach.

Translated to a strategy of self-care, hope, and the larger change needed to stem the tide of violence, one might consider this 5-percent strategy. Typically, one does *not* hear that "I don't have time to eat/go to work/pay my bills ..." etc. But it is common to hear "I don't have time to exercise/shop for healthy food/visit my friends ..." etc. Indeed, no individual can save the world or stop the global violence epidemic alone. But each of us can take a small step – perhaps just 5 percent out of 100 percent – to avoid burnout and still contribute to the larger arena of violence prevention. For example, it takes no extra time to rule out violent language in everyday conversation – *a small individual contribution to the whole of violence prevention*. Also helpful is this strategy: in the stress-filled day of work with victim/survivors, enter into an appointment book (or reserve for time at home) explicit time for reflection, meditation, exercise, yoga, a special meal, etc. – that is, time for self-care activities that can easily turn into more work unless explicitly planned otherwise.

Because the face of violence and its wake can be so overwhelming, it is not uncommon to hear people say "It's too big [or too awful] ... there's nothing I can do." But while this sense of helplessness is understandable, it can also be seen as an excuse to do nothing, and thus becomes a self-fulfilling prophecy that allows the global epidemic of violence to continue unabated.

Besides individual self-care efforts, increasing awareness of the emotional toll often exacted from work with victim/survivors has led to programs that move beyond the traditional supports routinely available through supervisory and informal social networks. These programs address in a systematic manner the concepts and issues illustrated in this chapter's examples. One such program offered in several communities across Massachusetts is the Advocate Education and Support Project sponsored by the Center for Violence Prevention and Recovery at the Beth Israel Deaconess Medical Center in Boston.

This program emerged from a collaborative process that began with services to the Victim Witness program of the county attorney general's office in Boston, and engaged a range of agencies dedicated to victim/survivor services – battered women, sexual assault victims, hospitals, and community health centers. Through its focus on domestic violence and sexual assault advocates, it engages workers from the diverse agencies serving this clientele who often feel overwhelmed and distressed by the demands of working with victim/survivors. Since the program is tailored specifically to the needs and experiences of advocates in the field of inter-personal violence, it meets a need that heretofore has only incidentally been able to address workers' need for support and burnout prevention when the urgent needs of victim/survivors by necessity command unmitigated front-line attention.

The typical program format of the 8-to-10 session Beth Israel Deaconess program includes three phases:

1 The personal and professional impact of work with victim/survivors; a review of sources and typical manifestations of secondary traumatic stress; and an examination of the boundary issues and controls available to the worker.
2 Developing specific strategies to minimize the psychological and social impact of the work – including personal, professional, organizational and community action levels.
3 Developing specific supports and strategies to improve the work environment. (See Part IV: Online resources.)

Social change and professional strategies complementing self-care and support

The following summary of social change strategies is adapted from the classic work of Chin and Benne (1969). These strategies are particularly relevant to the sociocultural sources of violence and abuse, and therefore prevention in the broader sense. Engaging in at least some of them may also alleviate the personal sense of "powerlessness" one can feel in the face of so much violence around the world.

Strategies based on reason and research

Foremost among these strategies are research findings, new concepts, and the clarification of language to closely represent reality as experienced by people, not merely as theorized by aca-demics. These strategies rest on the assumption that people are reasonable and when presented with evidence will take appropriate action to bring about needed change. For example, there is information available for early detection of violence potential in domestic, learning, and work environments. However, this strategy alone is usually not enough to move people toward change, such as enacting workplace policies that affect staff safety and injury prevention on the job.

Strategies based on re-education and attitude change

These approaches to change are based on the assumption that people are guided by internal-ized values and habits and that they act according to institutionalized roles and perceptions of self. This group of strategies includes an activity central to violence prevention by fostering learning and growth in peaceful, non-violent interaction among the persons who make up the system to be changed. Included are public education programs that avoid excusing violence on questionable grounds of "temporary insanity" or excessive drinking – this makes every potential victim of violence or abuse aware of available legal, health, and social service programs in the community.

Power-coercive strategies

The emphasis in these strategies is on political and economic sanctions in the exercise of power, along with such moral power moves as playing on sentiments of guilt, shame, and a sense of what is just and right. These strategies build on religious and civil institutions such as the United Nations emphasizing the basic human rights of freedom from violence and abuse. It is assumed that political action approaches will probably not succeed apart from re-education and attitude changes. New action, such as public rallies for greater police protection, fair laws for victims, or protests against harassment and violence based on sexual identity, usually requires "new knowledge, new skills, new attitudes, and new value orientations." It is now common for health and mental health professionals to recommend that victims of intimate partner violence, rape victims, and other survivors participate in support groups that assist them to address these kinds of social and political issues in the healing process (Chin, & Benne, 1969, p. 42; Hoff *et al.*, 2009, Chapter 12).

Professional strategies

In the United States, the *Surgeon General's Workshop on Violence and Public Health Report* (US Department of Health and Human Services, 1986) recommended that all licensed professionals be required to study and pass examination questions in violence prevention and the treatment of various victims of violence. As a complement to this public policy statement, individual professionals can exert leadership and advocacy within their own groups for curriculum and in-service program development to systematically address this topic. At present, such educational endeavors are incidental at best (Ross *et al.*, 1998, Tilden *et al.*, 1994; Woodtli, & Breslin, 2002). The American Association of Colleges of Nursing (AACN, 1999) has produced a position paper underscoring the need for the inclusion of violence content in all nursing education programs. The World Health Organization (WHO, 2004) has produced a similar document for Schools of Public Health worldwide, while others have produced developed guidelines for criminal justice professionals in North America and other countries.

References

AACN – American Association of Colleges of Nursing (1999). *Position Statement on Defining Scholarship for the Discipline of Nursing*. Washington, DC: AACN.

Adams, B. (2008). Letter to the editor. *Policy, Practice, & Nursing*, 9(1), 5.

Antonovsky, A. (1980). *Health, Stress, and Coping*. San Francisco: Jossey-Bass.

Ashley, J. (1976). *Hospitals, Paternalism, and the Role of the Nurse*. New York: Teacher's College Press.

Barbee, E. L. (1993). Racism in U.S. nursing. *Medical Anthropology Quarterly*, 7(4), 346–62.

Burgess, A., & Hartman, C. (eds.) (1989). *Sexual Exploitation of Patients by Health Professionals*. New York: Praeger.

Chin, R., & Benne, K. D. (1969). General strategies for effecting change in human systems. In W. G. Bennis, K. D. Benne, & R. Chin (eds.), *The Planning of Change* (2nd edn.), pp. 32–57. Austin, TX: Holt, Rinehart and Winston.

Cox, H. (1991a). Verbal abuse nationwide: Part I: Oppressed group behavior. *Nursing Management*, February, 32–5.

Cox, H. (1991b). Verbal abuse nationwide: Part II: Impact and modifications. *Nursing Management*, March, 66–9.

Dangarembga, T. (1988). *Nervous Conditions*. Harare, Zimbabwe: Zimbabwe Publishing House.

Ehrenreich, B., & English, D. (1973). *Witches, Midwives and Nurses: A History of Women Healers*. Old Westbury, New York: The Feminist Press.

Faludi, S. (1991). *Backlash*. New York: Crown Publishers.

Freire, P. (1989). *Oppressed Group Behavior*. New York: Continuum.

Gerberich, S. G., *et al.* (2004). An epidemiological study of the magnitude and consequences of work related violence: the Minnesota Nurses' Study. *Occupational and Environmental Medicine*, 61, 495–503.

Gordon, S. (1991). Fear of caring: The feminist paradox. *American Journal of Nursing*, 89(2), 45–6.

Haley, J. (1969). The art of being a failure as a therapist. *American Journal of Orthopsychiatry*, 39(4), 691–5.

Herman, J. (1981). *Father-Daughter Incest*. Cambridge: Harvard University Press.

Hoff, L. A. (1990). *Battered Women as Survivors*. London: Routledge.

Hoff, L. A. (1991). Human abuse and nursing's response. In P. Holden, & J. Littlewood (eds.), *Nursing and Anthropology*, pp. 130–47. London and New York: Routledge.

Hoff, L. A. (1994). Comments on race, gender and class bias in nursing. *Medical Anthropology Quarterly*, 8(1), 96–9.

Hoff, L. A., Hallisey, B. J., & Hoff, M. (2009). *People in Crisis: Clinical and Diversity Perspectives* (6th edn.). New York & London: Routledge.

Hoff, L. A., & Slatin, C. (2006). Workplace health and safety: A report of PHASE/MNA focus groups, a two part series. *Massachusetts Nurse*, 77(8–9).

Hunter, M. (1990). *Abused Boys: The Neglected Victims of Sexual Abuse*. Lexington, MA: Lexington Books.

James, M., & Jongeward, D. (1971). *Born to Win*. Reading, MA: Addison-Wesley.

Keddy, B. (1993). Feminism and patriarchy in university schools of nursing: An unsettling dualism. Conference address: Women's Issues and Nursing Education. Moncton, New Brunswick, Atlantic Region – Canadian Association of University Schools of Nursing. Unpublished.

Kettl, P., Siberski, J.L., Hirschmann, C., & Wood, B. (1993). Sexual harassment of health care students by patients. *Journal of Psychosocial Nursing*, 31(7), 11–13.

Lanza. J. L. (1992). Nurses as patient assault victims: An update, synthesis, and recommendations. *Archives of Psychiatric Nursing*, 6(3), 163–71.

Levin, P. F., Hewitt, J. B., & Misner, S. T. (1998). Insights of nurses about assault in hospital-based emergency departments. *Image; Journal of Nursing Scholarship*, 30(3), 249–54.

Lifton, R. J. (1967). *Life in Death*. New York: Simon and Shuster.

MacLeod, L. (1989). *Wife Battering and the Web of Hope: Progress, Dilemmas, and Visions of Prevention*. Ottawa: Health and Welfare Canada. National Clearinghouse on Family Violence.

McComas, J. (1993). Experiences of student and practicing physical therapists with inappropriate patient sexual behavior. *Physical Therapy*, 73(11), 762–9.

McKinlay, J. B. (1979). The case for refocusing upstream: The political economy of illness. In E. G. Jaco (ed.), *Patients, Physicians and Illness* (3rd edn), pp. 9–25. New York: Free Press.

McManiman, J. (2000). The invisibility of men's pain. In B. Everett & R. Gallop (eds.), *The Link Between Childhood Trauma and Mental Illness*, pp. 253–70. Thousand Oaks, CA: Sage.

O'Sullivan, M. *et al.* (2008). It's part of the job: Healthcare restructuring and the health and safety of nursing aides. In L. McKee, E. Ferlie, and P. Hyde (eds.), *Organizing and Reorganizing: Power and Change in Health Care Organizations*, pp. 99–111. Houndmills, Basingstoke, Hampshire, UK: Palgrave MacMillan.

Phillips, S. P., & Schneider, M. S. (1993). Sexual harassment of female doctors by patients. *New England Journal of Medicine*, 329(26), 1936–9.

Quintal, S. (2002). Violence against nurses: An untreated epidemic? *Journal of Psychosocial Nursing*, 40(1), 46–53.

Rachlis, M., & Kushner, C. (1994). *Strong Medicine: How to Save Canada's Health Care System*. Toronto: HarperCollins.

Reverby, S. (1987). *Ordered to Care*. Cambridge: Cambridge University Press.

Roberts, S. (1983). Oppressed group behaviour: Implications for nursing. *Advances in Nursing Science*, 5(4), 21–30.

Roberts, S. J. (2000). Development of a positive professional identity: Liberating oneself from the oppressor within. *Advances in Nursing Science*, 22(4), 71–82.

Ross, M., Hoff, L. A., & Coutu-Wakulcyzk, G. (1998). Nursing curricula and violence issues. *Journal of Nursing Education*, 37, 53–60.

Russell, D. (1990). *Rape in Marriage* (rev. ed.). New York: Collier Books.

Salvage, J. (1985). *The Politics of Nursing*. London: Heinemann Nursing.

Schechter, S. (1982). *Women and Male Violence*. Boston: South End Press.

Segal, L. (2000). *Why Feminism? Gender, Psychology, Politics*. New York: Columbia University Press.

Smith, G.R. (2008). Health disparities: What can nursing do? *Policy, Politics, & Nursing Practice*, 8, 285–91.

Tilden, V. P., Schmidt, T. A., Limandri, B. J., Chiodo, G. T., Garland, M. J., & Loveless, P. A. (1994). Factors that influence clinicians' assessment and management of family violence. *American Journal of Public Health*. 84(4), 628–33.

US Department of Health and Human Services (1986). *Surgeon General's Workshop on Violence and Public Health Report*. Washington, DC: Health Resources Service Administration.

Vance, C., Talbott, S., McBride, A., & Mason, D. (1985). An uneasy alliance: Nursing and the women's movement. *Nursing Outlook*, 33(6), 281–5.

Waring, D. (1990). *If Women Counted: A New Feminist Economics*. San Francisco: Harper San Francisco.

WHO – World Health Organization (2004). *Handbook for the Documentation of Interpersonal Violence Prevention Programmes*. Geneva: WHO.

Woodtli, A., & Breslin, E. (2002). Violence-related content in the nursing curriculum: A follow-up national survey. *Journal of Nursing Education*, 41(4), 340–8.

13 Comprehensive service issues

Health and criminal justice interface

Lee Ann Hoff and Marilynne Bell

- Interdisciplinary collaboration for primary, secondary, and tertiary care
- A Crisis Paradigm and psychosociocultural perspective on victimization

  - Steps of formal crisis management

- Community mental health and police roles
- Victimization Assessment Tool
- Illustration 1: comprehensive service – intimate partner violence

  - Prevention
  - Treatment of physical injury and obtaining forensic evidence
  - Crisis assessment, intervention, counseling, and coordination
  - Follow-up counseling and/or treatment
  - Mandated reporting of battering: a controversial issue

- Illustration 2: comprehensive service – sexual assault victims

  - Prevention
  - Assessment, treatment, and obtaining forensic evidence
  - Crisis management
  - Comprehensive assessment and counseling
  - Follow-up counseling and treatment
  - Teaching issues in this case
  - SANE Avalon Centre program – Halifax, Nova Scotia

- Psychiatric care of survivors: a cautionary note
- Human rights, gender issues, and medical /professional ethics

  - The Tarasoff case and "duty to warn"
  - Female genital mutilation (FGM), surgical restoration of "virgin status," and cultural relativism

Although interdisciplinary collaboration is a given in service to anyone with complex health problems, system loopholes may result in clients "falling through the cracks" and not getting the service they need. But in delivering care and treatment to both victim/survivors and perpetrators, *life itself* – of clients as well as that of providers – may depend on such collaboration. Complementing other chapters' discussion of particular situations across the spectrum of violence and abuse, this chapter delineates and summarizes health, mental health, and criminal justice roles. Case examples will illustrate various facets of comprehensive clinical service for an abused woman and a sexual assault victim. The examples build on essential content for delivering comprehensive service (discussed in Chapter 3), and the distinct but complementary functions of the healthcare team (see Table 3.1). They also address service for assailants and the children affected by parental abuse. A complementary service model is highlighted in a psychosociocultural Crisis Paradigm. The forensic and ethical issues in medicine are discussed only as general information for all front-line health and social service providers, with the understanding that detailed protocols such as the "Rape Crisis Kit" are available in designated medical emergency and trauma centers and conform to legal requirements of various countries and government jurisdictions.

Interdisciplinary collaboration for primary, secondary, and tertiary care

The unfortunate truth about this book's topic is that there is more than enough work to go around. A second truth is that power struggles among providers send exactly the wrong message to clients who because of abuse or violence feel disempowered and are struggling to regain their sense of self-mastery that is threatened by violence. Put another way, the very fact of collaboration among providers can serve as a model about how to get along and treat one another with respect even in the highly charged atmosphere of delivering care to an injured and usually acutely distressed victim/survivor or perpetrator. This principle applies not only to professional healthcare teams, but also within specialized services for victim/survivors.

Primary, secondary, and tertiary care for victim/survivors and assailants can be viewed as a continuum of services that correspond roughly to the essential features of a comprehensive medical and mental healthcare system. In such an integrated system, primary care would encompass education in violence prevention geared to the public as well as individual clients. Twenty-four hour crisis services might also be seen as primary care, depending on degree of injury and the psychological aftermath of abuse and violence. Hospital treatment of injuries and follow-up counseling or psychotherapy encompass both secondary and tertiary levels of care in the classical prevention schema presented in Chapter 3.

The humanitarian and financial costs of tertiary level care and treatment far outweigh the costs of public education about violence prevention aimed at whole populations (Hoff *et al.*, 2009, Chapter 1). The essential services are based on the Community Mental Health Acts of 1963 and 1965 mandated by the US government and have been extended to include addiction and rehabilitation services, and programs specific to victim/survivors. It is noteworthy that despite epidemiological and clinical data from national studies in Canada (Coretta, 2008; MacMillan, & Wathen, 2001) and the United States (Tjaden, & Thoennes 2000) there is still a debate about routine screening for violence in emergency and primary care settings (Furniss *et al.*, 2007; Rhodes, & Levinson, 2003). A rationale presented is the lack of evidence from "randomized controlled trials" (RCTs) to assure "evidence-based practice" (Wathen, & MacMillan, 2003). This argument presumes that RTCs are practitioners' only "valid" source of evidence, thus discounting reams of social science research, clinical experience, and the accounts of millions of victim/survivors about the devastating impact of violence on their health and social life (Rodriguez *et al.*, 1996; Weiss, 2000; WHO, 2004).

In contrast, given the known morbidity and mortality risks of hypertension and diabetes, for example, the first routine steps in primary care are asking the patient to "step on the scale" for current weight, and ascertaining vital signs. Moving on in the scale of value-laden topics: it is routine for primary care providers in health history protocols to ask about consumption of alcohol, despite the fact that some may understate or fail to disclose their daily/weekly consumption

– yet, the questions continue to be asked with the hope that the patient receives a message that someone cares about possible excess drinking and its health impact. No less should be expected vis-à-vis screening for violence issues. If nothing else, and the patient is not ready to disclose for whatever reason, at least a seed has been planted for possible future action.

Two factors help us understand these disparate approaches to screening in healthcare settings: (1) the continuing "mind-body" split in medical practice; and (2) the well-known fact of the long time it takes to bring about social and attitudinal change when deeply embedded values and powerful vested interests are involved (see Chapter 12). As noted in Chapter 6, rape as the "spoils of war" has been going on for centuries, but surely more research is not needed to rationalize action on this crime – as in RCTs. Certainly a question to consider is why we are still debating rather than acting on evidence we already have on the global epidemic of interpersonal and other violence and its impact on individuals, families, the economy, and whole nations.

A Crisis Paradigm and psychosociocultural perspective on violence

Chapters 1 and 2 comprise the foundation for a Crisis Paradigm presented here for its particular applicability to services for victim/survivors of abuse and violence. This book's diverse examples underscore the multidisciplinary perspective needed for comprehensive victim/survivor care. Of particular significance for this book is the development of the Crisis Paradigm from ethnographic research with battered women and their families (Hoff, 1990). Evidence from this study made very clear that writers on the subject (e.g. Caplan, 1964; Erikson, 1963) had correctly defined crisis as the acute emotional response to critical life events and life cycle transition states.

Significantly, earlier crisis theory described unanticipated events such as a life-threatening heart attack or diagnosis of cancer as something that "just happened" or "bad luck" with no readily definable cause, but which nevertheless evoked emotional turmoil and perhaps crisis. This theoretical framework left little room for understanding a crisis-producing event such as rape or life-threatening intimate partner violence which one cannot interpret as the "normal" ups and downs of life which most will encounter at one time or another, but which leave a considerable "above normal" emotional toll in their wake well beyond whatever physical injuries accompanied the assaults.

At the inception of the research from which the Crisis Paradigm emerged (Hoff, 1990), social and psychological literature commonly referred to the purported "psychopathology" of women who stayed with abusive partners, and a complementary psychopathology framework for excusing perpetrators (Stark *et al.*, 1979 (a sociological/medical team)). It seemed reasonable, then, in engaging abused women to share their stories, to use an established psychiatric/mental health framework to learn about their lives retrospectively, during, and following their experience of intimate partner abuse (see Hoff *et al.*, 2009, for a description of this Comprehensive Mental Health Assessment (CMHA) tool and see also Part IV: Online resources).

Revealed from this research process was the fact that the purportedly "progressive" mental health assessment protocol (the CMHA tool) based on civil rights of the mentally ill included the first ever routine assessment item on risk of assault/homicide, but did NOT include an item on the distress/crisis level ensuing from victimization by violence. This "incidental" discovery and "moment of truth" led to this conclusion: the assumed "objectivity" of mental health professionals could not be upheld, since established mental health practitioners obviously held the culture-wide value of treating "wife battering" as a "private" family matter. It included "flashbacks" to psychiatric hospital treatment of women with the presenting problem of serious depression; the entire treatment team knew incidentally that these women had experienced serious abuse by their male partners, but it was understood that their responsibility was to "treat" her depression, thus aiding and abetting the widespread acceptance of the women's psychopathology as the "cause" of her plight. Feminist psychiatrists such as Elaine Hilberman (1980) soon joined grassroots and feminist professionals in redefining psychological sequelae of intimate partner violence.

These developments led to a recasting of unanticipated critical events and life transition states *not* as emotional crisis itself, but rather as the *origins of potential emotional crisis*, and added *sociocultural* factors as a third major origin of crisis to account for violence and abuse not as *private* matters but as *social action for which the perpetrator was accountable* – thereby displacing the victim's purported psychopathology as explanation for abuse. Another development was the addition of the Victimization Assessment Scale to the CMHA tool (see Hoff & Rosenbaum, 1994). Its use is illustrated in Table 13.2 below, and builds on the "triage" questions included in Chapter 4. Research on violence risk during pregnancy by McFarlane *et al.* (1992) and many others, led to a policy by the Joint Commission on Accreditation of Healthcare Organizations (JCAHO, 1993) requiring victimization to be included in intake health history forms as a condition of accreditation in the United States.

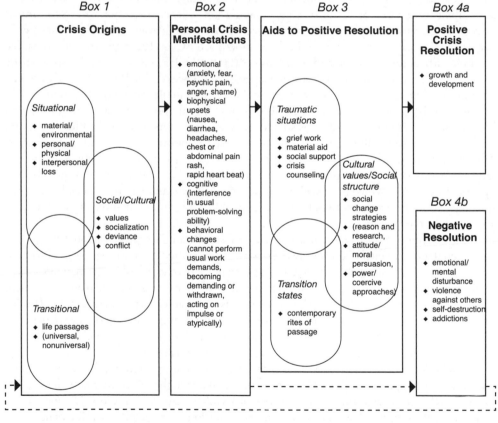

Figure 13.1 A Crisis Paradigm.
Source: Hoff (1990, 2009).

Crisis origins, manifestations, and outcomes, and the respective functions of crisis management have an interactional relationship. The intertwined circles represent the distinct yet interrelated "origins" of crisis and "aids to positive resolution," even though personal manifestations are often similar. The solid line from "origins" to positive resolution illustrates the *opportunity* for growth and development through crisis; the broken line depicts the potential *danger* of crisis in the absence of appropriate aids.

Besides studies of intimate partner and sexual assault, the Crisis Paradigm draws on other research and clinical experience with survivors of violence and critical life events (for example, Antonovsky, 1980), and work with survivors of man-made disasters (see Hoff *et al.*, 2009, Chapter 13). The inclusion of sociocultural origins of crisis extends the traditional focus of crisis intervention on situational and developmental life events, a framework found inadequate to guide practice with people intentionally injured through violence, prejudice, neglect, or disaster. It also shows the interrelationship between the three origins of crisis, and depicts 1) the *crisis process* experienced by the distressed person from origin through resolution and 2) the place of natural and formal crisis intervention in promoting growth and avoiding negative crisis outcomes. By its depiction of social change strategies that complement sociocultural origins of crisis, along with the potential negative outcomes of crisis without appropriate intervention, the Crisis Paradigm underscores this central feature of comprehensive care of victim/survivors: crisis care is *necessary*, but in cases of abuse extended over years (e.g. incest, torture, or repeated battering) is usually *not sufficient*. The Crisis Paradigm suggests a tandem approach to crisis care – that is, attending to the immediate problem while not losing sight of the social and public health strategies needed to address the complex sociocultural origins of crisis related to violence. This psychosociocultural perspective serves as the framework for the two illustrations of comprehensive care below that incorporate the basic steps of crisis care.

Steps of formal crisis management

1 Assessment (including risk of injury to self and others)
2 Planning
3 Implementation
4 Evaluation/follow-up

Table 13.1 summarizes the four components of comprehensive service by discipline. For the most part, these service components should be incorporated in primary, secondary, and tertiary care settings. Table 13.2 summarizes the four components by level of student: Beginning, Intermediate, Advanced (undergraduate), and Graduate or crisis/victimization specialist. The delineation by discipline and level of student can serve as a framework to plan formal and clinical instruction within various curriculum approaches to violence content: a single course; curriculum thread; series of short courses; or problem-based learning. (See online resources.)

Community mental health and police roles

Given their mission of protecting the public and authority to prevent injury and death whenever possible, police are often the first responders across a range of crisis situations – child abuse, intimate partner violence, sexual assault, and violence in learning and work environments. In that role, police themselves are often at high risk of injury, and thus are explicitly trained in how to protect themselves and others in hostile or highly charged situations. Even so, in domestic and other dangerous encounters, some observers are quick to criticize police for what they perceive as using excessive force.

Yet the unfortunate truth in some communities is that police are often performing by default and alone the high risk mental health work that should be carried out in collaborative arrangements with mental health professionals. Officers may resent this situation, and with justification, as mental health professionals are often unavailable for collaboration with police

Table 13.1 Comprehensive service components by discipline

Service component		Discipline
1	Prevention	All
2	Treatment of physical injury	Medicine, dentistry, nursing, physical therapy
3	Crisis management	
	a Identification/triage	All
	b Comprehensive crisis assessment	Crisis specialists, family medicine, nurse practitioner, psychiatric nursing, psychiatry, psychology, social work
	c Crisis counseling	Crisis specialists, mental health professionals
	d Referral	All, depending on mission and crisis situation
4	Follow-up counseling/treatment	Medicine, nursing, mental health professionals, physical therapy, occupational therapy, dentistry, specialists such as substance abuse counselors (depending on assessment and needs)

in cases of domestic violence or an out-of-control psychiatric patient (Earley, 2006; Hoff *et al.*, 2009, Chapter 12). On the other hand, a significant percentage of an average officer's time is spent in "service" or domestic calls. Officer training, therefore, should include appropriate collaboration with professional crisis specialists in potentially dangerous domestic scenes. If mobile crisis outreach teams are not available, police officers should have 24-hour access to telephone consultation regarding mental patients or other crisis situations (Hoff, 1993). In the absence of such services to police, if officers and others are injured, it may be easy to criticize the police for using excessive force when, for example, communication efforts failed to defuse a volatile situation. But such a response only underscores the importance of crisis training and the 24/7 availability of expert consultation for police in interpersonal violence situations (see Sully *et al.*, 2005 and Sully, 2002 for such programs in London, UK).

In instances of sexual assault, police officers have responded very enthusiastically to the success of Sexual Assault Nurse Examiner (SANE) programs. They have observed the meticulous attention SANEs give to collecting evidence in rape charges which greatly reduces officers' time spent for investigation, and increases the likelihood that victims will cooperate with law enforcement in witness statements because they have been treated with kindness and respect.

Even if officers are not physically injured in hostage or other crisis situations, they and their families can suffer psychological trauma that may require weeks or months for recovery. The issues discussed in Chapters 11 and 12 on workplace violence, vicarious traumatization, and burnout apply to police officers as well. In fact, police departments and hostage negotiation teams paved the way in the practice of debriefing and offering stress relief services to officers who are involved in shooting and other highly traumatic incidents – a practice now recommended as routine for abused or injured health and social service workers.

Table 13.2 Comprehensive service components by student level

	Service component	Focus at various student levels			
		Beginning	Intermediate	Advanced	Graduate and crisis specialist
1	Prevention	Personal and family life	Individual and families in crisis	Community and population groups at risk	Teaching and counseling; community education
2	Treatment of physical injury	Observe and assist as directed	Perform with immediate assistance of preceptor or supervisor	Perform with assistance or supervision on-site	Perform with preceptor available on-site
3	Crisis management				
a	Identification and triage	X	X	X	X
b	Comprehensive crisis assessment	O	O	Assist	Perform with supervision
c	Crisis counseling	O	O	Observe or Perform with supervision	Perform with supervision
d	Referral	X	X	X	Depends on particular needs and mission
4	Follow up counseling and/or treatment	O	O	O	According to needs assessment and mission

Key:
  X Do perform
  O Do *not* perform.

Victimization Assessment Tool

Once victimization status is identified, it should be followed by in-depth assessment (preferably by mental health professionals with backgrounds in victimology who are also sensitive to gender

Table 13.3 Victimization Assessment Tool

Key to risk	Level of victimization	Typical indicators
1	No experience of physical violence or abuse	No memory of violence recently or in the past
2	Experience of abuse/violence with minor physical and/or emotional trauma	Currently, verbal arguments that occasionally escalate to pushing and shoving or mild slapping. History *may* include past victimization that is no longer problematic or for which a solution is in process
3	Experience of abuse/violence with moderate physical and/or emotional trauma	Abused several times a month in recent years, resulting in moderate trauma/emotional distress (for example, bruises, no threat to life, no weapons). History *may* include past victimization that is still somewhat problematic (for example, a sexual abuse incident/overture by a parent or step-parent over 2 years ago)
4	Experience of abuse/violence with severe physical and/or emotional trauma	Violently attacked (for example, rape) or physically abused in recent years, resulting in physical injury requiring medical treatment. Threats to kill, no guns. History *may* include serious victimization (for example, periodic battering, incest, or other abuse requiring medical and/or psychological treatment)
5	Life-threatening or prolonged violence/abuse with very severe physical and/or emotional trauma	Recent or current life-threatening physical abuse, potentially lethal assault or threats with available deadly weapons. History *may* include severe abuse requiring medical treatment, frequent or ongoing sexual abuse, recent rape at gun- or knifepoint, other physical attack requiring extensive medical treatment

issues) to ascertain the extent of trauma and the victim/survivor's response (see also Burstow, 1992; Campbell, & Humphreys, 1993; Everett, & Gallop, 2000; Herman, 1992).

Illustration 1: comprehensive service – intimate partner violence

Mrs Sophia Penotti, three months pregnant, was brought by her husband to the local hospital emergency service for vaginal spotting. She was tearful on admission and appeared highly anxious, but on inquiry by both the triage nurse and examining physician, Mrs Penotti stated she was just sad and fearful about losing her baby. Examination revealed a contusion on Mrs Penotti's arm which she said occurred when she "stumbled and fell against a chair" during a recent spell of "nausea and dizziness." Mr Penotti appeared overly solicitous and had to be strongly persuaded to remain in the waiting area while Mrs Penotti was examined. Following examination the nurse spent about 10 minutes with Mrs Penotti discussing health issues such as smoking during pregnancy, diet, etc. The nurse also inquired further about her sadness, particularly since no serious physical complications of pregnancy were evident despite the spotting. Mrs Penotti denied anything that would have indicated abuse in the relationship with her husband. She was urged to see her regular pregnancy care provider for a follow-up appointment within a week, or sooner if more serious bleeding ensued.

As it turns out, Mrs Penotti and her husband had been having fierce arguments ever since she learned she was pregnant. During several of these arguments, Mr Penotti had struck his wife, but medical treatment was not pursued following any of the attacks. Since this was to be her fourth child, Mrs Penotti's husband wanted his wife to have an abortion; she adamantly refused to do so, not only on religious grounds, but because she finds most of her meaning in life in her role as a mother of her other three children, ages 5, 3, and 2 years.

Five months after this incident, Mrs Penotti, now eight months pregnant and semi-conscious, was brought by ambulance to the emergency department of the same hospital following ingestion of approximately 50 aspirin and several OTC (over the counter) sleeping pills approximately one hour earlier. Besides the systemic sequelae of the drug overdose, examination also revealed that Mrs Penotti had two loose teeth, various contusions, and strangle marks on her neck. Some fetal distress was also noted.

Distraught relatives who accompanied the ambulance informed staff that Mrs Penotti had come to their house earlier in the evening after another beating by her husband. She said that she was thinking of getting a divorce and going on welfare because "no matter what I do, he treats me like a dog." Her family had taken pains to talk to Mr Penotti urging him to stop his violence, and suggesting that they try one more time to "work things out." Mrs Penotti followed her family's advice, went home, tried to make up, but this time her husband nearly killed her by strangling. Having concluded that she had done everything she could to stop the violence, Mrs Penotti saw suicide as her only option. She was found by her family after they placed a follow-up call to the house and learned from the 5-year-old child (who had witnessed the violence) that "Mommy won't wake up." Following medical treatment and recovery, Mrs Penotti spent 10 weeks in a battered women's refuge, followed by ongoing casework through the welfare department. Divorce proceedings were started and she began rebuilding her life as a single parent of her four children.

The case of Mrs Penotti and her family illustrates a range of services on behalf of someone who has survived abuse. These services fall into four major categories:

1 Prevention
2 Treatment of physical injury
3 Crisis assessment and intervention
4 Follow-up counseling/treatment

For each category the role of various health disciplines is noted, together with suggestions of how these service components might have been applied at various times on behalf of Mrs Penotti and her family.

Prevention

In addition to the initial emergency visit with "spotting" as the presenting complaint, the risk factors in this family might have been detected, and life-threatening injuries prevented at several points within the health and social service systems:

- at routine pre-natal visits (medicine, midwifery, nursing);
- at any visits to emergency or pediatric services on behalf of the children (medicine, nursing);
- at routine or emergency dental visits (dental hygiene, dentistry);
- at visits to housing department (social work);
- at inquiries of pharmacist about which OTC medication would "help me sleep."

Treatment of physical injury and obtaining forensic evidence

This involves medicine, dentistry, nursing, physical therapy (depending on nature of injury). It includes not only precise medical records, but also photographs of injuries in the event of later criminal justice and court action either chosen by the victim, or as mandated in particular jurisdictions.

Crisis assessment, intervention, counseling, and coordination

This includes several steps, although not all disciplines necessarily implement each step.

1 Triage and assessment of life-threatening risk (all disciplines)

The legacy of considering violence among intimates and family members as a "private" issue may still serve as a barrier to prevention (as suggested above) and identification of persons at risk from violence and abuse. Intake workers need to be alert to the fact that many abused persons, particularly battered women, are reluctant to disclose their plight because of fear and/ or the legacy of "blaming the victim." Often they may present with psychosomatic complaints or anxiety, and may reveal abuse as the source of these symptoms only following *explicit inquiry by an empathetic health provider*.

It therefore cannot be overstated that screening questions be incorporated into whatever protocols are in use as part of *routine health assessments throughout the health and social service system*. Victim identification and preventive activity is unlikely to occur until all health professionals are committed to *asking routinely* about actual or potential abuse at various entry points to the human service system.

The screening protocol should include questions about suicide and assault potential and resource depletion, since these problems are often secondary to the primary problem of abuse and may signal the severity of trauma from victimization (Stephens, 1985). The probability of reducing life-threatening risk for all concerned is greatly increased through such questioning. For example, instead of suicidality, Mrs Penotti might have had fantasies of killing her husband. Or, if she retaliated with violence, her husband may have appeared for treatment (Ferris *et al.*, 1997). Therefore, *both women and men*, whether at risk as victims or assailants, should be screened. A triage tool is illustrated in Chapter 4, and applies generally across the clinical service scenarios of other chapters. Here are the triage questions that should have been applied to Mrs Penotti's case early on and which might have signaled crisis counseling and possible prevention of the near-fatal suicide attempt:

1 *Have you been troubled or injured by any kind of abuse or violence?* (e.g. hit by partner, forced sex). If injury is obvious (Mrs. Penotti's contusion): *Would you tell me about the dizziness and how you happened to stumble and fall against a chair?*
2 If yes: *Has something like this ever happened before? Describe.* [Mrs. Penotti acknowledges the fierce arguments, and that he "hit me once but promised not to do it again."]
3 *Do you have anyone you can turn to or rely on now to protect you from possible further injury?* [Mrs. Penotti: "Yes, I'm very close to my family ... they've talked to him, and they think I should try to work things out, because at least he pays the bills."]
4 *Do you feel so badly now that you have thought of hurting yourself/suicide?* [Mrs. Penotti: "Not right now, but I have thought about taking pills when things get bad."]
5 *Are you so angry about what's happened that you have considered hurting someone else?* [Mrs. Penotti: "Yes, I've thought about poisoning his food, but I don't think I'd get by with it."]

It is assumed, of course, that such inquiries occur within the context of a client/provider relationship in which respect, empathy, and rapport are paramount. Thus, depending on screening outcomes, the foundation is laid for appropriate referral, more in-depth assessment, and action to prevent further assaults, suicide, or retaliatory violence. Mrs Penotti's case underscores the need throughout human services for more attention to the *interactive* relationship between victimization, suicide, and assault/homicide potential. (See Hoff *et al.*, 2009, for details on risk assessment and suggestions for implementation, Chapters 3 and 11.)

It is possible, of course, that Mrs Penotti might still have denied the cause of her injuries during the earlier emergency visit, but that likelihood is decreased when health personnel throughout the system are prepared not only to detect incongruities between injuries and the woman's "story," but also how to do sensitive questioning around suspicious injuries and implement a follow-up plan that would not jeopardize her safety or leave a full eight months between visits. As it turned out, on admission for a near fatal suicide attempt, Mrs Penotti's level of victimization was 5 on the Victimization Assessment Tool (Table 13.3).

2 Comprehensive crisis and mental health assessment (crisis specialists, social work, clinical psychology, psychiatric nursing, family medicine, psychiatry)

In Mrs Penotti's case and similar instances, this facet of care would occur in the social work or psychiatric liaison service affiliated with emergency departments. See standard texts and Part IV: Online resources.

3 *Crisis counseling* (family medicine, psychiatric nursing, psychology, social work). See standard texts and Part IV: Online resources.
4 *Referral* is indicated in two instances:
   • by anyone who identifies a person at risk but whose mission does not include comprehensive assessment and crisis counseling (dental practitioner, pharmacist, physiotherapist);
   • by the disciplines which do crisis work (medicine, nursing, occupational therapy) but not the longer-term counseling or psychotherapy which may be indicated for some.

Follow-up counseling and/or treatment

This involves mental health professionals with sensitivity to and experience with abuse issues, occupational therapy, physical therapy, specialists such as substance abuse counselors, and survivors' support groups.

Depending on prior history and/or indications of serious depression and suicide risk, professional counseling may not be needed by battered women, though at the very least a peer support group, as offered in most refuges or in 12-step programs, is indicated.

Service for Mr Penotti includes collaboration between the criminal justice system and treatment programs for men who batter. (See Chapter 10, standard texts, and Part IV: Online resources.) Mrs Penotti's situation underscores the fact that the "natural crisis management" measures which she and her family took are not sufficient for a *public health* phenomenon such as violence, but must be supplemented by services from *formal* institutions.

The Crisis Paradigm (Figure 13.1) illustrates key elements of Mrs Penotti's service needs. The Medicine Wheel approach described in Chapter 8 complements most facets of this crisis model, and emphasizes the role of the entire community. The essence of the circle and the Medicine Wheel is that the end means a new beginning, to "mend the sacred hoop." The concept of crisis entails "danger [of the present] and opportunity" to move toward a future free of violence. While the Medicine Wheel approach may connect indigenous people to healing ceremonies and the sweat lodge, the crisis model cites "contemporary rites of passage" for people at risk. Both models also address not only the needs of the victim, but also the assailant. The Medicine Wheel's work with victims, assailants, and children occurs in a four-part community-embedded process focusing on Past, Today, Tomorrow, and Future, complementing the Crisis Care Process (Assessment, Planning, Implementation, Follow-up).

The delivery of these comprehensive service components to survivors of abuse and their assailants within a multifaceted service system demands the assumption of multiple roles by individual providers (Klevens *et al.*, 2008). In the EFPO (Education of Future Physicians for Ontario) Working Paper No. 9 (1993), consultation with clients revealed their perception of physicians within nine roles: Accountable Professional; Advocate; Collaborator; Communicator; Contextual Interpreter/Clinical Mediator; Humanist; Lifelong Learner/Scholar; Medical Expert; Partner in Healing.

With the exception of "Medical Expert," these roles are consonant with the expected roles of other health professionals, keeping in mind the distinct mission of each discipline. For example, nursing focuses holistically on health promotion and needs arising from the client's response to illness, trauma, etc.; occupational therapy and physical therapy focus on treatment and rehabilitation. In addition to the above roles, nursing, dental hygiene, occupational therapy, pharmacy, and physiotherapy emphasize *teaching* (geared especially toward prevention and self-care). For example, an abused woman at any entry point may need precise information about realistic dangers from her spouse and from self-medication, and how to detect life-threatening risk of assault, particularly if she has become jaded from repeated abuse or has begun to take her partner's violence for granted. The role of *counselor* and "ritual expert" applies to all mental health professionals, crisis specialists, or graduates such as in family medicine.

Mandated reporting of battering: a controversial issue

Illustration 1 raises the controversial question of mandatory reporting of domestic violence (as is required in *all* cases of child abuse or neglect). In the United States, such mandatory reporting laws for abused adults exist in four states: California, Colorado, Rhode Island, and Kentucky. Central to this controversy is the issue of empowerment as expressed by female emergency department patients (Rodriguez *et al.*, 2001). Nearly half of non-English-speaking patients opposed mandatory reporting on grounds of protecting autonomy and sociopolitical factors such as fear of deportation. Mandatory reporting might also be counter-productive in providing a "quick fix" or loophole in the important process of emergency department health professionals linking abused women to crisis and follow-up mental health services – as in, "I've reported it, so now it's someone else's responsibility."

A related issue concerns mandated treatment of perpetrators, and/or grounds for prosecution in cases of femicide. The details of these issues are in the province of the police and criminal justice systems and beyond the scope of this book (see Chapter 10 and Adams, 2007). It is important to emphasize, however, that abused women are at greatest danger after requesting a protective order; announcing they want a divorce, or beginning the process of gaining child custody. This fact is tied to the centrality of *power and control* in the dynamics of intimate partner violence. Thus, when confronted with the *State's* power to intervene, the perpetrator's violence (in a play to maintain control) may escalate to a more dangerous level, which may include murder. Secondly, while an abused woman's awareness of homicidal danger can save her life, in the vast majority of cases women are hesitant to engage the criminal justice system against their partners; primarily, they want the violence to stop so they and their children can live in safety and without terror. Thus, they need empathetic listening, support around their decisions, information about signs of lethal danger, and the *empowerment* arising from ownership of the decision process. As a result of progressive governmental action around victims' rights, such support and expert assistance is available through victim advocacy services attached to police and court systems – similar to the SANE program introduced in Chapter 6 and illustrated in the next section in cases of sexual assault.

Illustration 2: comprehensive service – sexual assault victims

Tanya is a 17-year-old with a past medical history of attention-deficit/hyperactivity disorder (ADHD), controlled on stimulant medication. She had dropped out of school in the past year as a consequence of getting involved in substance use with high school friends. This involved using alcohol, marijuana and then a brief foray into cocaine use. Her parents sought out assistance for her once they became aware of the problem. She was involved for 6 weeks in a residential community program for youth addressing addictions and attending school through that program. At the time of the assault she was out of the residential program, living at home with her parents, and had returned to the public high school. She was not yet sexually active, although she created an image of herself as very "street smart" with her peers.

She was downtown at dusk when she passed a man on the street. There were few people about as the after-work rush hour had passed and she was on her way to the bus stop. He had his pet dog with him and the dog went up to her. She started to pat the dog. The man made small talk and then when she was engaged in the conversation he moved into her space and physically restrained her. He then dragged her into an urban area with dense foliage and threatened her with a weapon if she did not have "sex" with him. She was terrified and yet she resisted him. The assault was brutal. He was verbally abusive, using sexualized pejorative labels to demean her (intended to disempower her and play into his own fantasy). The resulting physical trauma was extensive to her genital area. She had human bite marks on her breasts. He then told her he would seek her out and kill her if she told anyone. She realized this would be the only way to get away from him and agreed to his demand.

Tanya then went into a corner store a few blocks away, and the clerk called the police, who responded promptly. She was not afraid of the police as during her substance use she had met the community police officer. There was also a community police officer housed in her high school. So she saw the police as helpful rather than harmful.

The team that responded was composed of both a male and female police officer. They spoke with her and once they appreciated the issue they got a description of the perpetrator and location for the assault. The rapist was apprehended by another police team. Tanya was taken to the emergency department at the nearby hospital. The police had informed the hospital they were bringing in a sexual assault case, so the SANE was called and came to the hospital. Tanya's mother was notified by the police and came to the hospital. When Tanya's mother arrived she was agitated and upset for her daughter; Tanya then totally fell apart, started crying and physically shaking.

She was then assessed in a dedicated treatment area. A sexual assault (SA) victim may decide that she does not want to involve the police depending on the context and sequence of events. If the victim/survivor does not choose to file a report with the police immediately then she/he may decide to pursue a forensic exam and make a decision about charges at a later date. Through the SANE program they have the option of having the forensic evidence collected, frozen and stored for up to six months. If the victim/survivor decides to report the SA, the SANE coordinator will contact the police and provide the forensic evidence at that time. They will then proceed with the investigation. Tanya had already given the police her statement and expressed clearly that she wished to pursue charges at this time. Once Tanya agreed to a forensic examination, the chain of evidence would be transferred to the police. The SANE nurse completed a forensic examination. Tanya required wound cleansing and suturing of labial tears by the gynecology resident on call following the forensic exam.

Tanya was informed of the possible health risks associated with SA and she was given information including pregnancy prevention, STD prevention, STD testing and follow-up protocols. She was given an information package with various resources available to her through the hospital and in the community, and was asked to see her family physician within the next few days. She was given alternative contacts if she did not feel comfortable with her own physician. The SANE advised her that if she chose not to pursue charges at this time, the forensic evidence would be kept for six months and that she may lay charges now or in the future up to six months.

Tanya went home with her mother. Her first request was to have a shower and clean herself up. She saw her family physician (whom she trusted) two days later. The physician invited her to tell as much of the story as she was comfortable with. Her physician observed in the interview that Tanya appeared disconnected from the events she described and her affect was flat when she told her story. She startled easily when a door across the hallway was closed. Tanya had not returned to school, and was requesting that her mom stay at home with her. Her sleep was fitful and she was having intrusive memories from the SA. Tanya denied feeling suicidal, and said she did not want to use alcohol or marijuana to cope with the sexual assault and that she wanted help with maintaining the gains she had made over the prior year.

Prevention

The prevention of sexual assault encompasses the following:

- community programs on prevention strategies;
- educational programs in the schools;
- reducing the widespread tolerance for violence;
- conflict resolution through non-violent negotiation;
- criminal justice system public alerts, programming;
- police presence in the schools as identified interventionists;
- public education role for the community at large.

Assessment, treatment, and obtaining forensic evidence

This assessment was conducted by a SANE in Tanya's case. The other possible examiners would be an emergency room physician or nurse practitioner or a specialist physician, i.e. a gynecologist. In this instance Tanya was seen by a SANE from the Avalon Centre in Halifax, Nova Scotia. A forensic examination was completed with her consent. This should be conducted within 72 hours of the assault. It is preferable but not mandatory that the victim/survivor not shower, bathe or douche, clean her teeth, until after the exam is completed. The exam involves:

- taking a medical history;
- documenting details of the assault/abuse to help identify potential infections, injuries, and guide the treatment required;
- taking blood and urine samples to test for pregnancy and /or infections;
- an internal exam (vaginal, rectal and oral) that may be performed at this time.

SA follow-up may be with a primary care provider (family physician or nurse practitioner) depending on the victim's choice and comfort level or be provided by the SANE. Tanya chose to see her family physician and went with a checklist form notifying the healthcare provider of the SA and tests completed and a suggested follow-up protocol.

Crisis management

This includes:

- Identification and triage.
- Police typically are the first contact with the victim following the sexual assault (SA), taking her/his statement in a non-judgmental manner.
- Assessment of medical needs initially and provision of support for the victim, ensuring safety, and providing transport to the Emergency Medical facility
- SA Advocate program for victims. The police may make a referral to Victim Services.

Comprehensive assessment and counseling

Depending on level of training in crisis care, this can be done by the SANE nurse examiner, emergency room physician, family physician, social worker, a mental health professional, or a specialized sexual assault counselor such as at Avalon Centre (described in detail below).

Follow-up counseling and treatment

As with crisis counseling, follow-up therapeutic counseling might be done by any one of the following professionals: school nurse, SANE, nurse practitioner in community setting, family practice nurse, family physician/GP, mental health professionals, Victim Services personnel (criminal justice system). Adjunct services would be with an adolescent addictions counselor, and/or a social worker (available in certain contexts, i.e. when the victim/survivor is on social assistance).

Teaching issues in this case

Tanya's case reveals the following issues for teaching and learning: She is a vulnerable adolescent, suffers ADHD, abuses substances, has difficulty with impulse control, and is not likely to have good boundaries. Also evident is some family dysfunction prior to the SA, and defiant behaviors related to substance abuse. Her past history puts her at risk for victim-blaming by family, police, and healthcare providers.

SANE Avalon Centre program – Halifax, Nova Scotia

The Avalon Centre houses and coordinates the SANE program. Based on the SANE model introduced in Chapter 6, the program was developed as an outcome of a collaborative needs assessment from the Metro Wide Sexual Assault Response Initiative (2000) comprised of representatives from community groups, police, health providers, hospital administrators for women and child health programming and the Department of Health. The Halifax program is unique in that the service operates out of the Avalon Centre, a community-based non-governmental organization (NGO) that coordinates and administers the SANE program out of their offices. The provision of timely, sensitive comprehensive care to sexual assault victims is their mandate. They have also developed their program on the basis of a *collaborative woman-centered approach*. This approach embraces underlying principles and philosophies that inform their engagement with the individual woman client, family or community to identify needs (see WHO 2008).

Prior to this, a service had historically been offered by a team of metro-based primary care physicians, all women, who set in motion a coordinated response program. The limitation in that program was physician availability and response timeliness given competing practice responsibilities and possible lengthy court-related responsibilities. With a dedicated SANE program these issues are resolved. Also, in the emergency room setting, physicians were often deferring SA victim assessments, as they are time-consuming and once in the process of a forensic exam there needs to be continuity in the chain of evidence with police taking the samples collected.

An on-call SANE is available 24/7 to respond to SA cases, providing immediate care and conducting a forensic examination at the emergency rooms of three regional hospitals, including the pediatric hospital for persons 13 years of age and older. The SANE program is a dedicated inclusive service, providing continuity from initial encounter to testimony in court. The advantage of the association with the Avalon Centre is multifaceted. The Centre's location does not have an identifiable stigma, compared with a hospital setting where someone in the waiting room may know the victim or her/his family, hence compromising confidentiality. The Center is also a resource for associated services with the provision of phone guidance, educational materials and an on-site counseling service with professional counselors familiar with the immediate and long-term psychological, emotional and physical outcomes of sexual assault. The Avalon Centre provides information/education programs, and plays an activist role in the community. Also, if the victim chooses to participate in a forensic exam, the facility will freezer store the forensic evidence for up to six months such that the victim does not have to make a decision about laying criminal charges in the acute phase after the SA, but has that option up to six months after the event.

Overall, women experience systematic injustices in gaining redress for SA because of low reporting rates, higher filtering rates before they reach criminal prosecution than for other offences, low conviction rates, and a remarkably higher rate of success on appeals. This continues to be a problem for victims of SA. Some programs have tried to address these issues. In this community police SA sensitivity training has been mandatory since 2002. When possible the police try to have a female officer in attendance on SA cases. The inherent risk is that this can lead to burnout for female police officers. Similar issues exist for SANEs. A pro-active preventive initiative should be considered when setting up these services (see Chapter 12).

Sexual Assault Response Team (SART) programs have been started in many communities and include many team players. SARTs often oversee coordination and collaboration of services and programs related to immediate response to SA cases, ensure a victim-centered approach to service delivery as well as looking at prevention strategies. In communities with SART programs SANEs are an integral member working closely with other members of the community sexual assault response teams, crisis programs, law enforcement officers, crown prosecutors, and judges (often providing sensitivity training) and child protection services to meet the various needs of victim/survivors and hold the offenders/assailants accountable for their crimes.

Psychiatric care of survivors: a cautionary note

The issue of psychiatric referral did not arise in the Tanya case above but may in the future. For all practitioners and students throughout the health and social service system a cautionary note is indicated in considering their role in the decision to refer to mental health professionals.

In the consultation process used to develop this book, "psychiatric survivors" provided some of the most poignant examples of client/provider interaction within the healthcare system. Members of the various chapters of Psychiatric Survivors of Ontario, for example, note the origin of their organization's title: after having first survived violence and abuse from intimates, family members, or strangers, they then survived the psychiatric system intended to serve them. The concerns of this group, while a minority among clients, are shared by many psychiatrists, other therapists, and policy analysts, as documented by the reform efforts underway in Ontario and elsewhere (Helfrich *et al.*, 2008; Herman, 1992; Hoff, 1993; Marks, & Scott, 1990; Scheper-Hughes, & Lovell, 1986). Contemporary psychiatric practitioners and social analysts support a key position of community activists: "Victim-blaming" and ascribing causality of abuse to the alleged psychopathologies of victims, while at the same time excusing assailants on psychiatric grounds is now a discredited legacy (Burstow, 1992; Hilberman, 1980; Hoff, 1990; Mirchinson, 1993; Stark *et al.*, 1979).

Perhaps there are few instances of misguided use of a psychopathology framework more suspect than in the diagnosis of "borderline personality disorder" in which a psychiatric diagnosis is applied with little or no explicit attention to the client's history of childhood sexual abuse (Everett, & Gallop, 2000). Other misuses of a "personality disorder" diagnosis include veterans of war trauma or violent men whose childhood histories of abuse have never been identified or treated (Hoff *et al.*, 2009, Chapter 12; Semiz *et al.*, 2007). A return to earlier principles of social psychiatry might correct the overwhelming dominance of ascribing a "disorder" label to increasing numbers of life problems, including, for example, ascribing "anti-social personality disorder" to someone engaging in violent and abusive behaviors – a pattern that minimizes a key theme of this book: the importance of *accountability* for one's actions, while acknowledging that cognitive impairment from mental illness might excuse one in certain instances, as discussed in Chapter 11.

Survey, interview, and focus group data for this book revealed the remnants of a psychopathology approach by a curricular emphasis on teaching victim/survivor issues in psychiatric courses. A recommendation therefore bears considering: while health educators (especially in medicine, nursing, occupational therapy, clinical social work and psychology) must address the needs of women in psychiatric settings whose care at victimization crisis points was inadequate, several foci should be emphasized in the treatment of these women (regardless of which curriculum design is selected):

- explicit assessment for victimization history;
- counseling and therapy by persons with a critical analysis, an understanding of the sociocultural underpinnings of sexual assault and woman abuse, and experience with victim/survivors as recommended by grassroots community groups;
- cautious use of psychotropic drugs;
- linkage to other survivors and community-based support groups with special expertise in victim/survivor care.

The widespread trend of addressing woman abuse issues primarily in courses such as psychiatric nursing needs re-examining. This practice reinforces a psychopathology paradigm while obscuring violence as the *power and control* issue it really is. Instead, various healing therapies are recommended on behalf of those whose psychopathologies might have been *prevented*, especially by crisis intervention and peer support at entry points such as prenatal and emergency services.

Clearly, if crisis concepts and intervention strategies are *first* introduced in a psychiatric course, a *tertiary preventive level* (and the assumption of psychopathology) is implied, rather than the current emphasis on *primary care* and preventive intervention that are so important in situations of abuse and violence. Since most health professions students will already have experienced life crises of their own, and will confront the crises of others in their *first* clinical experience (which is rarely, if ever, in a psychiatric setting), the concept of crisis and its relation to victimization should be introduced in concert with concepts of stress and coping, regardless of the general curriculum design. This implies that the time allotted to psychiatric courses could be reduced or refocused, as some of the psychosocial concepts traditionally reserved for these courses will have been addressed earlier (e.g. in courses on family health) as essential content for *all* clinical situations.

Human rights, gender issues, and medical/professional ethics

The Tarasoff case and "duty to warn"

In 1969 a graduate student at the University of California disclosed to his psychotherapist his intention to kill his estranged girlfriend. The therapist informed the police of the possible danger this man posed, but did not warn the girlfriend of her potential danger. Later, the client killed the young woman as he had planned. The victim's parents filed a civil suit for her wrongful death, and the court found the University of California and its student counseling service to be liable for its failure to warn the identified victim (VandeCreek, & Knapp, 2001). By extension, this principle applies to those working in programs for violent men in which appropriate engagement with victims is a key aspect of practice (Adams, & Cayouette, 2002; Adams, 2007; Callahan, & Jennings, 2002).

This landmark case set a precedent for all mental health practitioners in the United States and Canada, requiring them to incorporate "duty to warn" potential victims of homicide in their professional ethics protocols for practice. Implementing this ethical duty, however, implies that practitioners have evidence-based knowledge of the signs of assault and/or homicide risk potential, such as discussed in Chapter 11. In other words, casual reference to "murderous anger" with no specific plan, means, or history of assault does not qualify as grounds to forego usual client/therapist confidentiality and pick up the phone to call a potential victim. But in holistic context and in-depth assessment of risk factors, a rating of 3 or above on the Assault/homicide risk assessment (Table 11.1), would warrant a warning to such a prospective victim. The ethical principle here is that the life of an at-risk person supersedes the ordinary ethical norm of client/

therapist confidentiality – as, for example, in the case of an adolescent at grave risk of suicide who says "But you can't tell my parents." Skilled therapists will know how to deal with such a situation without betraying an adolescent's trust while also engaging the parents – keeping in mind that the adolescent's latent message may be *precisely* to get a message across to parents which he/she has been unable to do alone (see Hoff *et al.*, 2009, Chapter 9).

Female genital mutilation (FGM), surgical restoration of "virgin status," and cultural relativism

In Canada, the United States, and some other countries, medical professionals can be charged with assault for performing FGM (some substituting "modification" for the term "mutilation"); furthermore, parents requesting the operation in the US and Canada can be charged with aiding and abetting the assault. Based on the World Health Organization (WHO) definition, FGM is also grounds for claiming political asylum in some countries.

Historically, societies in which FGM has been a widely accepted cultural ritual have resisted Westerners' attempts to abolish the practice. Education by persons within one's own cultural group is a more acceptable approach to this issue as illustrated by this example from the 1985 United Nations Women's Conference in Nairobi: a Sudanese physician lectured on the serious health and childbirth problems associated with FGM (especially in its most radical form) complete with anatomical illustrations from her obstetrics/gynecology (OB/GYN) practice with women who had had the procedure. Immigrant physicians in the US and Canada who are approached by their fellow immigrants requesting performance of the procedure on their daughters state that they find it helpful to simply explain to parents that Canadian and US physicians are professionally forbidden to perform the procedure (see Oboler, 2001).

Besides FGM, gender-based violence takes other intricate forms. In June 2008, *The New York Times* reported on the violence against Muslim women living in Europe in an article titled "Muslim women and virginity: the consequences when 2 worlds collide". According to the author, Sciolino (2008), the issue of violence against Muslim women has been particularly charged in France, where a renewed and fierce debate has occurred about a prejudice that was supposed to have been buried in Western countries with the twentieth century's sexual revolution: the importance of a woman's virginity.

The uproar came after a court in France annulled a marriage of two French Muslims because the groom found his bride was not the virgin she had claimed to be. The bride, a nursing student in her 20s, confessed and agreed to the annulment. The court ruling cited breach of contract, and no reference to religion. Consequently, Sciolino describes, some feminists, lawyers and doctors warned that the court's acceptance of the centrality of virginity in marriage would encourage more Frenchwomen from Arab and African Muslim backgrounds to have their hymens restored. "There is much debate about whether the procedure is an act of liberation or repression" (Sciolino, 2008). On one hand, the specialists who perform the procedure argue that they are empowering women by giving them a viable future and preventing them from being abused – or even killed – by their fathers or their brothers, based on the falsehood that they are only worthy of respect if they are virgins when they marry. On the other, there are gynecologists and obstetricians who oppose the procedures of hymen restoration on moral, cultural, and health grounds (Sciolino, 2008). Overall, these issues illustrate the concept of cultural relativism as discussed in Chapter 2, i.e. justifying and excusing certain practices on grounds that "this is part of our culture" in contrast to interpretation using a universal human rights perspective including bodily integrity and freedom of sexual expression regardless of gender (Torry, 2000).

In conclusion, no one person has to do everything in this complex arena, but system-wide, everyone needs at least general knowledge of the "big picture," a hopeful attitude and belief in the possibility of change, and the skills specific to one's particular role in a team approach to violence prevention and comprehensive care. The idea and essentials of such care can then move beyond a mere abstract concept to the *reality* that even small steps may be life-saving for victim/survivors and their assailants – not to mention the health and social welfare of whole nations.

References

Adams, D. (2007). *Why Do They Kill? Men Who Murder Their Intimate Partners*. Nashville: Vanderbilt University Press.

Adams, D., & Cayouette, S. (2002). Emerge: A group education model for abusers. In E. Aldarondo, & F. Mederos (eds.), *Programs for Men Who Batter: Intervention and Prevention Strategies in a Diverse Society*, pp. 4-1–4-23. New York: Civic Research, Inc.

Antonovsky, A. (1980). *Health, Stress, and Coping*. San Francisco: Jossey-Bass.

Burstow, B. (1992). *Radical Feminist Theory: Working in the Context of Violence*. Thousand Oaks, CA: Sage.

Callahan, D., & Jennings, B. (2002). Ethics and public health: Forging a strong relationship. *American Journal of Public Health*, 92(2), 169–76.

Campbell, J. C., & Humphreys, J. H. (1993). *Nursing Care of Survivors of Family Violence*. St. Louis: Mosby-Year Book.

Caplan, G. (1964). *Principles of Preventive Psychiatry*. New York: Basic Books.

Coretta, C. M. (2008). Domestic violence: A worldwide exploration. *Journal of Psychosocial Nursing & Mental Health Services*, 46(3), 26–35.

Earley, P. (2006). *Crazy: A Father's Search Through America's Mental Health Madness*. New York: Berkley Books.

Editorial (2007). Intimate partner violence: Doctors' roles should be integrated with the needs of patients and society. *British Medical Journal*, 334, 706–7.

EPFO – Educating Future Physicians for Ontario (1993). Survivors of violence against women: Some views on their expectations of physicians. *Educating Future Physicians for Ontario Working Paper 9*. Ottawa: Ontario Medical Association.

Erikson, E. (1963). *Childhood and Society* (2nd edn.). New York: Norton.

Everett, B., & Gallop, R. (2000). *Linking Childhood Trauma and Mental Illness: Theory and Practice for Direct Service Practitioners*. Thousand Oaks, CA: Sage.

Ferris, L. E., *et al.* (1997). Guidelines for managing domestic abuse when male and female partners are patients of the same physician. The Delphi Panel and Consulting Group. *Journal of American Medical Association*, 278, 851–67.

Furniss, K., McCaffrey, M., Vereene, P., & Rovi, S. (2007). Nurses and barriers to screening for intimate partner violence. *American Journal of Maternal Child Nursing*, 32(4), 238–43.

Helfrich, C. A., Fujiura, G. T., & Rutkowski-Kmitta, V. (2008). Mental health disorders and functioning of women in domestic violence shelters. *Journal of Interpersonal Violence*, 23(4), 437–53.

Herman, J. (1992). *Trauma and Recovery: The Aftermath of Violence*. New York: Basic Books.

Hilberman, E. (1980). Overview: The "wife beater's wife" reconsidered. *American Journal of Psychiatry*, 137, 1336–47.

Hoff, L. A. (1990). *Battered Women as Survivors*. London: Routledge.

Hoff, L. A. (1993). Review essay: health policy and the plight of the mentally ill. *Psychiatry*, 56(4), 400–19.

Hoff, L. A., Hallisey, B. J., & Hoff, M. (2009). *People in Crisis: Clinical and Diversity Perspectives* (6th edn.). New York & London: Routledge.

Hoff, L. A., & Rosenbaum, L. (1994). A victimization assessment tool: Instrument development and clinical implications. *Journal of Advanced Nursing*, 20(4), 627–34.

JCAHO – Joint Commission on Accreditation of Healthcare Organizations (1993). *Accreditation Manual for Hospitals*. 2 v. Oakbrook Terrace, IL: JCAHO.

Kim, S., & Kim, J. (2001). The effects of group intervention for battered women in Korea. *Archives of Psychiatric Nursing*, 15(6), 257–64.

Klevens, J., Baker, C. K., Shelley, G. A., & Ingram, E. M. (2008). Exploring the links between components of coordinated community responses and the impact on contact with intimate partner violence services. *Violence against Women*, 14(3), 346–58.

Leth, P. M., & Banner, J. (2008). Forensic medical examination of refugees who claim to have been tortured. *The American Journal of Forensic Medicine and Pathology*, 26(2), 125–30.

MacMillan H. L., & Wathen C. N. with the Canadian Task Force on Preventive Health Care, (2001). *Prevention and Treatment of Violence against Women: Systematic Review & Recommendations*. CTFPHC Technical Report No. 01–4. London, ON: Canadian Task Force.

Marks, I., & Scott, R. (eds.). (1990). *Mental Health Care Delivery: Innovations, Impediments and Implementation*. Cambridge: Cambridge University Press.

McFarlane, J., Parker, B., Soeken, K., & Bullock, L. (1992). Assessing for abuse during pregnancy: Severity and frequency of injuries and associated entry into prenatal care. *Journal of the American Medical Association*, 267(23), 3176–8.

Mitchinson, W. (1993). The medical treatment of women. In S. Burt (ed.), *Changing Patterns: Women in Canada* (391–415). Toronto: Stewart, McLelland.

Oboler, R. S. (2001). Law and persuasion in the elimination of female genital modification. *Human Organization*, 60(4), 311–18.

Rhodes, K. V., & Levinson, W. (2003). Interventions for intimate partner violence against women: Clinical applications. *Journal of American Medical Association*, 289(5), 601–5.

Rodriguez, M. A., Szkupinski, Q. S., & Bauer, H. M. (1996). Breaking the silence: Battered women's perspectives on medical care. *Archives of Family Medicine*, 5, 153–8.

Rodriguez, M. A., McLoughlin, E., Nah, G., & Campbell, J. C. (2001). Mandatory reporting of domestic violence injuries to the police: What do Emergency Department patients think? *Journal of the American Medical Association*, 286(5), 580–3.

Scheper-Hughes, N., & Lovell, A.M. (1986). Breaking the circuit of social control: Lessons in public psychiatry from Italy and Franco Basaglia. *Social Science and Medicine*, 23(2), 159–78.

Sciolino, E. (2008, June 11). Muslim women and virginity: 2 worlds collide. *The New York Times*, 1, A13.

Semiz, U. B., Basoglu, C., Ebrinc, S., & Cetin, M. (2007). Childhood trauma history and dissociative experiences among Turkish men diagnosed with antisocial personality disorder. *Social Psychiatry and Psychiatric Epidemiology*, 42(11), 865–73.

Stark, E., Flitcraft, A., & Frazier, W. (1979). Medicine and patriarchal violence: The social construction of a "private" event. *International Journal of Health Services*, 9, 461–93.

Stephens, B. J. (1985). Suicidal women and their relationships with husbands, boyfriends, and lovers. *Suicide and Life-Threatening Behavior*, 15(2), 77–90.

Sully, P. (2002). Commitment to partnership: Interdisciplinary initiatives in developing expert practice in the care of survivors of violence. *Nursing Education in Practice*, 2, 92–8.

Sully, P., Greenway, K., & Reeves, S. (2005). Domestic violence, policing and health care: Collaboration and practice. *Primary Health Care Research and Development*, 2005(6), 31–6.

Thayer, L. (2004). Hidden hell: Women in prison. *Amnesty Now*, Fall, 10, 10–13.

Tjaden, P. Thoennes, N. (2000). *Full Report of the Prevalence, Incidence and Consequences of Violence against Women*: Washington, DC: National Institute of Justice.

Torry, W. I. (2000). Culture and individual responsibility: Touchstones of the culture defense. *Human Organization*, 59(1), 58–71.

VandeCreek, L., & Knapp, S. (2001). *Tarasoff and Beyond: Legal and Clinical Considerations in the Treatment of Life-Endangering Patients* (rev. edn.). Sarasota, FL: Professional Resource Press.

Wathen, C. N., & MacMillan, H. L. (2003). Interventions for violence against women: Scientific review. *Journal of American Medical Association*, 289(5), 589–99.

Weiss, E. (2000). *Surviving Domestic Violence: Voices of Women Who Broke Free*. Salt Lake City, Utah: Agreka Books.

Wies, J. R. (2008). Professionalizing human services: A case of domestic violence shelter advocates. *Human Organization*, 67(2), 221–33.

WHO – World Health Organization (2004). *Handbook for the Documentation of Interpersonal Violence Prevention Programmes*. Geneva: WHO.

WHO (2008). *Guidelines for Medico-Legal Care for Victims of Sexual Violence*. Geneva: WHO.

Part IV

Online resources

Please visit the *Violence and Abuse Issues* companion website at:
http://www.routledge.com/textbooks/9780415465724

Index

Entries in **bold** indicate a table or a figure

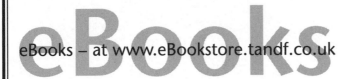